History Communication Skill Stations

For Internal Medicine Examinations

History Taking and Communication Skill Stations

For Internal Medicine Examinations

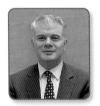

Wanis H Ibrahim MB ChB FRCP (Edin) FRCP (Glasg) FRCPI FCCP F (Pulm)
Senior Consultant Internist & Pulmonologist
Hamad General Hospital, Professor of Clinical Medicine
Qatar University and Weill Cornell Medicine-Qatar, Doha/Qatar

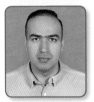

Mushtaq Ahmed CABM FRCP (Glasg) HERMES
Consultant Pulmonologist, Hamad General Hospital,
Assistant Professor of Clinical Medicine, Weill Cornell Medicine-Qatar
Doha/Qatar

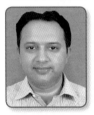

Muhammad A Waheed CABM MRCP (UK)
Consultant Physician
Northampton General Hospital
Northampton, UK

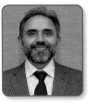

Rayaz A Malik BSc (Hons) MSc MBChB PhD FRCP
Professor of Medicine and Consultant Endocrinologist,
Weill Cornell Medicine-Qatar, Doha/Qatar
Central Manchester Teaching Hospitals, University of Manchester, UK

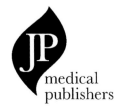

JP
medical
publishers

London • New Delhi

© 2020 Jaypee Brothers Medical Publishers

Published by Jaypee Brothers Medical Publishers,
4838/24 Ansari Road, New Delhi, India

Tel: +91 (011) 43574357   Fax: +91 (011)43574390

Email: info@jpmedpub.com, jaypee@jaypeebrothers.com
Web: www.jpmedpub.com, www.jaypeebrothers.com

JPM is the imprint of Jaypee Brothers Medical Publishers.

ISBN: 978-1-909836-99-0

British Library Cataloguing in Publication Data
A catalogue record for this book is available from the British Library

Library of Congress Cataloging in Publication Data
A catalog record for this book is available from the Library of Congress

Development Editor: Harsha Madan
Editorial Assistant: Keshav Kumar
Cover Design: Seema Dogra

Preface

The most common reason for a candidate to fail their clinical examinations is a lack of proper preparation for the examination, irrespective of their clinical experience and original medical school attended. Preparing for a clinical examination is like preparing to go to battle.

"If you know the enemy and know yourself, you need not fear the result of a hundred battles. If you know yourself but not the enemy, for every victory gained you will also suffer a defeat. If you know neither the enemy nor yourself, you will succumb in every battle."

—Sun Tzu, The Art of War

It is no surprise that a cardiology fellow adept at diagnosing and managing patients with cardiac problems fails the history taking or communication skill station of a simple cardiac case or a neurology fellow fails to elicit the full spectrum of neurology symptoms. Feedback from candidates who have failed is often that the case was simple and frequently encountered in their day-to-day clinical practice, but the examiner was unfair. Yet, the real reason for failure is the lack of a systematic approach to elicit the history, especially on social aspects and patient concerns. Success for any postgraduate clinical examination requires broad and detailed medical knowledge, alongside the ability to take a clear and focused history, whilst listening to and allowing the patient to air their concerns. Stress in the 'real examination' will expose not only significant skill and knowledge gaps, but also your inability to listen with empathy.

History taking and communication skills should become second nature to all candidates preparing for their clinical examinations (practice makes perfect). There is no better way to prepare than by presenting your case to a registrar or a consultant. Close to the examination, seek exam-oriented consultant supervision during the ward round and mock examinations. Revision courses help to familiarise candidates with the common examination cases and scenarios, alongside esoteric cases, but are never sufficient alone to pass the clinical examinations. Revising large swathes in medical textbooks without context to the patient or commonly encountered scenarios in the examination is guaranteed route to failure. Clinical acumen and common sense cannot be derived from the textbooks. Many of the large medical textbooks are detailed, extremely wordy, and include a plethora of information that can be positively detrimental for the clinical examinations. Books dedicated to history taking and communication skill stations familiarise and prepare the candidate with the commonest examination scenarios. The examiners are looking for logical and common-sense clinical answers, not the latest theories on the molecular basis of disease; there simply is not enough time for such detailed discussions. Furthermore, examiners are briefed not to stray into their own areas of expertise. As international clinical examiners and organizers of a range of postgraduate clinical board examinations, we advise that candidates need to be concise and direct, but at all times must show empathy if they are to succeed in their history taking and communication skill stations. It is no secret that many non-English candidates will struggle with these two stations. This book includes all the possible scenarios that are typically and frequently encountered in postgraduate clinical examinations. It provides a 'model answer' for each scenario and a typical conversation between the doctor and patient, with the most likely primary and differential diagnosis alongside up-to-date information relevant to the topic.

The book is intended for candidates preparing for postgraduate clinical examinations emphasising history taking and communication skills, e.g. MRCP (UK & Ire) PACES, Arab Board, and Arabian Gulf Boards and for medical students preparing for their final clinical examinations. This book is complementary to 'Short Cases in Clinical Exams of Internal Medicine' by Professor Wanis H Ibrahim.

Wanis H Ibrahim

Important note

This publication is intended to provide postgraduate medical doctors and medical students with the necessary information to pass their clinical examinations. The authors of this book have made every effort and care to ensure the information provided in this book is accurate. However, since medical knowledge is constantly changing, neither the authors nor the publisher can assume any responsibility for any consequences arising from the use of the information contained in this book.

Acknowledgements

The authors are indebted to the following colleagues from Hamad Medical Corporation for their great assistance during the preparation of this book—Dr Mansoor Hameed from the Pulmonary Division, Dr Elrazi Awadelkarim, Dr Haseeb Chaudhary, Dr Ibrahim Abubeker, Dr Ahmed Mohie, and Dr Mohamed Ibrahim from the Internal Medicine Department, Dr Ahmed Al-Mohammed and Dr Dhabia Al-Mohannadi from the Internal Medicine Residency program, Dr Kamran Mushtaq and Dr Mohammed Elbadri from the Gastroenterology Section. Special thanks go to Dr Mohammed Danjuma, Dr Claret Charles Isabrye and Dr Akhnuwkh Jones for their review and valuable comments during the preparation of this book.

Contents

List of abbreviations

2-h PG:	2-hour plasma glucose	EEG:	Electroencephalography
ACEI:	Angiotensin-converting enzyme inhibitor	ELISA:	Enzyme-linked immunosorbent assay
AF:	Atrial fibrillation	ERCP:	Endoscopic retrograde cholangiopancreatography
AIDS:	Acquired immune deficiency syndrome	ESRD:	End-stage renal disease
AIN:	Acute interstitial nephritis	EUS:	Endoscopic ultrasound
AKI:	Acute kidney injury	FDA:	Food and drug administration
ALP:	Alkaline phosphatase	FEV1:	Forced expiratory volume in 1 second
ALT:	Alanine transaminase		
AMA:	Anti-mitochondrial antibody	FVC:	Forced vital capacity
ANA:	Anti-nuclear antibody	FPG:	Fasting plasma glucose
ARB:	Angiotensin receptor blocker	GB:	Gall bladder
AST:	Aspartate transaminase	GDM:	Gestational diabetes mellitus
BIPAP:	Bilevel positive airway pressure	GERD:	Gastroesophageal reflux disease
BMI:	Body mass index	GFR:	Glomerular filtration rate
CAD:	Coronary artery disease	GIST:	Gastrointestinal stromal tumour
CAT:	COPD assessment test	GIT:	Gastrointestinal tract
CD4:	Cluster of differentiation 4	GLP-1:	Glucagon-like peptide-1
CDI:	Clostridium difficile infection	GN:	Glomerulonephritis
CHF:	Congestive heart failure	GOLD:	Global initiative for chronic obstructive lung disease
CKD:	Chronic kidney disease		
CNS:	Central nervous system	GP:	General practitioner
COPD:	Chronic obstructive pulmonary disease	GUT:	Genito-urinary tract
		HAART:	Highly active antiretroviral therapy
COX:	Cyclooxygenase	HBeAg:	Hepatitis B e-antigen
CPAP:	Continuous positive airway pressure	HBIG:	Hepatitis B immunoglobulin
		HBsAg:	Hepatitis B surface antigen
CSF:	Cerebrospinal fluid	HBV:	Hepatitis B virus
CT scan:	Computed tomography scan	Hct:	Hematocrit
CVS:	Cardiovascular system	HCV:	Hepatitis C virus
CXR:	Chest X-ray	HONK:	Hyperglycaemic non-ketotic state
DAPT:	Dual anti-platelet therapy	HP:	Hypersensitivity pneumonitis
DM:	Diabetes mellitus	HPI:	History of presenting illness
DNAR:	Do not attempt resuscitation	HSCT:	Haematopoietic stem cell transplantation
DPI:	Dry powder inhaler		
DPP4:	Dipeptidyl peptidase 4	HTN:	Hypertension
DVLA:	Driver and vehicle licensing agency	ICP:	Intracranial pressure
DVT:	Deep venous thrombosis	IFG:	Impaired fasting glucose
ECG:	Electrocardiogram	IGT:	Impaired glucose tolerance

IL5:	Interleukin 5		PEFR:	Peak expiratory flow rate
ILD:	Interstitial lung disease		PEG:	Percutaneous endoscopic gastrostomy
IPF:	Idiopathic pulmonary fibrosis			
LABA:	Long-acting beta agonist		PEJ:	Percutaneous endoscopic jejunostomy
LAMA:	Long-acting muscarinic agent			
LKM:	Liver-kidney-muscle		PET scan:	Positron emission tomography scan
LTOT:	Long-term oxygen therapy			
MDI:	Metered dose inhaler		PFT:	Pulmonary function testing
MEN:	Multiple endocrine neoplasia		PLMS:	Periodic limb movement syndrome
MODY:	Maturity-onset diabetes of the young		PND:	Paroxysmal nocturnal dyspnoea
			PPI:	Proton pump inhibitor
MRCP:	Magnetic resonance cholangiopancreatography		PUD:	Peptic ulcer disease
			RA:	Rheumatoid arthritis
MRI:	Magnetic resonance imaging		RLS:	Restless leg syndrome
MS:	Multiple sclerosis		RRMS:	Relapsing remitting MS
NAFLD:	Non-alcoholic fatty liver disease		SABA:	Short-acting beta agonist
NASH:	Non-alcoholic steatohepatitis		SGLT2:	Sodium–glucose cotransporter 2
NSAID:	Nonsteroidal anti-inflammatory drug		SLE:	Systemic lupus erythematosus
			SLICC:	Systemic Lupus International Collaborating Clinics
OGTT:	Oral glucose tolerance test			
OHS:	Obesity hypoventilation syndrome		STEMI:	ST elevation myocardial infarction
OSA:	Obstructive sleep apnoea		TB:	Tuberculosis
OSCE:	Objective structured clinical examination.		TIA:	Transient ischaemic attack
			TN:	Trigeminal neuralgia
PACES:	Practical assessment of clinical examination skills		TSH:	Thyroid-stimulating hormone
			UAS:	Upper airway stimulation
PCI:	Percutaneous coronary intervention		UVPPP:	Uvulopalatopharyngoplasty
			VHL:	von Hippel–Lindau
PCR:	Polymerase chain reaction			

Introduction

The value of history taking

Despite the advent in modern medical technology and the wide availability of sophisticated laboratory and imaging tests, proper history taking, and physical examination remain the most valuable diagnostic tools in clinical medicine and the cornerstone of clinical practice. Ninety percent of all correct diagnoses can be made through a combination of patient history, physical examination and basic tests, excluding imaging studies. Medical history alone can contribute to the final diagnosis in up to 80% of cases and a proper history can limit expensive and anxiety-producing investigations. Taking a proper history involves carefully listening to what the patient has to say, followed by relevant and systematic questions. Doctors, who communicate effectively, can more accurately diagnose their patient's problems and in turn their patients better understand their disease and adhere to treatment.

History taking and communication skill stations in clinical examinations

Clinical examinations are an integral part in the assessment of a doctor's clinical competence. History taking and communication skill stations are a key determinant of success or failure in all national or international clinical examinations. Whilst the time allocated for each station may differ slightly, the overall objective is the same—'can this doctor take an adequate history and communicate effectively?'

Timing for communication skill station for the PACES examination:
- 5 minutes to read the scenario and make notes
- 14 minutes to communicate with the patient/surrogate
- 1 minute to collect your thoughts
- 5 minutes for discussion with examiners.

Timing for communication skill station for the Arab Board OSCE Examination:
- 3 minutes to read the scenario
- 10 minutes with the patient/surrogate.

Plate 1

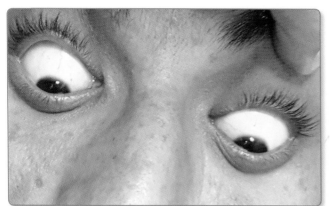

Figure 2 Patient with jaundice (Part 1).

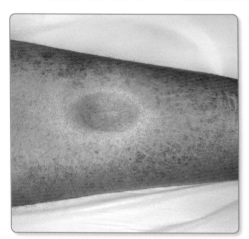

Figure 1 Pitting oedema of the legs (Part 2).

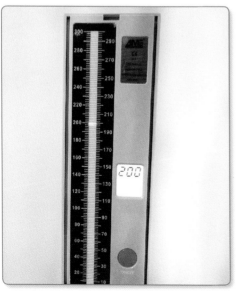

Figure 2 High blood pressure (Part 2).

Plate 2

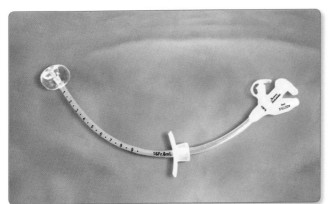

Figure 1 PEG tube (Part 4).

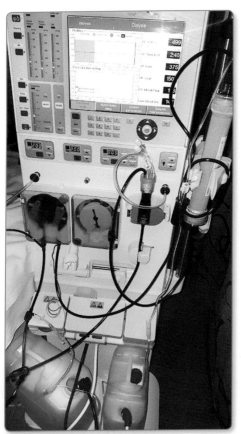

Figure 2 Haemodialysis machine (Part 4).

Part 1

History taking station

Important rules regarding history taking station

- Candidates should read the scenario carefully and make a plan before entering the station. Think about what questions to ask and write your plan on a paper.
- While reading the scenario, candidates often feel that the information given on the paper is not sufficient to point to a particular disease or problem. Do not panic; more information will come during patient/surrogate interview.
- Follow the systematic manner of history taking. Use the following five step approach for history taking (see the steps of history taking below):
  - *Introduction and greeting*
  - *Obtain the history*
  - *Explain the diagnosis and plan of management to the patient*
  - *Ask about and respond to patient's concerns/questions*
  - *Summarise, check understanding, and close the interview.*

- Make note of any positive points in the history provided by the surrogate. Most of the time, such information is relevant to the problem.
- Do not forget to enquire about and respond to patient's concerns.
- Do not forget to ask about the effect of the illness on certain aspects of patient's life such as job, psychological status, sexual life, daily activity, and family.
- Do not forget menstrual history in females.
- Do not forget to explain to the patient the problem, summarise the interview, and properly close the discussion.
- During examinations, candidates often forget important aspects in the history. Develop your own way of remembering important points. For instance, use the mnemonic "MOTHERS" while enquiring about social history.
- Some candidates feel that time given for the history taking station is not enough. This is usually due to lack of adequate preparation. Frequent practice of history taking scenarios under the supervision of a registrar/colleague/consultant will overcome this problem.

Steps to follow in the history taking station

The following are ideal steps to be followed by candidates in history taking stations (as well as in real patient encounters). Candidates often forget important steps such as summarisation, confirmation of patient's understanding, and proper closure of the interview.

1. Establish rapport and good doctor-patient relationship

- Introduce yourself, address the patient with respect, and shake hands with the patient (be aware of social and religious reasons preventing some patients from shaking your hand).
- Inform the patient the purpose of the meeting.
- Sit at the same level as the patient and remove barriers (**Figure 1**).

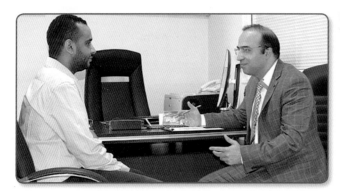

Figure 1 Sit at the same level as the patient and avoid barriers.

- Be a good listener—avoid unnecessary interruptions.
- Make sure you avoid 'speech diarrhoea'—talking too much and interrupting the patient.
- Start with an open-ended question.

2. Obtain the history

Personal history

Confirm the name and age.

Chief complaints and their duration

- I understand that you have been referred by your GP because of (symptom). Could you tell me more about that?
- Could you kindly tell me what has been the problem recently?
- *Avoid*: What brought you in this time? Or why are you here today?

History of presenting illness

- Define the chief complaints (each symptom has its own way of analysis; please see "how to analyse chief symptoms).
- Review the system(s) involved as associated symptoms.
- Determine disease progress, investigations, and treatment given.
- Establish effects of the disease on different aspects of the patient's life:
    - Function and activity
    - Sexual life
    - Psychology
    - Family—divorce/separation/care.
    - Finance and work

Past medical history

- Similar symptom(s) in the past.
- *Common diseases*: Diabetes mellitus (DM), hypertension (HTN), heart disease, cancer, kidney disease, and respiratory diseases
  (If there are any of these diseases, you must establish details of each disease such as level of control, complications, follow-up, and the level of patient's education regarding the disease).
- Previous hospitalisations/transfusions/medical procedures.

Past surgical history

Previous surgery/complications.

Menstrual history

- Menarche
- *Menstrual periods*: Regular—amount
- Use of oral contraceptive pills
- Pregnancies and abortions.

Dietary history

Vegetarian/normal diet/risk control diet.

Family history

- Similar illness
- Other illnesses
- Inherited disorders
- Malignancy.

Drug history

- Chronic drugs
- Over-the-counter drugs [such as non-steroidal anti-inflammatory drugs (NSAIDs)/anabolic steroids]
- Drug allergies.

Social history

Social history can be remembered using the mnemonic "**MOTHERS**":
- **M**arital status
- **O**ccupation
- **T**ravel
- *Habits*: Smoking, alcohol, and drug abuse
- *Exposure*: Birds/animals/pollution/sick people
- *Rupees/Riyals*: Financial status/housing
- **S**exual history.

Review of systems (Table 1)

(Pay attention to the forgotten systems by candidates such as constitutional, skin, and endocrine).
- Explain the problem, the plan of management, and follow-up plan to the patient
- Respond to the patient's concerns/questions
- Summarise, check understanding, and close.

Eliciting a history of alcohol consumption

- How much does the patient drink?
  - One unit equals 8 g of alcohol (10 mL of pure ethanol)
  - *Safe limits:* 14 units/week
- Which type of alcohol?
  - One unit equates to a 25-mL measure of spirit
  - One unit equates to half a pint of beer
  - A 175-mL glass of wine contains two units
- Ask about symptoms suggestive of alcoholism (**CAGE** questions):
  - Have you ever felt you needed to *cut down* on your drinking?
  - Have people *annoyed* you by criticising your drinking?
  - Have you ever felt *guilty* about drinking?
  - Have you ever felt you needed a drink first thing in the morning *(eye-opener)* to steady your nerves or to get rid of a hangover?
  - (Answering "yes" to any two of these questions suggests that the patient has a serious alcohol dependence problem.)

3. **Explain the problem, the plan of management, and follow-up plan to the patient.**
4. **Respond to the patient's concerns/questions.**
5. **Summarise, check understanding, and close.**

Table 1 Review of systems			
Constitutional	**Dermatology**	**Neurological system**	**Cardiovascular**
Fatigue	Rashes	Loss of consciousness	Chest pain/discomfort/ tightness
Fever	Bruising/bleeding	Dizziness	
Weight loss/gain	Itchiness	Hearing abnormalities/ tinnitus	Palpitations
		Visual problems	Shortness of breath
Endocrine	Colour changes		Orthopnoea
Heat or cold intolerance	Hair and nail changes	Seizures	Paroxysmal nocturnal dyspnoea
Sweating		Weakness	
Polydipsia		Numbness	Leg oedema
Polyphagia		Tingling	
		Tremor	
		Sphincter problems	
Respiratory	**Gastrointestinal**	**Genitourinary**	**Musculoskeletal**
Cough	Change in appetite	Loin pain	Muscle or joint pain
Sputum	Weight loss	Frequency	Stiffness
Haemoptysis	Jaundice	Urgency	Swelling of joints
Shortness of breath	Mouth ulcers	Dysuria	Back pain
Wheezing	Dysphagia	Haematuria	
Nocturnal apnoea	Heartburn	Incontinence	
Snoring	Nausea and vomiting	Weak stream	
	Haematemesis	Urethral discharge	
	Diarrhoea	Erectile dysfunction	
	Constipation		
	Rectal bleeding		

Further reading

Beresford TP, Blow FC, Hill E, et al. Comparison of CAGE questionnaire and computer-assisted laboratory profiles in screening for covert alcoholism. Lancet 1990; 336:482–485.

Department of Health and Social Care. UK Chief Medical Officers' Low Risk Drinking Guidelines, 2016. [online] Available from https://assets.publishing.service.gov.uk/government/uploads/system/uploads/attachment_data/file/545937/UK_CMOs__report.pdf [Last accessed October, 2019].

Ewing JA. Detecting alcoholism. The CAGE questionnaire. JAMA 1984; 252:1905–1907.

How to analyse chief symptoms

Fatigue

Common scenarios

- Anaemia:
  - Non-steroidal anti-inflammatory drug-induced gastrointestinal tract (GIT) loss
  - Gastrointestinal tract malignancy
  - Malabsorption (celiac)
- Adrenal insufficiency (association with type 1 diabetes mellitus)
- Myasthenia gravis:
  - Diurnal variation of fatigue associated with muscle weakness
- Hypothyroidism:
  - Weight gain, dry skin, and hair loss
- Obstructive sleep apnoea
- Chronic fatigue syndrome

Fatigue is a nonspecific symptom that denotes a feeling of tiredness and lack of energy and can be caused by many diseases that involve different systems. In postgraduate clinical examination, common causes of fatigue include anaemia (most commonly from GIT loss), chronic fatigue syndrome (CFS), obstructive sleep apnoea (OSA), and to lesser extent diseases of other systems such as myasthenia gravis, heart failure, hypothyroidism, depression, and drugs (Candidates often forget to ask about symptoms suggestive of OSA such as heavy snoring and nocturnal apnoea).

Important points to elaborate in the history of fatigue

- **What does the patient mean exactly by fatigue?**
  Does he/she mean excessive tiredness or weakness? Weakness may suggest a neuromuscular disorder. Sometimes, patients may use these two terms interchangeably to mean lack of energy and increased tiredness.

- **Onset of fatigue**
  New-onset fatigue that was not there before and tends to worsen with time usually indicates an organic/physical cause and should be investigated.

- **How long have you had the fatigue?**
  Longer duration may suggest chronic fatigue syndrome.

- **Is it worse with time?**
  Fatigue that worsens with time usually indicates an organic cause.

- **Is it related to exertion or only at rest?**
  Fatigue that worsens with physical activity and improves with rest suggests organic (e.g. anaemia) rather than psychological cause.

- **Is there any diurnal variation of the fatigue?**
  This is a very important question that is often forgotten by candidates and it may be the clue to the diagnosis of mysathenia. Fatigue in patients with myasthenia gravis tends to worsen at the end of the day.

- **What are the aggravating and relieving factors of fatigue?**
  Can you tell me if there is anything that makes your fatigue worse? Exertion may point to anaemia or other chronic diseases such as kidney disease, muscle disease,

connective tissue disease, etc. Diurnal changes may point to myasthenia gravis. In CFS, the fatigue may worsen with physical or mental activity, but does not improve with rest.

Important associated symptoms in a patient with fatigue

- **Dizziness:** Particularly postural, may suggest anaemia or adrenal insufficiency.
- **Muscle pain:** May suggest muscle disease.
- **Change in appetite:** May suggest hyper-/hypothyroidism, diabetes, cancer, etc.
- **Change in weight:** Weight loss with fatigue usually suggests serious disorders such as cancer, thyrotoxicosis, chronic infections, or connective tissue disorders.
- **Symptoms that may suggest endocrinopathies (hyper-/hypothyroidism, adrenal insufficiency, and Cushing's syndrome):** Hot/cold intolerance, weight gain, weight loss, palpitations, postural dizziness, etc.
- **Symptoms of blood loss:** Melena, haematemesis, and fresh bleeding per rectum.
- **Fever:** May suggest chronic infections.
- **Heavy snoring, nocturnal apnoea, and morning headaches:** Suggest OSA.

Review of systems

As fatigue can be caused by diseases of many body systems, it is crucial that you perform a detailed and thorough review of all systems.

Fatigue may be the sole manifestation of adrenal insufficiency; therefore, you should ask about increased pigmentation, abdominal symptoms, and the presence of other autoimmune diseases.

Past history, menstrual history, dietary history, family history, drug history, social history, and review of systems: Should be covered as described in the "steps to follow in history taking".

Chronic fatigue syndrome

The diagnosis CFS should be considered after excluding other possible causes and the symptoms have persisted for 4 months in an adult. Careful history, physical examination, and necessary laboratory investigations have to be done before diagnosing a patient with CFS. There is no single test to confirm the diagnosis of CFS. Red flag symptoms/signs that should point to other diagnosis include:
- Localising/focal neurological signs
- Signs and symptoms of inflammatory arthritis or connective tissue disease
- Signs and symptoms of cardiorespiratory disease
- Significant weight loss
- Sleep apnoea
- Clinically significant lymphadenopathy.

Further reading

Rosenthal TC, Majeroni BA, Pretorius R, et al. Fatigue: an overview. Am Fam Physician 2008; 78:1173–1179.
National Institute for Health and Care Excellence (NICE). Chronic fatigue syndrome/myalgic encephalomyelitis (or encephalopathy): diagnosis and management. Clinical guideline [CG53], 2007. [online] Available from https://www.nice.org.uk/guidance/cg53/chapter/1-Guidance#presentation [Last accessed October, 2019].

Weight loss

> **Common scenarios**
>
> - Hyperthyroidism
> - Type 1 diabetes mellitus
> - Malabsorption syndromes (celiac)
> - Malignancy (GIT)
> - Acquired immunodeficiency syndrome (AIDS)
> - Anorexia nervosa

Weight loss can be intentional or unintentional. Many conditions can cause significant weight loss and include psychological diseases (depression, anorexia nervosa, and bulimia nervosa), chronic infections, malignancies, poor nutrition, and hyperthyroidism.

Important points to elaborate in the history of weight loss

- **How much weight has the patient lost?**
  See the classification of significant weight loss in **Table 2**.

- **Intentional or unintentional**
  Ask whether weight loss is intentional or unintentional.

- **How is the patient's appetite?**
  Conditions that cause weight loss with increased appetite include:
  - Hyperthyroidism
  - Diabetes mellitus
  - Bulimia nervosa
  - Insulinoma
  - Anxiety/depression.

- **Dietary history**
  Ask details about the patient's dietary history.

- **Use of slimming pills**
  Do you use any slimming pills or over-the counter tablets that may reduce weight? A number of over-the counter medications may cause weight loss.

- **Recent change in psychological status**
  Depression/anxiety may lead to weight loss.

- **Associated symptoms**
  - How is your appetite?

Table 2 Classification of severity of weight loss		
	Significant weight loss	**Severe weight loss**
1 week	1–2%	>2%
1 month	5%	>5%
3 months	7.5%	>7.5%
6 months	10%	>10%

- Palpitations, sweating, heat intolerance, eye problems, rash, and hyperthyroidism
- Review carefully the GIT system
- Review all the systems with particular attention to the GIT system, endocrine system, and cardiovascular and respiratory systems.

Past history, menstrual history, dietary history, family history, drug history, social history and review of systems
- Pay attention to past history or family history of neoplasms
- Pay attention to smoking history and dietary history.

Further reading

Blackburn GL, Bistrian BR, Maini BS, et al. Nutritional and metabolic assessment of the hospitalized patient. J Parenter Enteral Nutr 1977; 1:11–22.
Vanderschueren S, Geens E, Knockaert D, et al. The diagnostic spectrum of unintentional weight loss. Eur J Intern Med 2005; 16:160–164.

Joint pain

Common scenarios

- Rheumatoid arthritis (RA)
- Reactive arthritis
- Gout
- Systemic lupus erythematosus (SLE)
- Behçet's disease

- **What is the duration of joint pain?**
  Acute symptoms last from hours to 2 weeks.
  Chronic symptoms last beyond 2 weeks. Septic arthritis usually presents acutely and typically involves a single large joint.

- **Which joints are affected? And how many are affected?**
  The size (small or large) and kind of joints involved provide major diagnostic clues. Spondyloarthropathies typically involve the spine, including sacroiliac joints and medium/large joints, such as the shoulders, hips, knees and ankles. RA and lupus typically involve smaller joints such as the wrists, fingers, and toes.
  Number of joints affected are also important: pauciarticular pattern (two to four joints) and polyarticular pattern (five or more joints). Spondyloarthropathies are typically pauciarticular, whereas RA is usually polyarticular. Some spondyloarthropathies, such as psoriatic arthritis, may also present in a polyarticular manner.

- **Is it only pain (arthralgia) or is it associated with swelling and redness?**
  Two broad categories of arthritis are recognised: (1) Inflammatory and (2) Non-inflammatory (degenerative arthritis). The following symptoms usually suggest inflammatory type—presence of joint swelling, erythema, prolonged morning stiffness (>1 hour), and pain at rest. Involvement of weight bearing joints and pain that is mainly on movement are suggestive of non-inflammatory type of arthritis, such as osteoarthritis.

- **Is it symmetrical or asymmetrical?**
  A symmetric presentation suggests an underlying inflammatory arthritis.

- **Does it involve the axial joints?**
  - Ankylosing spondylitis
  - Spondyloarthropathies.

- **Is there morning stiffness?**
  If there is morning stiffness, ask about the duration of this stiffness. Non-inflammatory arthritis typically causes less than 1 hour of morning stiffness. Prolonged morning stiffness (>1 hour) is suggestive of inflammatory conditions.

- **Is it migratory arthritis?**
  In migratory arthritis, symptoms shift from one joint to another and do not stay in one joint for very long. Diseases that are typically associated with migratory arthritis are:
  - Rheumatic fever
  - Systemic lupus erythematosus
  - Infectious arthritis such as gonococcal arthritis
  - Whipple's and Lyme disease.

- **Is it aggravated by activity or rest? And does it wake the patient from sleep?**
  Joint pain that comes on at rest and wakes the patient from sleep usually indicates inflammatory arthritis.

Presence of extra-articular symptoms (particularly eyes and skin)

Symptoms of uveitis/conjunctivitis (eye redness and pain)

- Ankylosing spondylitis
- Behçet's disease
- Rheumatoid arthritis
- Conjunctivitis.

Skin rash/nodules

- Psoriatic arthritis
- Systemic lupus erythematosus
- Rheumatoid arthritis (nodules)
- Henoch-Schonlein purpura.

Gastrointestinal tract symptoms

Diarrhoea

- Reactive arthritis
- Inflammatory bowel disease
- Whipple's disease.

Mouth ulcers

- Behçet's disease
- Systemic lupus erythematosus
- Crohn's disease.

Urethral/genitourinary tract

Symptoms of urethritis may suggest reactive arthritis.

Fever

Septic arthritis/reactive arthritis/other rheumatologic disorders.

Past history of chronic diseases

- Kidney disease, hypothyroidism, etc. (may lead to crystal-induced arthritis).
- Gout and pseudogout.

Family history
Family history of rheumatologic and autoimmune diseases.

Drug history
Use of steroids and immunosuppressant medication.

Sexual history
- Gonococcal infection
- Human immunodeficiency virus (HIV)
- Hepatitis B virus (HBV), hepatitis C virus (HCV) (ask about previous transfusions and drug abuse). They all may cause arthritis.
- *Chlamydia trachomatis*: Reactive arthritis.

Social history
Candidate should obtain a detailed social history with a focus on the effect of the symptoms on his/her functional capabilities, job, financial and family status.

Travel history
- Lyme disease (exposure to ticks in endemic areas)
- Reactive arthritis.

Review of systems

Rheumatoid arthritis and SLE can involve multiple organs such as lungs, heart and haematological and nervous systems. Ask carefully about symptoms of urethritis and conjunctivitis for possibility of reactive arthritis (Reiter's disease) (Can't see, can't pee, and can't bend his knee).

Further reading

Dearborn JT, Jergesen HE. The evaluation and initial management of arthritis. Prim Care 1996; 23:215–240.
Pujalte GG, Albano-Aluquin SA. Differential diagnosis of polyarticular arthritis. Am Fam Physician 2015; 92:35–41.

Sudden loss of vision

Common scenarios
- Transient ischaemic attack (TIA)
- Giant cell arteritis
- Vitreous haemorrhage (diabetic retinopathy)
- Optic neuritis

History of presenting illness

- **Is the visual loss monocular or binocular?**
  The differential diagnoses of sudden vision loss are vast. In general, monocular vision loss usually indicates an ocular problem. Binocular vision loss is usually cerebral in origin.

- **Is it just a single episode or were there previous episodes?**
  Recurrent episodes of loss of vision may suggest TIA.

- **Was the onset acute or chronic?**

- **What is the duration?**

- **How has it progressed?**

- **Is it painful or painless?**

- **Is the pain worse when you move your eyes?**
  Optic neuritis usually occurs in multiple sclerosis and visual loss is associated with pain on eye movement. The most common reason for painless sudden visual loss is ischaemia.

- **Does it involve the entire visual field or a part and which part?**

- **Are there any other visual symptoms?**
  Floaters, flashing lights, halos around lights, distorted colour vision and jagged/mosaic patterns (scintillating scotoma) may point to certain causes of sudden visual loss such as retinal detachment or vitreous haemorrhage.

- **Is there any history of eye trauma?**
  In addition to diabetic retinopathy, vitreous haemorrhage can also be caused by eye trauma.

Review of systems
- Ask about jaw or tongue claudication (giant cell arteritis).
- Temporal headache (giant cell arteritis).
- Proximal muscle pain and stiffness (giant cell arteritis).
- Headache (ocular migraine and giant cell arteritis).
- Review the cardiovascular system carefully for palpitations [atrial fibrillation (AF)], coronary artery disease (CAD), intermittent claudication, and rest pain.

Past medical history
- Ask about previous ophthalmic history (e.g. contact lens use, severe myopia, recent eye surgery or injury).
- Ask about previous strokes (TIA).
- *Ask about diabetes mellitus*: DM can cause thrombosis/TIA and vitreous haemorrhage and both can lead to sudden visual loss.
- Ask about other risk factors for vascular disease, e.g. hypertension and haematologic disorders (sickle cell, polycythaemia, Waldenström macroglobulinemia, or multiple myeloma can cause a hyperviscosity syndrome).
- Ask about heart disease and AF.

Drug history
- Oral contraceptive pills
- Ergot alkaloids for migraine
- *Anticoagulants/antiplatelets*: Vitreous haemorrhage.

Family history
- Migraine headaches
- Thrombophilia.

Social history

Smoking history.

Further reading

Chan S. Sudden loss of vision. Hong Kong Med J 2010; 16:155.
Du Toit N. Sudden loss of vision. S Afr Fam Pract 2013; 55:235–240.
Sharma N, Ooi JL, Sharma D, et al. Sudden loss of vision – a case study. Aust Fam Physician 2013; 42:48–50.

Dyspepsia

Common scenarios

- Dyspepsia in old people with alarm symptoms
- Chronic mesenteric ischaemia

History of presenting illness

- **What does the patient mean exactly by dyspepsia?**
  Although epigastric pain is the predominant symptom of dyspepsia, the definition may also include other symptoms such as heartburn, nausea or bloating.

If the main symptom is pain, then assess the pain using the mnemonic:

LIQOR AAA
Location of symptom, **I**ntensity of symptom, **Q**uality of symptom, **O**nset of symptom/precipitating factors, **R**adiation of symptom, **A**ssociated symptoms, **A**lleviating factors, and **A**ggravating factors.

DOCS ARE FIT
Duration, **O**nset, **C**haracter, **S**ite, **A**ssociated Symptoms, **R**adiation, **E**xacerbating and relieving factors, **F**requency, **I**ntensity, and **T**iming.

Ask about the relationship of the symptoms to food and which type of food aggravates the symptoms [gallbladder (GB) disease, peptic ulcer disease (PUD), mesenteric ischaemia, chronic pancreatitis, etc.].

The candidate must ask about the alarm symptoms for dyspepsia

- Unintentional weight loss
- Older age group >60 years
- Progressive dysphagia/ progressive symptoms
- Odynophagia
- Unexplained iron deficiency anaemia
- Persistent vomiting
- Palpable mass or lymphadenopathy
- Family history of upper gastrointestinal cancer.

Review of systems

- Ask about dysphagia.
- Symptoms suggestive of gastroesophageal reflux disease (GERD) (heartburn, acidity and regurgitation).
- Vomiting, haematemesis, melena, and change in bowel habit.

Past history

- Past history of PUD, GB disease.
- Past history of AF, DM, HTN, and CAD pointing toward chronic mesenteric ischaemia.

Family history

- Family history of GIT malignancies or other malignancies.
- Family history of PUD.

Drug history

- Use of NSAIDs/steroids—PUD
- Use of warfarin—chronic mesenteric ischaemia [ask about international normalised ratio (INR) levels].

Social history

- Smoking history
- Alcohol use.

Further reading

Moayyedi PM, Lacy BE. Andrews CA, et al. ACG and CAG Clinical Guideline: management of dyspepsia. Am J Gastroenterol 2017; 112:988–1013.
Talley NJ, Vakil NB, Moayyedi P. American Gastroenterological Association technical review on the evaluation of dyspepsia. Gastroenterology 2005; 129:1756–1780.

Headache

Common scenarios

- Migraine
- Cerebral venous sinus thrombosis
- Giant cell arteritis
- Idiopathic intracranial hypertension
- Pheochromocytoma
- Trigeminal neuralgia
- Cluster headache
- Headache in immunocompromised patient

History of presenting illness

Headache like any other pain should be analysed using the LIQOR AAA.

Migraine headache

- Usually throbbing or pulsatile
- Commonly on one side
- Aggravated by menstrual periods, alcohol, lack of sleep, certain foods such as chocolate, cheese, coffee, etc.
- May be preceded by migraine aura such as problems with vision, dizziness, lip, and facial numbness, etc.
- Usually lasts for hours and sometimes for days.
- Associated with nausea and vomiting, photophobia, phonophobia, or depression.
- Relieved by migraine treatment such as triptans and indomethacin.
- In addition, patients tend to prefer resting in a quiet dark room.

Headache due to increased intracranial pressure

- Usually generalised "all over" headache.
- Tends to be of maximal intensity in the morning.
- Usually dull and deep.
- Aggravated by coughing, bending forward, sneezing and Valsalva manoeuvre.
- May be relieved by rest.
- Associated with projectile vomiting.
- May be associated with changes in the level of consciousness, seizure, personality changes, limb weakness, or numbness.

Hypertension headache

- Usually causes throbbing headache.
- The headache is usually occipital.
- Usually more intense on awakening.
- May persist for days.
- May be associated with palpitations, blurring of vision, confusion, seizure, or deterioration of level of consciousness.

Cluster headache

- Unilateral, often severe headache.
- Attacks usually come in clusters, i.e. occur daily (often at the same time) for some weeks followed by a period of remission.
- *Typical sites include:* Orbital, supraorbital, or temporal regions.
- Typically associated with autonomic symptoms such as ptosis, meiosis, lacrimation, conjunctival injection, rhinorrhoea, and nasal congestion.
- Attacks typically last for minutes to less than 2 hours.

Trigeminal neuralgia

- Recurrent brief episodes of unilateral electric shock-like pains.
- Onset is sudden.
- Duration is very short (seconds).
- *Location*: In the distribution of one or more divisions of the fifth cranial (trigeminal) nerve (most commonly V2 and V3, very rare in V1 distribution).

- The pain usually occurs in paroxysms.
- Trigeminal neuralgia pain is classically triggered by light touch of the face in V1, V2, and V3 areas.
- *Other triggering factors include:* Brushing teeth, chewing, talking, grimacing, or smiling.
- Trigeminal neuralgia typically occurs after the age of 50 years.
- If trigeminal neuralgia is diagnosed before the age of 50 years, a secondary cause has to be excluded such as demyelinating disease [multiple sclerosis (MS)] or cerebellopontine angle tumours and an MRI brain is mandatory before diagnosing idiopathic trigeminal neuralgia.

Tension headache

- Frequent headache episodes.
- Duration is minutes to days.
- Bilateral pain, pressing, and tightening (e.g. "band-like").
- Mild-to-moderate intensity.
- No nausea/vomiting.
- No more than one of photophobia or phonophobia.
- Not aggravated by routine activities.
- May or may not be associated with pericranial tenderness on manual palpation.

Headache due to pheochromocytoma

- Sudden onset.
- Short duration.
- Unlike migraine, it is bilateral affecting any part of the head. The occipital, nuchal-occipital, and frontal-occipital regions are the predominant locations.
- Throbbing, pulsating.
- Frequently associated with palpitations and excess sweating.
- Apprehension and/or anxiety, often with a sense of impending death, tremor.
- Sudden increase in both systolic and diastolic blood pressure before and after the onset of headache.

Review of systems

- Other neurological symptoms.
- *Trigeminal neuralgia in young*: Ask about other symptoms of MS.
- *Symptoms of pheochromocytoma*: Palpitation, sweating, anxiety and nervousness.
- *Symptoms suggestive of increased intracranial pressure (ICP)*: Projectile vomiting, personality changes and seizure/weakness/numbness.
- Ask about alarm/red flag symptoms of headache (See below).

Past medical history

- Ask about history of HTN.
- Ask about history of migraine.
- Ask about previous strokes, brain lesions.
- Ask about previous head trauma.
- Ask about diseases that cause immunosuppression.
- *Recurrent sinusitis*: Can lead to cerebral venous thrombosis, brain abscess, or meningitis.

Family history

- Family history of migraine.
- Family history of cancer.

Drug history

- *Use of oral contraceptive pills*: Cerebral venous sinus thrombosis, migraine.
- Drugs for migraine.
- Steroids.
- *Other drugs that may cause increased ICP*: Isoretinoic acid, tetracyclines, steroids, etc.

Social history

- Smoking (risk of malignancy).
- *Alcohol*: Subdural haematoma, bleeding.
- Change in personality.
- *Travel history*: Malaria, meningitis.
- *Sexual history*: HIV, neurosyphilis.

What are the red flag symptoms/signs of headache?
- New-onset headache.
- Severe headache (worst headache in patient's life)/thunderclap headache.
- Associated symptoms such as fever, weight loss.
- Development of focal neurological signs such as weakness, seizure, or confusion.
- Headache in immunocompromised patient/HIV (toxoplasmosis, tumours)
- New headache in a pregnant woman (preeclampsia, cerebral venous sinus thrombosis).
- Headache in older age groups (see below).
- Other symptoms of increased ICP such as projectile vomiting, worsening with stooping, cough, exertion, or sexual activity.

Headache in older patients (above age of 50 years)

New onset headache in older people may suggest serious underlying conditions such as:
- Brain tumour
- Giant cell arteritis
- Trigeminal neuralgia
- Chronic subdural haematoma.

Further reading

Bryans R, Decina P, Descarreaux M, et al. Clinical Practice Guideline for the Management of Headache Disorders in Adults. (2012) [online] Available from https://www.researchgate.net/publication/262636337_Clinical_Practice_Guideline_for_the_Management_of_Headache_Disorders_in_Adults. [Last accessed October, 2019].

Headache Classification Committee of the International Headache Society (IHS). The international classification of headache disorders, 3rd edition (beta version). Cephalalgia 2013; 33:629–808.

Watanabe M. Headache in pheochromocytoma. In: Martin JF (Ed). Pheochromocytoma: A New View of the Old Problem. New York: IntechOpen; 2011.

Loss of consciousness/seizure/confusion

> **Common scenarios**
> - New-onset seizure
> - Syncopal attack
> - Hypoglycaemia
> - Loss of consciousness in alcoholic patient

History of presenting illness

- Was it witnessed by someone else?
- Was it sudden?
- What were the circumstances before the episode? What was the patient doing?
- Did the patient become unaware of the surrounding?
- Was the attack preceded by an aura?
- Was the attack preceded by headache?
- How many times has it happened?
- How long did the attack last?
- Did the patient sustain any head trauma before the attack?
- Did the patient bite his/her tongue/injure him/herself during the attack?
- Did the patient lose sphincter control during the attack?
- Any jerky movements with the attack? If yes, where did they start and how did they proceed?
- Any other neurological symptoms such as weakness, tingling/numbness, headache, and double vision?
- How did the attack end?
- Did it end spontaneously, or with administration of glucose, or benzodiazepines, etc.?
- What happened after the attack?
- Did the patient experience any confusion or weakness?
- Was blood sugar and/or electrolytes checked?

Review of systems

- Ask about other neurological symptoms.
- Ask about cardiovascular symptoms, e.g. palpitation and chest pain (arrhythmia can lead to loss of consciousness).
- Review other systems.

Past history

- Past history of similar episodes
- Past history of epilepsy
- Past history of diabetes (if yes enquire about details of diabetic control)
- Past history of neurological, cardiac, and renal diseases
- Past history of depression or psychiatric diseases (drugs/suicide)
- Previous accidents or head trauma.

Family history

- Family history of epilepsy
- Family history of neurological disease.

Drug history

- Drug history (particularly in the elderly).
- Currently prescribed and over-the-counter medications.
- Is there any withdrawal or sudden discontinuation of any medication (such as benzodiazepines and neuropsychiatric medications) before the incident? Drug withdrawal is an important cause of loss of consciousness, seizure and confusion. Check drug interaction.

Social history

- Details of alcohol intake
- Drug abuse
- Living condition
- Recent travel.

Causes of loss of consciousness/seizure/syncope/acute confusion

- *Structural brain lesion*:
  - *Parenchyma*: Space-occupying lesion/abscess/oedema/trauma
  - *Vascular*:
    - *Arteries:* Ischaemic stroke, haemorrhagic stroke
    - *Veins*: Cerebral venous thrombosis.
  - *Meninges*: Meningoencephalitis
  - *Hypoperfusion states*:
    - Carotid stenosis
    - Severe aortic stenosis
    - *Severe hypotension*: Shock, postural and drugs.
- *Metabolic and systemic causes (look for organs in the body other than brain)*:
  - *Thyroid:* Hypothyroidism/hyperthyroidism
  - *Lungs*: Hypercapnia
  - *Liver*: Hepatic encephalopathy
  - *Kidneys*: Uremic encephalopathy
  - *Blood*:
    - Hypoglycaemia/hyperglycaemia
    - Hypocalcaemia/hypercalcaemia
    - Hyponatraemia/hypernatraemia
    - Thiamine deficiency.
- *Cardiac causes*:
  - Arrhythmias
  - Myocardial infarction/cardiac arrest.
- *Drugs and drug withdrawal*:
  - Alcohol intoxication/withdrawal
  - Drugs and drug withdrawal
  - Toxic agents.
- *Idiopathic epilepsy*.

Further reading

Palaniswamy C, Aronow WS, Agrawal N, et al. Syncope: approaches to diagnosis and management. Am J Ther 2016; 23:e208–17.

Breathlessness/dyspnoea

> ## Common scenarios
> - Exertional breathlessness due to anaemia from use of aspirin/clopidogrel/NSAIDs
> - Hypersensitivity pneumonitis (extrinsic allergic alveolitis)
> - Chronic breathlessness from respiratory muscle weakness
> - Congestive heart failure

History of presenting illness

- **How long do you have breathlessness?**

- **How was the onset of breathlessness? Was it acute or chronic?**
  Duration and onset of breathlessness is very important. Acute breathlessness/
  dyspnoea usually develops over hours to a few days. Chronic breathlessness usually
  has duration more than 4 weeks.
  Conditions that may cause acute breathlessness include:
  - Pulmonary embolism
  - Asthma exacerbation/chronic obstructive pulmonary disease (COPD)
  - Pneumonia
  - Acute pulmonary oedema
  - Acute myocardial infarction
  - Acute aortic dissection
  - Pneumothorax
  - Acute hypersensitivity pneumonitis.
  Conditions that may cause chronic breathlessness:
  - Chronic heart failure
  - Interstitial lung diseases
  - Anaemia
  - Respiratory muscle weakness from neuromuscular disorders
  - Obesity
  - Pulmonary arterial hypertension
  - Chronic thromboembolic pulmonary hypertension.

- **Is it at rest, exertion, or both?**

- **How severe is the dyspnoea?**

Modified medical research council dyspnoea scale

- *Grade 0:* I only get breathless with strenuous exercise.
- *Grade 1:* I get shortness of breath when hurrying on level ground or walking up a slight hill.
- *Grade 2:* On level ground, I walk slower than people of the same age because of
  breathlessness or have to stop for breath when walking at my own pace.
- *Grade 3:* I stop for breath after walking about 100 yards or after a few minutes on level
  ground.
- *Grade 4:* I am too breathless to leave the house, or I am breathless when dressing.

- **Is there associated paroxysmal nocturnal dyspnoea (PND)? (Do you wake up from
  sleep because of difficulty in breathing?)**
  Paroxysmal nocturnal dyspnoea (PND) is typically associated with heart failure. It
  can also happen with asthma. Unlike heart failure, in asthma, dyspnoea is usually not
  related to exertion and PND does not usually improve with sitting forward.

- **Is there associated orthopnoea? (Do you feel breathless when you lie flat?)**
  Orthopnoea occurs because of redistribution of interstitial oedema when the patient lies in the supine position. It is characteristic of left ventricular failure. Patients with orthopnoea tend to sleep in the upright position and use multiple pillows to keep them sitting. Absence of orthopnoea argues against presence of significant left ventricular failure.

- **Is there associated ankle swelling?**
  Presence of ankle oedema may be due to heart failure, cor pulmonale, nephrotic syndrome, liver disease, calcium channel blockers, and pregabalin.

- **Are there associated palpitations?**

- **Is there associated syncope?**

- **Is there associated postural dizziness?**

- **Is there any associated chest pain?**

- **Is there associated abdominal distension?**

- **Are there associated symptoms of anaemia such as blood loss, fatigue, etc.?**

Review of systems

- Review cardiovascular system
- Review respiratory system
- Ask about melena/haematemesis/blood loss.

Menstrual history

- History of recurrent abortions (pulmonary embolism/antiphospholipid).
- Use of oral contraceptive pills (pulmonary embolism).

Past medical history

- Similar illness in the past
- History of heart disease
- *History of pulmonary disease*: COPD, asthma, interstitial lung disease (ILD), etc.
- History of HTN
- History of DM
- History of anaemia
- Dietary history
- Vegetarian/diet associated with anaemia.

Drug history

- Cardiac or respiratory medications (e.g. amiodarone)
- Non-steroidal anti-inflammatory drugs/aspirin/clopidogrel causing anaemia
- Allergy and anaphylaxis.

Social history

- Smoking
- Alcohol
- *Occupation (current and past)*: Occupational lung disease, past occupations for asbestos-related lung disease.

- Keeping birds or pets (hypersensitivity pneumonitis/allergic diseases)
- Travel history
- *Housing condition*: Which floor? (Is there an elevator in the building?)
- *How does dyspnoea affect the patient's life*: Job, finance, family, daily activity and sexual activity.

Further reading

Berliner D, Schneider N, Welte T, et al. The differential diagnosis of dyspnea. Dtsch Arztebl Int 2016; 113:834–845.
Mahler DA, Wells CK. Evaluation of clinical methods for rating dyspnea. Chest 1988; 93:580–586.

Cough

Common scenarios

- Drug-induced cough [angiotensin-converting enzyme (ACE) inhibitors and sitagliptin]
- Upper airway cough (post-nasal drip, allergic rhinitis)/GERD-induced cough
- Hypersensitivity pneumonitis (birds, farmers, etc.)
- Occupational lung diseases

History of presenting illness

- How long have you had the cough?
- Is it dry or with phlegm?
- History of wheezing.
- History of dyspnoea, orthopnoea, or PND
- Hoarse voice
- Have you coughed up blood?
- Is there any leg swelling?
- Do you suffer nasal or throat symptoms such as itchy nose, frequent sneezing, itchy throat, or desire to clear throat? (These symptoms suggests allergic rhinitis or post-nasal drip as the cause of chronic cough).
- Do you have acidity or heartburn? (GERD is an important cause of chronic cough).
- *Diurnal variation of cough:* GERD/asthma.
- *Seasonal variation of cough:* Exposure to different allergens such as pollens in certain seasons.

Review of systems

- *Cardiac symptoms*: Breathlessness, PND, orthopnoea, chest pain, and leg swelling.
- *Respiratory*: Wheezing, sputum
- *Gastrointestinal tract symptoms*: GERD, dysphagia
- *General*: Fever, weight loss.

Past history

- Similar illness in the past
- *History of pulmonary disease*: COPD, asthma, ILD, etc.
- History of heart disease
- History of HTN
- History of DM
- Previous hospital admissions and vaccination.

Family history
- Family history of asthma or allergic rhinitis.
- Family history of communicable diseases.

Drug history
- Use of ACE inhibitor or sitagliptin
- Hydralazine
- Amiodarone
- Alpha-blockers
- Non-steroidal anti-inflammatory drugs
- Pioglitazone.

Social history
- History of smoking
- History of alcohol use
- *Recent and past occupation*: Exposure to chemicals or pollution causing lung diseases and asbestos exposure (enquire carefully about remote exposure to asbestos/previous jobs).
- Keeping pets or birds.
  (Respiratory history is never complete without asking about occupation and keeping pets or birds).

Further reading
Irwin RS, French CL, Chang AB, et al. Classification of cough as a symptom in adults and management algorithms: CHEST Guideline and Expert Panel Report. Chest 2018; 153:196–209.

Chest pain

Common scenarios
- Angina and ischaemic heart disease
- Pulmonary embolism
- Aortic dissection
- Oesophageal spasm
- Lung cancer

Differentiating the cause of chest pain

Anginal pain
- Usually central/retrosternal
- Burning, tightening, or heaviness
- Radiates to left shoulder, arm and jaw
- Aggravated by exertion and emotional stress (sometimes meals)
- Relieved by sublingual nitroglycerin/rest
- Can last up to 10 or 20 minutes
- May be associated with dyspnoea, nausea, vomiting and dizziness.

Myocardial infarction pain
- Crushing type
- Lasts more than 20 minutes
- Not relieved by rest
- Associated with dyspnoea, nausea, vomiting and dizziness.

Prinzmetal's angina (variant angina/angina inversa)
- Caused by coronary vasospasm rather than atherosclerosis
- The pain is similar to angina pain
- Comes on at rest and very rarely on exertion
- Usually episodic
- Usually occurs while resting and during the night or early morning hours
- Usually severe
- Can be relieved by taking nitroglycerin
- Associated with ST-elevation but normal troponins
- Risk factors include heavy cigarette smoking, use of cocaine, use of migraine medications such as triptans, and exposure to severe cold weather.

Pulmonary embolism/pleuritic pain
- Sharp/stabbing
- Worsened with inspiration
- Associated with palpitations
- Lasts for days.

Acute aortic dissection
- Tearing pain
- Sudden onset
- Radiates to the back
- Very severe
- Persistent
- Associated with high blood pressure
- May lead to stroke or paraplegia.

Oesophageal spasm
- Retrosternal
- Usually squeezing
- May radiate to the back
- Aggravated by swallowing of food
- There may be a long history of GERD
- May be relieved by sublingual nitroglycerin.

Gastroesophageal reflux
- Burning
- Retrosternal and epigastric
- Aggravated by certain types of food (spicy, sour), and lying supine
- Relieved by antacids and proton pump inhibitor (PPI).

History of presenting illness
Chest pain should be analysed with LIQOR AAA.

Enquire about associated symptoms
- *Dyspnoea, PND and orthopnoea*: Cardiac
- *Palpitation*: Pulmonary embolism
- Syncope
- Dizziness
- *Gastrointestinal tract symptoms*: Heartburn/acidity.

Review of systems
Review carefully the cardiovascular, respiratory, and GIT systems.

Menstrual history

- History of recurrent abortions (pulmonary embolism/antiphospholipid)
- Use of oral contraceptive pills (pulmonary embolism).

Past medical history

- Heart disease
- *Coronary risk factors*: Diabetes, hypertension and dyslipidaemia
- Previous pulmonary embolism or deep vein thrombosis (DVT)
- History of GERD, oesophageal disease, or peptic ulcer.

Family history

- Heart disease
- Pulmonary embolism/DVT.

Drug history

- *Migraine tablets*: Triptans and ergot alkaloids may cause coronary vasospasm
- Use of cardiac medications or other medications.

Social history

- Smoking
- Alcohol
- *Drug abuse*: Cocaine (may cause spasm), use of NSAIDs
- Occupation
- How does the pain affect patient's life? Job, finance, family, daily activity and sexual activity.

Further reading

Kelly BS. Evaluation of the elderly patient with acute chest pain. Clin Geriatr Med 2007; 23:327–349.
Lenfant C. Chest pain of cardiac and noncardiac origin. Metabolism 2010; 59:S41–S46.

Palpitation

> ## Common scenarios
>
> - Hyperthyroidism
> - Pheochromocytoma
> - Atrial fibrillation
> - Panic attacks and anxiety

History of presenting illness

- How does the patient feel the heartbeat? Is it fast or slow?
- Does the patient feel a regular or irregular heartbeat?
- How long does the attack last?
- Is there anything you do that ends the attack? (Example: an attack of palpitations that ends by holding breath, taking deep breath, cough, or drinking cold water may suggest

supraventricular tachycardia whereas the one that ends by taking sweets/food may suggest hypoglycaemia).
- Have you ever felt dizzy or lost consciousness when the attack comes on?
- Is it associated with chest pain?
- Is it associated with difficulty in breathing?

Review of systems

- Enquire about symptoms of hyperthyroidism
- Enquire about symptoms of anaemia
- Enquire about symptoms suggestive of pheochromocytoma
- Enquire about symptoms of anxiety and psychiatric diseases.

Past history

- Past history of heart disease
- Past history of hypertension
- Past history of diabetes (hypoglycaemia and predisposition to cardiac disease)
- Past history of thyroid disease.

Family history

- Family history of sudden death (long QT interval, Brugada syndrome)
- Family history of heart disease or thyroid disease.

Drug history

Enquire about drugs that can cause palpitations such as calcium channel blockers, amiodarone, and levothyroxine.

Social history

- Smoking history
- Alcohol intake
- Drug abuse
- Excessive intake of coffee.

Further reading

Abbott A. Diagnostic approach to palpitations. Am Fam Physician 2005 15;71:743–750.

Diarrhoea

Common scenarios

- Chronic diarrhoea with steatorrhoea due to malabsorption syndromes (celiac disease)
- Acute or persistent diarrhoeal illness due to pseudomembranous colitis
- Inflammatory bowel disease
- Diarrhoea in kidney transplant patient
- Traveller's diarrhoea

History of presenting illness

- **How long have you had the diarrhoea?**
    - Acute—14 days or fewer in duration
    - Persistent—more than 14 days but fewer than 30 days in duration
    - Chronic—more than 30 days in duration.

- **Can you describe how does the stool look like?**
- **How frequent do you pass stool per day?**
- **Do you wake up at night with an urge to pass stool?** (suggests organic cause rather than irritable bowel)
- **Is there any blood in the stool?**
- **Is there any mucus or pus in the stool?**
- **Is it associated with flushing of the face or neck?**
  Carcinoid syndrome can cause chronic diarrhea and is associated with recurrent facial flushing

- **Is it related to certain types of food?**
    - Gluten in celiac disease
    - Milk or milk products in lactose intolerance.

- **Are there any symptoms suggestive of malabsorption (steatorrhoea, weight loss, flatulence, and abdominal distension)?**
  Steatorrhoea is a result of fat malabsorption and typically manifests with the passage of pale, bulky, and offensive stools. Due to the fat content, stools often float on top of the water and are difficult to flush. Patients may also observe oil droplets in the toilet after defecation.

- **Is it associated with heat intolerance, palpitations, or other symptoms of thyrotoxicosis?**

- **Has the patient received any antibiotic prior to the onset of diarrhoea?** (This question is often forgotten by candidates)
  Drug-induced diarrhoea and Clostridium difficile infection are important causes of diarrhoea following antibiotic ingestion.

- **Is there any recent history of camping or travel?**
  People who go camping are at risk of exposure to water sources contaminated with organisms.
    - Bacteria are the most common cause of traveller's diarrhoea with the most common pathogen being enterotoxigenic *Escherichia coli*, followed by *Campylobacter jejuni*, *Shigella* species, *Salmonella* species, and *Aeromonas* species.
    - *Viral causes of traveller's diarrhoea include:* Norovirus, rotavirus, and astrovirus.
    - Protozoal causes include *Giardia* and *Entamoeba*.
- **How long after return from travel did the diarrhoea start?**
    - Bacterial toxins generally cause symptoms within a few hours.
    - Bacterial and viral pathogens have an incubation period of 6–72 hours.
    - Protozoal pathogens have an incubation period of 1–2 weeks (rarely present in the first few days of travel).
- **Enquire about history of contact with sick people**
- **Enquire about history of contact with animals**
    - Exposure to young dogs or cats is associated with *Campylobacter* organisms.
    - Exposure to turtles is associated with *Salmonella*.
- **Ingestion of contaminated/rotten food**

Review of systems

- Enquire about symptoms of malabsorption
- Enquire about symptoms of *thyrotoxicosis* (may be associated with increased stool frequency).
- Enquire about symptoms of carcinoid (may manifest with diarrhoea).

Past medical and surgical history

- Similar diarrhoeal illness before
- History of colonic disease/malabsorption syndrome/food intolerance
- Past history of thyroid disease
- Past history of diabetes
- *Past colonic surgery*: Blind loop syndrome and bacterial overgrowth
- Bariatric surgery
- Organ transplant (there are important causes of diarrhoea to consider in organ transplanted patients).

Family history

Similar illness in the family or in contacts.

Drug history

Recent use of antibiotics/laxatives.

Social history

- Recent travel
- Recent camping
- Eating habits
- Sick contacts
- *Alcohol*: Chronic pancreatitis
- *Sexual history*: HIV enteropathy.

Stool diagnostic studies may be useful in cases of dysentery (passage of grossly bloody stools), moderate-to-severe disease, and symptoms lasting more than 7 days to clarify the aetiology and enable directed therapy. They are not routinely indicated in patients with mild watery diarrhoea or travel-associated diarrhoea.

There is no evidence for empiric antimicrobial therapy for routine acute diarrhoeal infection, except in cases of travel-associated diarrhoea where the likelihood of bacterial pathogens is high enough to justify the potential side effects of antibiotics.

Antibiotics for travel-associated diarrhoea include:

- Azithromycin 1,000 mg single dose
- Levofloxacin 500 mg single dose
- Ciprofloxacin 750 mg single dose.

Further reading

Centres for Disease Control and Prevention (CDC). Travelers' Diarrhea (2018). [online] Available from https://wwwnc.cdc.gov/travel/yellowbook/2020/preparing-international-travelers/travelers-diarrhea. [Last accessed October, 2019].

Riddle MS, DuPont HL, Connor BA. ACG Clinical Guideline: Diagnosis, treatment, and prevention of acute diarrheal infections in adults. Am J Gastroenterol 2016; 111:602–622.

Dizziness/vertigo

Common scenarios

- Anaemia
- Postural hypotension
- Adrenal insufficiency
- Autonomic neuropathy
- Peripheral versus central vertigo

History of presenting illness

- **What does the patient exactly mean by dizziness?**
  Patients may use the term dizziness to describe a range of sensations such as vertigo, presyncope, disequilibrium/unsteadiness, or lightheadedness.
- **Was the onset sudden or gradual?**
- **How long have you had the dizziness?**
- **How severe is the dizziness?**
- **What triggers the dizziness?**
  - *Head movement:* Inner ear disease such as benign positional vertigo or vestibular disorders
  - *Standing or sitting from recumbent position:* Postural hypotension
  - *Fasting:* Hypoglycaemia.

Important associated symptoms

- *Vertigo:* False sense that you or your surroundings are spinning or moving.
- *Palpitations or chest pain:* It may suggest cardiac cause such as ischaemia or arrhythmia.
- *Bleeding:* GIT bleeding
- *Increased skin pigmentation and GIT symptoms:* Adrenal insufficiency
- *Sweating, nervousness, palpitations, and presyncope:* Hypoglycaemia
- *Limb weakness, numbness, diplopia, imbalance, facial deviation, or swallowing difficulties:* Posterior circulation stroke or intracranial haemorrhage.
- *Peripheral numbness and burning:* Somatic small fibre and autonomic neuropathy
- *Nausea and vomiting:* It may suggest the presence of peripheral or central vertigo or adrenal insufficiency.
- *Ear symptoms:* Hearing loss may suggest Ménière's disease.

Review of systems

Candidate should analyse all systems with particular attention to central nervous system (CNS), cardiovascular system (CVS), GIT and endocrine systems.

Menstrual history

Menorrhagia.

Dietary history

- *Vegetarians*: May develop vitamin B12 deficiency
- *Poor nutritional intake*: It may lead to anaemia and dizziness.

Past history

- History of diabetes
- History of HTN
- History of heart disease
- History of stroke
- History of GIT or other bleeding diseases
- Recent surgery.

Drug history

Medications are implicated in about a third of causes of dizziness. It is very important to enquire about drugs taken by the patient including over-the-counter medications, e.g. NSAIDs which may cause GIT bleeding.

Family history

Family history of chronic diseases.

Social history

- Effects of dizziness on work and other aspects of patient's life
- Smoking history
- Alcohol history
- *Occupation*: Such as exposure to sun.

Further reading

Kerber KA, Baloh RW. The evaluation of a patient with dizziness. Neurol Clin Pract 2011; 1:24–33.
Kerber K. Vertigo and dizziness in the emergency department. Emerg Med Clin North Am 2009; 27:39–50.

Abnormal body movement

Common scenarios
- Restless leg syndrome
- New-onset seizure
- Drug-induced (levodopa, metoclopramide, or antipsychotic) movement disorders
- Periodic limb movement disorder

History of presenting illness

- **Is the onset of the abnormal movement sudden or gradual?**

- **For how long does the abnormal movement last?**
  Old definition of status epilepticus is 30 minutes of continuous seizure activity or a series of seizures without a return to full consciousness. Newer definition: 5 continuous minutes of generalised seizure activity or two or more separate seizure episodes without return to baseline.

- **Can you describe the abnormal movements?**
  - *Tremor*: Rhythmic oscillations caused by intermittent muscle contractions.
  - *Tics*: Paroxysmal, stereotyped muscle contractions, commonly suppressible, might be simple (single muscle group) or complex. Temporarily suppressible.
  - *Myoclonus*: Shock-like, arrhythmic twitches. Not suppressible.

- – *Chorea*: Dance-like, unpatterned movements, approximate a purpose (e.g. adjusting clothes, checking a watch). Often rapid and may involve proximal or distal muscle groups.
  - – *Athetosis:* Writhing movements, mostly of arms and hands. Often slow.
  - – *Dystonia*: Sustained or repetitious muscular contractions, with abnormal posture.
  - – *Hemiballismus*: Wild, large-amplitude, and flinging movements on one side of the body, commonly affecting proximal limb muscles but can also affect the trunk.
  - – *Seizure*: Uncontrolled physical convulsion, minimal twitch, gazing without response, or a combination of symptoms.
  - – *Epilepsy*: Recurrent, unprovoked seizures.
  - – *Restless leg syndrome*: A strong voluntary and irresistible urge to move the legs because of abnormal sensations in the legs, particularly when in bed and partially relieved by movement.
  - – *Periodic limb movement*: These are repetitive involuntary limb movements that occur during sleep.

- **When does this abnormal movement happen?**
  - – *Before sleep or at rest*: Restless leg syndrome
  - – *During sleep*: Periodic leg movement syndrome
  - – *Any time*: Seizure.
- **Which part of the body is involved in the abnormal movements?**
  For example, arms, legs and face of one side of the body, generalised or starts in one place and then spreads.

- **What are the precipitating factors?**
  - – *Flashing light*: Seizure
  - – *New stroke*: Seizure or hemiballismus.

- **Was it associated with loss of consciousness?**
- **Was it associated with urine or stool incontinence?**
- **Was it preceded by an aura?**
- **Was it associated with tongue biting or body injury?**
- **Is there any history of head trauma?**
- **What happened before, during, and after the incident?**

Review of systems

- *Cardiac symptoms:* Palpitations (arrhythmia)
- *Renal symptoms:* Frothy urine, reduced urine output, and change in urine colour. CKD is a risk factor for restless leg syndrome and systemic lupus erythematosus (SLE) may cause chorea and renal failure
- *Thyroid symptoms:* Hyperthyroidism may cause chorea
- Symptoms of increase sleepiness and fatigue in case of restless leg syndrome.

Past history

- Similar illness in the past
- History of epilepsy
- History of heart disease
- History of HTN
- History of DM
- History of stroke
- History of Parkinsonism or movement disorders
- History of head trauma
- History of systemic neoplasms, infections, and metabolic disorders.

Menstrual history

Pregnancy.

Family history

Family history of similar illness, epilepsy, or malignancy.

Drug history

Ask about drugs that might precipitate or worsen abnormal movements such as levodopa, metoclopramide, and antipsychotic medications.

Social history

- History of alcohol use
- History of drug abuse (hepatitis)
- Recent travel.

Further information not covered (at end of history taking)
Ask the patient the following question: Is there anything else that you feel is important and would like to discuss?

Further reading

Khalil A, Malik S. Movement disorders and tremors. InnovAiT 2013; 6:416–424.
Stanford Medicine 25. Types of involuntary movements. [online] Available from https://stanfordmedicine25.stanford.edu/the25/im.html [Last accessed October, 2019].

Abnormal liver function/jaundice

Common scenarios
- Non-alcoholic fatty liver disease
- Painless jaundice from cancer of head of pancreas
- Anabolic steroid/other drug-induced cholestasis
- Alcoholic liver disease (accompanying depression)
- Primary biliary cirrhosis

History of presenting illness

Analysis of Jaundice (Figure 2)
- Onset of jaundice (sudden/gradual)
- Duration
- *Progression*: Progressive/improved/stayed same
- Was it observed by patient/colleague/family or diagnosed by a doctor?
- Does the yellow discolouration involve only the eyes or both skin and eyes? (This is an important differentiating point between true jaundice and conditions such as carotenaemia resulting from excessive ingestion of carotene in carrots and green vegetables. Carotenaemia causes yellowish discolouration of the skin but spares sclera and mucus membranes).
- Is there any skin itching? *(obstructive jaundice)*
- Is there any associated fever? (cholangitis/cholelithiasis with bile duct stone)

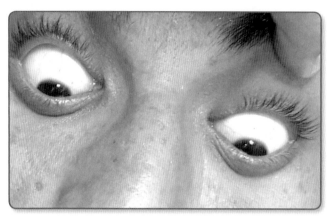

Figure 2 Patient with jaundice. (*See colour plate 1*)

- What is the colour of stool and urine? (dark urine or pale stool indicates obstructive jaundice)
- Is there any change in your appetite or weight loss? (hepatobiliary malignancy)
- Do you have nausea/vomiting? (acute hepatitis)
- Do you have abdominal pain? (painless cholestatic jaundice suggests underlying malignancy)
- Do you feel abdominal distension? (ascites/malignancy)
- Melena/haematemesis.

Review of systems

- Ask about fatigue (primary biliary cirrhosis/chronic liver disease/anaemia)
- Ask about fever (infectious cause)
- *Analysis of GIT*: As above
- *Rheumatologic system*: Joint pain/body pain (autoimmune hepatitis/haemolytic anaemia)
- *Joint pains involving metacarpophalangeal joints*: Haemochromatosis
- *Increase skin pigmentation*: Haemochromatosis.

Past history

- Past history of liver disease/stones
- Past history of jaundice
- History of GB stones
- History of cancer
- Past history of blood transfusions
- Autoimmune diseases (autoimmune hepatitis)
- Haemolytic anaemia
- *Obesity and overweight*: Non-alcoholic fatty liver disease (NAFLD*)*.

Menstrual history

- Amenorrhoea (autoimmune hepatitis/primary biliary cirrhosis)
- Use of oral contraceptive pills (may predispose to cholestasis and liver tumours)
- *Decreased libido and infertility*: Haemochromatosis.

Family history

- *Family history or contacts with jaundice or liver disease*: Hepatitis A, E
- Family history of liver diseases/GIT malignancies
- Family history of autoimmune diseases (autoimmune hepatitis)
- Family history of haemolytic anaemia.

Drug history

- Enquire about use of anabolic steroids in young men/bodybuilders
- Take details of drug history including over-the-counter medications.

Social history

- Details of alcohol intake
- Smoking
- Drug abuse particularly intravenous drug abuse (hepatitis/HIV)
- *Travel history*: Hepatitis A, E, and other infections causing hepatitis
- *Details of sexual history*: Hepatitis/HIV.

Further reading

Limdi J, Hyde G. Evaluation of abnormal liver function tests. Postgrad Med J 2003; 79:307–312.

Part 2

History taking scenarios

Scenario no. 1

A patient with bilateral leg swelling

Candidate copy

Please read the GP referral letter for Mr Ahmed. The time distribution for this station is as follows:

    You have (---) minutes to take a history from the patient.
    You have (---) minutes to collect your thoughts.
    You have (---) minutes for discussion with the examiners.

Please do not examine the patient

> **Dear Doctor,**
>
> Thank you for seeing Mr Ahmed, a 42-year-old who has been complaining of increasing leg swelling over the past few weeks. His complete blood count, kidney function test, and electrolytes were all normal.
>
> Yours faithfully,

> Please interview the patient and based on the history, construct a differential diagnosis and plan of investigation. Provide an explanation to the patient and answer any questions he may have.

Surrogate copy

Chief complaint and history of present illness (HPI)

- You have swelling in both legs for the last 6 weeks. It is made worse when you stand for a long time and reduces to some extent when you lie down.
- There is no leg pain.
- There is no redness over the swelling.
- You feel that your shoes are becoming tight.

Review of systems

- You do not have breathing problems or chest pain.
- You do not have liver disease.
- You have not noticed any swelling in your tummy.
- You do not have any kidney disease.

- You do not have any problems with passing urine.
- You do not have frothy urine.

Past history and drug history
- You have *high blood pressure.*
- If asked about medications for blood pressure, state that you were taking valsartan 80 mg daily but because your blood pressure was uncontrolled your doctor added *amlodipine* 10 mg daily 3 months ago.
- You had a road traffic accident 15 years ago for which you required a blood transfusion.

Social history
- You *smoke 20 cigarettes* per day for the past 15 years.
- You do not drink alcohol.
- You work as a supervisor in a construction company.
- You are happily married with two kids.

Your questions to the doctors and concerns
> *Doctor:* I read on Google that heart failure is a cause of leg swelling. Do I need an angiogram or echocardiogram?

Steps in history taking in a patient with leg swelling

Step 1: Introduction, greeting and confirmation of patient identity
- Good morning Mr Ahmed (shakehands with the patient), pleased to meet you.
- I am Dr X working in the medical outpatient clinic.
- Can I confirm that I am talking to Mr Ahmed?
- I have just read the referral letter from your GP who is concerned about the swelling in your legs.
- Can you tell me more about that?
- Allow the patient to speak.
- Avoid interruptions.
- Avoid medical jargon [e.g. oedema, cardiac, renal, periorbital, abdomen, chronic obstructive pulmonary disease (COPD), etc.]
- *Use open-ended questions at the beginning such as:* Anything else?

Step 2: Elaborating important points in the history of leg swelling

History of presenting illness
- Does it involve one leg or both legs?
- Is it getting worse, staying the same, or decreasing since it started?
- Is the swelling painless or painful?
- Is there any swelling in other parts of the body?

Presence of periorbital swelling may suggest nephrotic syndrome.
Abdominal distension may suggest ascites.
Presence of scrotal oedema (more extensive pathology).

Review of systems
- *Cardiac symptoms:* Chest pain, exertional dyspnoea, paroxysmal nocturnal dyspnoea (PND), orthopnoea
- *Renal symptoms:* Frothy urine, reduced urine output, change in urine colour
- *GIT symptoms:* Abdominal pain
- *Thyroid symptoms:* Cold intolerance, fatigue, menorrhagia
- *Symptoms of obstructive sleep apnoea:* Heavy snoring, increased sleepiness and fatigue, witnessed apnoeic attacks during sleep.

Past history

- Similar illness in the past.
- History of heart disease.
- History of hypertension (HTN).
- History of diabetes mellitus (DM).
- History of liver disease.
- History of kidney disease.
- *History of pulmonary disease*: COPD, ILD, obstructive sleep apnoea
- History of blood transfusion or IV drug abuse (viral hepatitis causing chronic liver disease).
- History of thyroid disease.
- Previous surgery, hospital admissions, and vaccination.

Menstrual history in females

Pregnancy may cause leg oedema.

Family history

- Family history of heart, lung, liver or kidney disease.
- Family history of thrombosis/clots.

Drug history

- Calcium channel blockers
- Minoxidil
- Hydralazine
- Alpha blockers
- *Nonsteroidal* anti-inflammatory drugs (NSAIDs)
- Pioglitazone in diabetic patients.

Social history

- History of smoking.
- History of alcohol use (liver and heart disease).
- History of drug abuse (hepatitis).
- *Occupation*: Sedentary, exposure to pollution causing lung disease.

Further information not covered (at end of history taking)

Ask the patient the following question: Is there anything else that you feel is important and would like to tell me about?

Step 3: Explaining to the patient the diagnosis and plan of management

Mr Ahmed, after reviewing your history, there are some potential reasons to explain your leg swelling. As you do not have symptoms other than the leg swelling, I think the most probable cause of your leg swelling is the medication called amlodipine that was recently started to control your blood pressure. This drug is well-known to cause leg swelling, especially at the high dose of 10 mg. I am going to prescribe an alternative tablet called a thiazide diuretic that will help to control your blood pressure, without causing leg swelling. Meanwhile, please continue to take the valsartan as before. I would also recommend that you keep your legs elevated during sleep and avoid prolonged standing or sitting. Smoking can cause serious problems in your lungs and heart and this, in turn, may lead to swelling of the legs. Therefore, I would strongly suggest that you quit smoking as soon as possible and I will refer you to one of my colleagues who specialise in helping people quit smoking. Another important issue is the blood pressure control. Uncontrolled blood pressure can affect the heart and kidneys, which can lead to leg swelling. I would recommend that you take your blood pressure medications regularly and have a regular check-up of your blood pressure to keep it under control with a target of <140/90 mmHg.

Your GP ordered some blood tests which were all normal. I am going to request a urine test to look for protein in your urine. If the swelling does not improve after stopping amlodipine, I will arrange for a scan of your heart.

I am going to arrange another appointment with myself in 2 weeks to review the urine tests and to see how you are getting on with the new tablet.

Check patient understanding and agreement on plan of management.

Does that make sense to you?

Step 4: Ask about and address patient's concerns

Do you have any questions or concerns at this moment?

Patient's concern: Doctor; I read that heart failure can cause leg swelling. Could you order a scan of my heart?

Reply: It is true that heart failure can cause leg swelling, but that is usually associated with difficulty in breathing and other symptoms which you do not have. It is, therefore, less likely that your leg swelling is due to heart failure. However, I am going to see you again after stopping the amlodipine and if I do not see improvement in the swelling, I will order some more tests and heart scan will be one of them.

After answering each concern, confirm the agreement by saying; "Is that alright? Or does that make sense to you?"

Step 5: Summarise the discussion, confirm patient's understanding, and close the meeting

Mr Ahmed, I would like to summarise our discussion to be sure the information provided is clear to you. The most probable cause for your leg swelling for the time-being is the drug amlodipine. I am going to stop the amlodipine and give you an alternate tablet to help control your blood pressure. I am also going to arrange for some urine tests and will see you in 2 weeks to see how you are getting on and arrange further tests if necessary. Meanwhile, I am going to provide you with my contact number in case you have any further questions or concerns regarding your condition. Does that sound good to you? You can get information from the internet regarding leg swelling caused by amlodipine. Thank you and see you soon.

Discussion

Problem

Leg oedema (**Figure 1**).

Diagnosis

Drug-induced leg oedema (amlodipine).

Other plausible diagnosis

- **Congestive heart failure (CHF)**
  The patient is hypertensive and does not have other symptoms of heart failure.

- **Cor pulmonale from COPD**
  Patient's age and history are against this diagnosis and he does not have other symptoms.

- **Chronic liver disease from previous blood transfusion**
  Absence of abdominal distension is against this diagnosis.

Oedema is a frequently encountered problem in clinical practice. Many candidates do not find a problem in remembering cardiac, hepatic, renal causes, and protein malnutrition/loss. However, drugs which are an important cause of leg oedema are

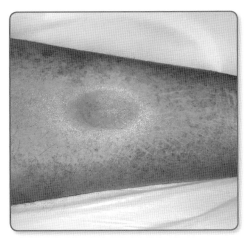

Figure 1 Pitting oedema of the legs. (*See colour plate 1*)

usually forgotten by candidates. Oedema is commonly bilateral but may be confined to one limb more than the other. The aetiology of each is usually different.

Causes of bilateral leg oedema

- Congestive heart failure
- Cor pulmonale
- Chronic liver disease
- Nephrotic syndrome
- Hypothyroidism
- Protein malnutrition/loss
- Drugs.

Causes of unilateral leg swelling

- Deep venous thrombosis
- Lymphedema
- Cellulitis.

Patients with heart failure often have other symptoms in addition to peripheral oedema such as exertional dyspnoea, PND, and orthopnoea. The mechanism of oedema in CHF is the elevated venous pressure secondary to right heart failure.

Patients with liver cirrhosis tend to develop ascites first. Leg oedema may develop later in the course of the disease. (*Remember the common causes of ascites without pitting leg oedema in the exam are: abdominal malignancy, tuberculosis, liver cirrhosis and Budd-Chiari*).

Many medications can cause pedal oedema. These include arteriolar vasodilators such as calcium channel blockers, oestrogens, minoxidil, and hydralazine. Other drugs that increase sodium reabsorption such as NSAIDs, pioglitazone, and rosiglitazone can also cause peripheral oedema. Calcium channel blocker-induced leg oedema is most commonly seen with the dihydropyridine subclass. The oedema appears to be dose and time-dependent. Because medication-induced oedema is caused by capillary HTN, diuretics are not an effective treatment. The addition of angiotensin converting enzyme inhibitors (ACEIs) and angiotensin-receptor blockers may be effective.

Patients with the nephrotic syndrome typically present with periorbital and peripheral oedema with or without ascites. The factors responsible for oedema in nephrotic syndrome include the reduced transcapillary oncotic pressure due to severe hypoalbuminaemia as well as increased sodium retention.

Lymphedema is usually nonpitting. The causes of lymphedema include damage or obstruction of the lymphatic channels by cancer, filariasis, radiation or surgery.

Further reading

Messerli FH. Vasodilatory edema: a common side effect of antihypertensive therapy. Curr Cardiol Rep 2002; 4:479–482.

O'Brien JG, Chennubhotla SA, Chennubhotla RV. Treatment of oedema. Am Fam Physician 2005; 71:2111–2117.

Trayes K, Studdiford J. Edema: diagnosis and management. Am Fam Physician 2013; 88:102–110.

Scenario no. 2

A patient with uncontrolled blood pressure

Candidate copy (Figure 2)

Please read the GP referral letter for Mr Ali. The time distribution for this station is as follows:

>   You have (---) minutes to take a history from the patient.
>   You have (---) minutes to collect your thoughts.
>   You have (---) minutes for discussion with the examiners.

Please do not examine the patient

> **Dear Doctor,**
>
> Thank you for seeing Mr Ali, a 55-year-old who has persistently high blood pressure. Despite being on 3 antihypertensive agents, his average blood pressure reading is 180/95. Besides his hypertension, he has type 2 diabetes mellitus (controlled), coronary artery disease, and obesity. His complete blood count, kidney function test, and electrolytes are all within the normal range.
>
> Yours faithfully,

> Please interview the patient and based on the history construct a differential diagnosis and plan of investigation. Provide an explanation to the patient and answer any questions he may have.

Surrogate copy

Chief complaint, HPI and review of systems (ROS)

- You have been referred because your blood pressure is difficult to control despite being on three medications.
- Your main complaint is feeling *lethargic and tired* for more than 3 years.
- You do not vomit blood.
- You do not have black stool.
- Your weight has increased recently, and you have less energy.
- You did not notice any change in your skin colour.
- You do not feel any palpitations.

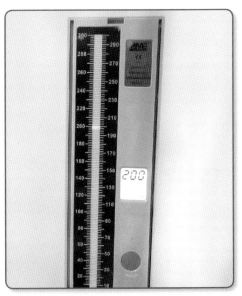

Figure 2 High blood pressure. (*See colour plate 1*)

Questions you answer only if asked by candidates
- You are feeling *sleepy all the time.*
- You tend to *fall asleep frequently* when with your family and friends and during social events.
- Your wife is complaining that *you snore loudly* at night and she now sleeps in another room because of your snoring.
- Your wife tried to wake you up multiple times as she thought you were *choking and your breathing stopped frequently while sleeping.*

Past history
- You have high blood pressure for 10 years. For the first 7 years, your blood pressure was controlled on perindopril 10 mg; however, for the last 3 years your GP has found difficulty in controlling your blood pressure. He added amlodipine 10 mg and indapamide 2.5 mg, but your blood pressure is still uncontrolled.
- You were admitted 2 years ago because of a heart attack and you underwent stenting of the arteries of your heart.
- You have had diabetes for the last 7 years, which is well-controlled on metformin and sitagliptin.
- You were admitted last year to the hospital with a fractured femur due to a *road traffic accident* as you had *fallen asleep while driving.*
- You do not have kidney disease.

Social history
- You do not smoke.
- You work as an accountant in a bank.
- You previously received a warning letter from your manager as he found you *asleep at work.*

- You are married and you have *reduced interest in your sex life with problems in erection.*
- *Drug history:* As above
- You do not take steroids or NSAIDs.

Your main concerns (please ask at the end of discussion)
- Is there any treatment for obstructive sleep apnoea?
- It will be very difficult for me to stop driving as I use my car to drive to work.

Steps in history taking in a patient with uncontrolled hypertension

Step 1: Introduction, greeting, and confirmation of patient identity
- Good morning Mr Ali (shakehands with the patient), pleased to meet you.
- I am Dr X working in the medical outpatient clinic.
- Can I confirm that I am talking to Mr Ali?
- I have just read the referral letter from your GP who is concerned that your blood pressure is not well-controlled despite being on three medications.
- Can you tell me more about that?
- Allow the patient to speak.
- Avoid interruptions.
- Avoid medical jargon (e.g. kidney, Cushing's, pheochromocytoma, obstructive, apnoea, etc.)
- *Use open ended questions such as:* What else?

Step 2: Elaborating important points in the history of a patient with uncontrolled HTN

History of presenting illness
- *Medication adherence:* Are you taking your blood pressure tablets regularly?
- Identifying possibility of secondary causes of HTN.
- Obstructive sleep apnoea (usually forgotten and overlooked as a cause of uncontrolled HTN):
  - Do you snore loudly at night?
  - Did your wife tell you that your breathing stopped/interrupted when sleeping?
  - How many times do you wake up at night to pass urine?
  - Do you suffer from restless sleep, with frequent wake ups during the night?
  - Do you suffer daytime fatigue/tiredness?
  - Do you suffer problems with memory and concentration?
  - Do you suffer morning headache?
  - Do you have problems with your sexual function (impotence and decreased desire)?
  - What size is you neck collar?
  - Do you feel acidity and a burning stomach after food?
- *Symptoms suggestive of kidney disease:*
  - Change in urine amount, colour, frothy urine or blood in the urine.
  - History of kidney stones (hyperparathyroidism/MEN).
- *Symptoms suggestive of pheochromocytoma:*
  - Palpitations
  - Flushing
  - Sweating
  - Tremor
  - Panic
  - Facial pallor
  - Headache.
- *Symptoms suggestive of Cushing' syndrome:*
  - Acne
  - Easy bruising
  - Fatigue/muscle weakness
  - Oral thrush.

Review of systems

- *Cardiac symptoms*: Chest pain, dyspnoea, PND, orthopnoea
- *Renal symptoms*: Frothy urine, reduced urine output, change in urine colour
- *GIT symptoms*: Gastroesophageal reflux disease (GERD)
- *Thyroid symptoms*: Cold intolerance, fatigue
- *Symptoms of obstructive sleep apnoea:* Heavy snoring, increased daytime sleepiness and fatigue, and witnessed apnoeic attacks during sleep.

Past history

- History of heart disease
- History of HTN
- History of DM
- History of kidney disease such as polycystic kidneys
- History of endocrine diseases.
- History of obstructive sleep apnoea
- History of thyroid disease
- History of weight gain
- History of depression or psychological disease.

Menstrual history in females

Not applicable in this case.

Family history

- Family history of kidney disease
- Family history of hypertension
- Family history of endocrine problems.

Drug history

- Use of NSAIDs
- *Use of steroids:* May cause or worsen HTN.

Social history

- History of smoking
- History of alcohol use
- *Occupation:* Sedentary/operating heavy machinery
- *Driving:* It is very important to ask about *driving and any previous accidents because of falling asleep.*

Further information not covered (at end of history taking)

- *Ask the patient the following question:* Is there anything else that you feel important and would like to tell me about?

Step 3: Explaining to the patient the diagnosis and the plan of management

Mr Ali, after reviewing your history, there are some possible reasons to explain why your blood pressure is not well-controlled. From your symptoms, I think the most likely cause of your uncontrolled blood pressure is a condition called 'obstructive sleep apnoea.' Apnoea means to stop breathing. In OSA, you may stop breathing for short periods of time while sleeping. Even when you are trying to breathe, there may be little or no airflow into the lungs. These pauses in airflow (obstructive apnoeas) can occur on and off during sleep and cause you to wake up from a sound sleep. Frequent apnoeas can cause many problems. The lack of undisturbed sleep can make you feel tired the next day and cause you to fall asleep while driving which may result in car accidents. These periods of stopping breathing can, with time, cause high blood pressure (hypertension), heart disease, stroke, DM, or early death. Therefore, I would strongly recommend that we perform an urgent sleep study to see if you have OSA.

Does this make sense to you?—Pause to allow patient to ask.

Obstructive sleep apnoea is diagnosed by a sleep study (called polysomnography). During a sleep study, your breathing, heart rate, and oxygen levels will be monitored.

A sleep study is often done at a sleep centre where you will be scheduled to stay overnight. Alternatively, a home sleep apnoea test may also be used to diagnose OSA.

Patient: Is there any treatment for OSA?

Reply: Sleep apnoea can be effectively treated, and there are a number of ways to do so. The type of treatment recommended will depend on the reason for and severity of the sleep apnoea. If your OSA is because of being overweight, then weight loss can make the apnoea go away completely.

Continuous positive airway pressure (CPAP) is a device that can treat OSA. It is a machine that works like a compressor and blows air into a mask that is worn snugly over the nose and/or mouth or in the nostrils (nasal pillows) during sleep. The flow of air acts like a splint to keep your upper airway from collapsing and helps to prevent obstruction and the apnoea from occurring. The air pressure is adjusted to a setting that best controls the apnoea. Often a person will also notice much less snoring when wearing CPAP.

There are devices and surgeries can be done to treat OSA. The type of device or surgery will depend on what has caused the apnoea. Some oral appliances or devices that are worn in the mouth during sleep may keep your airway open. Most oral devices work by either bringing the jaw forward or keeping the tongue from blocking the throat. Oral appliances are most likely to help a person who has mild sleep apnoea and who is not overweight.

As I mentioned earlier OSA carries a high risk of car accidents if you are driving a vehicle. You may fall sleep whilst driving and harm yourself or others. Therefore, it is very important that you stop driving until your OSA is confirmed and treated effectively. You must tell the Driver and Vehicle Licensing Agency (DVLA).

I would also advise that you reduce or quit alcohol as it may worsen OSA. You need to avoid alcohol for at least 4 hours before going to bed.

The snoring and apnoea in patients with OSA may get worse when they sleep on their backs. If you sleep on your back, you can use a pillow or sew a small ball into your pyjama bottoms to force yourself to sleep on your side.

I am going to arrange an urgent appointment with a sleep specialist and a sleep study for you. I will ask a colleague who specialises in nose and throat disease to examine you for any possibility of nose or throat problems that might be responsible for your OSA. I will also request some blood tests of thyroid and kidney function. For weight reduction, an appointment with the obesity specialist will be arranged as there are alternative drugs called GLP-1 agonists and SGLT-2 inhibitors for diabetes which can also help you lose weight. I will arrange another appointment with myself in 2 weeks to see the results of the sleep study and the blood and urine tests. I hope by that time I will be able to give you more answers.

Check patient understanding and agreement on plan of management.

Does that make sense to you?

Step 4: Ask and address patient's concerns

Do you have any questions or concerns at this moment?

Patient's concerns in this case: Is there any treatment for OSA?

Reply: Answered above

Doctor: It will be very difficult for me to stop driving as I use my own car to drive to work.

Reply: I understand this is difficult Mr Ali, but continuing to drive with the possibility of OSA can be very dangerous and harmful to yourself as well as others. People with OSA tend to fall asleep very easily while driving and this could result in a more serious accident than your previous one where you broke your leg.

Furthermore, not informing the DVLA can put you at risk of legal liabilities. In the meantime, until we confirm the diagnosis and treat your OSA, I would sincerely advise you to use public transport.

After answering each concern, confirm the agreement by saying; "Is that okay or does that make sense to you?"

Step 5: Summarise the discussion, confirm patient's understandings, and close the meeting

Mr Ali, I would like to summarise our discussion to be sure the information provided is clear to you. The most likely explanation for your blood pressure is a condition called OSA. I am going to arrange further blood and urine tests as well as a sleep study and an urgent appointment with a sleep specialist and ear nose and throat doctor. I will see you in 2 weeks to give you more answers about the test results and diagnosis. Meanwhile, please stop driving or operating heavy machinery until your OSA is confirmed and effectively treated. I am going to provide you with my contact number in case you have any further questions or concerns regarding your condition. Does that sound good to you? You can also have some information from the web regarding OSA. Thank you and see you soon.

Discussion

Problem

Resistant hypertension.

Diagnosis

Obstructive sleep apnoea.

Other plausible diagnoses

- Renal disease
- Cushing's syndrome
- Pheochromocytoma
- Hyperaldosteronism.

Resistant hypertension is defined as blood pressure that remains above goal despite the concurrent use of three different classes of antihypertensive agents. Ideally, one of the three agents should be a diuretic and all agents should be prescribed at their optimal dose.

Uncontrolled hypertension should be differentiated from resistant hypertension. Patients with uncontrolled hypertension include those who lack blood pressure control secondary to poor adherence and/or an inadequate treatment regimen, as well as those with true treatment resistance.

Potentially reversible causes of hypertension may contribute to treatment resistance including obstructive sleep apnoea, renal parenchymal disease, renal artery stenosis, and primary aldosteronism, which should be assessed for and treated appropriately. Recent studies indicate that primary aldosteronism is a much more common cause of hypertension than previously reported and may be present in about 20% of patients with resistant hypertension.

There may also be pseudo-resistance where there is a lack of blood pressure control secondary to poor medication adherence or white coat hypertension.

Causes of uncontrolled blood pressure

- Poor adherence
- White-coat effect
- Obesity
- Excessive dietary sodium intake
- Heavy alcohol intake

Table 1 Common and uncommon secondary causes	
Common secondary causes	**Uncommon secondary causes**
• Obstructive sleep apnoea	• Pheochromocytoma
• Renal parenchymal disease	• Cushing's disease
• Primary aldosteronism	• Hyperparathyroidism
• Renal artery stenosis	• Aortic coarctation
	• Intracranial tumour

- Nonsteroidal anti-inflammatory agents, decongestants, liquorice, erythropoietin, amphetamine-like stimulants, steroids, and oral contraceptives
- Presence of secondary causes (**Table 1**).

Further reading

American Thoracic Society. What is obstructive sleep apnea in adults? Patient Education/Information Series. [online] Available from: https://www.thoracic.org/patients/patient-resources/resources/obstructive-sleep-apnea-in-adults.pdf. [Last accessed October, 2019].

Calhoun DA, Jones D, Textor S, et al. Resistant hypertension: diagnosis, evaluation, and treatment. A scientific statement from the American Heart Association Professional Education Committee of the Council for High Blood Pressure Research. Hypertension 2008; 51:1403–1419.

Scenario no. 3

A patient with chronic cough

Candidate copy

Please read the GP referral letter for Mr Abdul.
The time distribution for this station is as follows:
    You have (---) minutes to take a history from the patient.
    You have (---) minutes to collect your thoughts.
    You have (---) minutes for discussion with the examiners.

Please do not examine the patient

> **Urgent referral**
> **Dear Doctor,**
> Thank you for seeing Mr Abdul, a 43-year-old who has been complaining of cough for the last 3 months that is distressing him. His chest and heart examination are unremarkable
> Yours faithfully,

> Please interview the patient and based on the history construct a differential diagnosis and plan of investigation. Provide an explanation to the patient and answer any questions he may have.

Surrogate copy

Chief complaint and HPI

- You suffer cough for the last 3 months. It is distressing and prevents you from sleeping. You have tried different cough syrups but without benefit.
- The cough is dry without sputum.
- You feel *irritation and itchiness in your throat.*
- You also feel an *itchy nose* and occasionally it becomes runny.
- Sometimes, you feel the *desire to clear your throat.*
- There is no fever.
- You have never coughed blood.
- You do not suffer difficulty with breathing.

Review of systems

- You do not have breathing problems or chest pain.
- You do not have wheezing.
- You have not lost weight.
- You have not noticed any change in your voice.
- You do not have headache.
- You sometimes feel acidity and burning in your stomach after food.

Past history

- You had high blood pressure for the past 1 year.
- You have type 2 diabetes mellitus.
- If asked about medications for blood pressure and diabetes, state that you take perindopril 10 mg once daily for the past 6 months, metformin 1,000 mg twice daily, sitagliptin 100 mg and empagliflozin 25 mg once daily. Your blood pressure and blood sugar are controlled.
- You have never suffered asthma.
- You have never suffered allergic rhinitis.

Family history

Your *sister has allergic rhinitis and asthma.*

Social history

- You quit smoking 5 years ago and you *smoked 20 cigarettes per day for 10 years.*
- You do not drink alcohol.
- You work as a laboratory technician in a chemistry laboratory.
- You are happily married with 2 kids.
- No contact with sick people.
- Only if asked: *You keep a parrot at home,* and you take care of it and clean its cage.

Your main concerns

You are concerned as one of your best friends, who you used to smoke with, has been diagnosed with lung cancer and you would like to have a CT scan of the lungs.

Steps in history taking in a patient with chronic cough

Step 1: Introduction, greeting, and confirmation of patient identity

- Good morning Mr Abdul (shakehands with the patient), pleased to meet you.
- I am Dr X working in medical outpatient clinic.
- Can I confirm that I am talking to Mr Abdul?

- I have just read the referral letter from your GP who states that you are complaining of a cough.
- Can you tell me more about that?
- Allow the patient to speak.
- Avoid interruptions.
- Avoid medical jargon (e.g. GERD, ACEI, hypersensitivity pneumonitis, sputum, COPD, etc.)
- *Use open ended questions such as:* What else?

Step 2: Elaborating important points in the history

History of presenting illness

- How long have you had the cough?
- Is it dry or with phlegm?
- Do you have any wheezing? (May suggest asthma)
- Is there a history of dyspnoea, orthopnoea or PND? (May suggest CHF)
- Hoarse voice? (May suggest lung cancer)
- Did you ever cough up blood? (Lung cancer, bronchiectasis, bronchitis)
- Leg swelling? (May suggest CHF)
- Do you suffer from an itchy nose, frequent sneezing, itchy throat or desire to clear throat? (May suggest allergic rhinitis and post-nasal drip)
- Do you have stomach acidity or heart burn? (GERD is an important cause of chronic cough)
- *Diurnal variation of cough:* GERD/asthma
- *Seasonal variation of cough:* (Exposure to different allergens such as pollen in spring season).

Review of systems

- *Cardiac symptoms:* Breathlessness, PND, orthopnoea, chest pain, leg swelling
- *Respiratory:* Wheezing, sputum
- *GIT symptoms:* GERD, dysphagia
- *General:* Fever, weight loss (TB, cancer, bronchiectasis).

Past history

- Similar illness in the past.
- *History of pulmonary disease:* COPD, asthma, ILD, etc.
- *History of heart disease:* Heart failure
- *History of HTN:* Heart failure, antihypertensive medications that can cause cough
- *History of DM:* Heart disease, sitagliptin use, ACEI
- Previous hospital admissions and vaccination.

Menstrual history in females

Not applicable in this patient.

Family history

- Family history of asthma or allergic rhinitis
- Family history of communicable diseases.

Drug history

- ACEI
- Sitagliptin.

Social history

- History of smoking
- History of alcohol use
- *Recent and past occupation:* Exposure to chemicals or pollution causing lung diseases, asbestos exposure
- Keeping pets or birds.

(Respiratory history is never complete without asking about details of occupation and keeping pets or birds)

Further information not covered (at end of history taking)

Ask the patient the following question: Is there anything else that you feel important and would like to tell me about?

Step 3: Explaining to the patient the diagnosis and the plan of management

Mr Abdul, after reviewing your history, there are some possible reasons to explain why you should have a cough. The drugs you are currently taking for your hypertension and diabetes, namely the perindopril and sitagliptin can both cause cough. As an initial step in your management, I would suggest that we discontinue these two medications and replace them with alternatives that do not cause cough. I will arrange to see you in 4 weeks after stopping the perindopril and sitagliptin. In case that the cough is gone by that time, there is no need to proceed for further investigations. However, if the cough persists, then I will order some further tests including a chest X-Ray and arrange an appointment for you in the cough clinic. There are other possible causes for your cough e.g. nose allergy (allergic rhinitis), reflux of the stomach acid and to lesser extent exposure to chemicals at the laboratory where you work. However, before proceeding to further testing of these diseases, we should stop these two medications and observe the response. It is also important to note that birds can lead to serious lung diseases and therefore, I would suggest that you take certain precautions when dealing with the parrot at home such as using a mask when coming in contact with it particularly when cleaning its cage.

Check patient's understanding and agreement on plan of management.

Does that make sense to you?

Step 4: Ask and address patient's concerns

Do you have any questions or concerns at this moment?

Patient concerns: Doctor; being an ex-smoker, I am bit worried about the possibility of cancer in my case. Can you order a CT scan of my chest?

Reply: I understand your concern. Cancer can occur in people who are smokers or quit smoking particularly if they have quit less than 15 years ago. However, as you do not have other serious symptoms that suggest cancer, I think cancer is a remote possibility in your case for the time being. Furthermore, a CT scan exposes you to a lot of radiation and the risks outweigh the benefits in your case. Additionally, I will arrange another appointment in 4-week time and see your response to stopping the two medications.

After answering each concern, confirm the agreement by asking; "Is that alright? Or does that make sense to you?"

Step 5: Summarise the discussion, confirm the patient's understanding, and close the meeting

Mr Abdul, I would like to summarise our discussion to be sure the information provided is clear to you. The most probable cause for the cough is the Perindopril and Sitagliptin. I am going to prescribe alternative medications for your blood pressure and diabetes and will arrange to see you gain in 4 weeks. Meanwhile, I am going to provide you with my contact number in case you have any further questions or concerns regarding your condition. Does that sound good to you? You can also get information from the internet on these 2 drugs. Thank you and see you soon.

Discussion

Problem

Chronic cough.

Diagnosis

Drug-induced cough (ACEI and sitagliptin).

Other plausible diagnosis

- **Allergic rhinosinusitis**
  Patient has itchy nose and throat, desire to clear throat.
- **Gastroesophageal reflux disease**
  He suffers acidity.
- **Occupational**
  Patient is working as a laboratory technician in a chemistry laboratory.
- **Hypersensitivity pneumonitis (Extrinsic allergic alveolitis)—from birds**
  Patient keeps a parrot and cleans it and the cage.

Classification of cough according to its duration

- *Acute cough:* <3 weeks in duration.
- *Subacute cough:* Between 3 and 8 weeks in duration.
- *Chronic cough:* >8 weeks in duration.

Common causes of chronic cough

- Upper airway cough syndrome (UACS), secondary to rhinosinus diseases.
- Asthma
- Nonasthmatic eosinophilic bronchitis (NAEB)
- Gastroesophageal reflux disease
- Drug-induced cough (ACEI or sitagliptin)
- Smoking
- *Other causes include:* COPD, bronchiectasis, heart failure, and hypersensitivity pneumonitis.
  In a patient with chronic cough who is taking sitagliptin or ACEIs, these drugs should be discontinued first to see if they are responsible for the cough. Patients should be followed in the clinic within 4–6 weeks after the initial evaluation and referral to a well-recognised cough clinic should be considered for refractory chronic cough.
  Angiotensin-converting enzyme inhibitor-induced cough is usually dry and hacking seen in around 10% of patients treated with an ACEI. It usually begins within 1–2 weeks of starting therapy (it can be delayed up to 6 months). It typically resolves within 1–4 days of discontinuing therapy, (can take up to 4 weeks).
  Sitagliptin can cause chronic cough, rhinorrhoea, dyspnoea, and fatigue. Symptoms typically develop within 1–8 weeks of starting and resolve within 1 week of stopping the drug.

Red flag symptoms for chronic cough

- Haemoptysis
- Smoker >45 years of age with a new cough, change in cough, or voice disturbance.

- Adults aged 55–80 years who have a 30 pack year smoking history and currently smoke or who have quit within the past 15 years.
- Prominent dyspnoea, especially at rest or at night.
- Hoarseness
- *Systemic symptoms:*
  - Fever
  - Weight loss
  - Peripheral oedema with weight gain
- Trouble swallowing when eating or drinking
- Vomiting
- Recurrent pneumonia
- Abnormal respiratory examination and/or abnormal chest radiograph.

Further reading

Baraniuk JN, Jamieson MJ. Rhinorrhea, cough and fatigue in patients taking sitagliptin. Allergy Asthma Clin Immunol 2010; 6:8.

Irwin RS, French CL, Chang AB, et al. Classification of cough as a symptom in adults and management algorithms: CHEST Guideline and Expert Panel Report. Chest 2018; 153:196–209.

Scenario no. 4

Anaemia

Candidate copy

Please read the GP referral letter for Ms Rahma.
The time distribution for this station is as follows:
    You have (---) minutes to take a history from the patient.
    You have (---) minutes to collect your thoughts.
    You have (---) minutes for discussion with the examiners.

Please do not examine the patient

> **Dear Doctor,**
>
> Thank you for seeing Ms Rahma, a 28-year old who has no significant past medical history apart from irritable bowel syndrome. She has been complaining of increasing fatigue and lethargy over the last 6 months. Blood tests have revealed iron deficiency anaemia with Hb 8 g/dL.
>
> Yours faithfully,

> Please interview the patient and based on the history construct a differential diagnosis and plan of investigation. Provide an explanation to the patient and answer any question she may have.

Surrogate copy

Chief complaints and HPI

- You complain of fatigue and body weakness for the last 6 months
- You also suffer stomach pain for 2 years
- This has worsened with time
- The fatigue becomes worse when you walk or perform minimal exercise
- You are finding difficulty in doing the shopping and you need to rest frequently
- It gets better when you sleep or lie down
- It is better at night
- You feel dizzy when you stand up
- No muscle pain
- No fever.

Questions to be answered only if you are asked

- The pain in your tummy is *diffuse* and gets worse after eating
- The pain is not relieved by passing stool
- You have *lost 7 kg in weight* over the last 6 months
- There is no particular food that causes the abdominal pain
- You also have frequent bouts of *loose motion* (3–5 times every day)
- The loose motion can *wake you up from sleep*
- The *stool is bulky*
- The *stool is difficult to flush*
- You do not have urgency to pass stool after eating
- You do not have constipation
- No blood in the stool
- No black stool
- No vomiting
- No history of mouth ulcer
- No joint pain
- You do not prefer any particular weather.

Review of systems

As mentioned above.

Past history

You have been told in the past that you have irritable bowel syndrome (IBS). You have tried different medications but they did not work.

Dietary history

You eat a normal diet with red meat 3 times per week.

Menstrual history

You have regular menses with a normal amount.

Drug history

- You are taking spasmolytic drugs but you do not feel they help.
- You are not taking NSAIDs or any other medication.

Family history

Your *younger sister was also told she had IBS* because of recurrent abdominal pain and diarrhoea.

Social history

- You are single.
- You work as an accountant.
- You do not smoke or drink alcohol.
- You have not travelled or been camping for ~2 years.

Your concerns

- You were diagnosed with IBS and reassured, but why do you have anaemia?
- This question to be asked only if candidate did not mention this diagnosis: Do I have celiac disease?

Steps in history taking in a patient with anaemia

Step 1: Introduction, greeting, and confirmation of patient identity

- Good morning Ms Rahma (shakehands with the patient), pleased to meet you.
- I am Dr X working in the medical outpatient clinic.
- Can I confirm that I am talking to Ms Rahma?
- I have just read the referral letter from your GP who has informed me that you complain of fatigue.
- Can you tell me more about that?
- Allow the patient to speak.
- Avoid interruptions.
- Avoid medical jargon (e.g. celiac, steatorrhoea, melena, haematemesis, etc.)
- *Use open ended questions such as:* What else?

Step 2: Elaborating important points in the history

History of presenting illness and review of systems

Fatigue is a nonspecific symptom that denotes feeling of tiredness and lack of energy and can be caused by many diseases that involve different systems. In postgraduate clinical examinations, common causes of fatigue include anaemia (most commonly from GIT loss), chronic fatigue syndrome, obstructive sleep apnoea and to a lesser extent diseases of other systems e.g. myasthenia gravis, heart failure, hypothyroidism, vitamin D deficiency, depression, and drugs.

Important points to elaborate in the history of fatigue include:

- **What does the patient exactly mean by fatigue?**
  Does he/she mean excessive tiredness or weakness? Weakness may be a problem with strength and points to a neuromuscular disorder. Sometimes, patients may use these two terms exchangeably to mean lack of energy and increased tiredness.

- **Onset of fatigue**
  New onset fatigue that was not there before and tends to worsen with time usually indicates an organic/physical cause and requires further investigation.

- **How long have you had the fatigue?**
  Longer duration may suggest chronic fatigue syndrome.

- **Has it worsened over time?**
  Fatigue that worsens over time usually indicates an organic cause.

- **Is it related to exertion or does it occur at rest?**
  Fatigue that worsens with physical activity and improves with rest suggests organic (such as anaemia) rather than psychological cause.

- **Is there any diurnal variation of the fatigue?**
  Fatigue in patients with myasthenia gravis tends to worsen at the end of the day.

- **What are the aggravating and relieving factors of fatigue?**
- **Important associated symptoms to be elaborated in a patient with fatigue include:**
  - *Dizziness*: Postural, may suggest anaemia or blood loss.
  - *Muscle pain*: May suggest muscle disease.
  - *Change in appetite*: May suggest hyperthyroidism, diabetes, cancer, etc.
  - *Change in weight*: Weight loss with fatigue usually suggests serious disorders such as cancer or thyrotoxicosis, chronic infections or connective tissue disorders.
  - Symptoms that may suggest endocrinopathies (hyper/hypothyroidism–adrenal insufficiency–Cushing's syndrome).

These symptoms include hot/cold intolerance, weight gain, weight loss, palpitation, postural dizziness, etc.

Symptoms of blood loss

Melena, haematemesis, fresh bleeding per rectum, and use of NSAIDs.
- *Fever*
  May suggest chronic infections.

Review of systems

As fatigue can be caused by diseases of many body systems, it is crucial that you perform a thorough review of all systems when encountered with such symptom.

Analysis of abdominal pain

- Abdominal pain like any pain in the body should be analysed using the mnemonic "LIQOR triple A" (**L**ocation, **I**ntensity, **Q**uality, **O**nset, **R**adiation, **A**ggravating factors, **A**lleviating factors, **A**ssociated symptoms).
- Associated symptoms of abdominal pain should screen all the GIT symptoms including:
  - Appetite
  - Difficulty in swallowing
  - Is there a history of weight loss?
  - Is there any particular food that causes abdominal pain?
- Do you have loose motion?
- How many times do you pass stool per day?
- Does loose motion wake you up from sleep? (This points to organic causes rather than IBS)
- Ask about symptoms of *malabsorption* in case of diarrhoea.
- Is the *stool bulky?*
- Is the *stool difficult* to flush?
- Do you feel urgency to pass stool after eating? (This is typical of IBS)
- Do you have constipation beside diarrhoea? (IBS-alternating diarrhoea and constipation)
- Ask about any particular food that can worsen the condition (food intolerance such as gluten and lactose intolerance)
- Is there blood in the stool?
- What colour is the stool?
- Is there vomiting?
- Do you have recurrent mouth ulcers? *(May suggest Crohn's disease)*
- Do you feel joint pain or swelling? (May suggest CT disease)

Past history

You have been told that you have irritable bowel syndrome. How was the diagnosis made? What symptoms did you have at the time?

Many patients who are diagnosed as IBS turn out to have other diagnoses (IBS is a diagnosis of exclusion; you have to exclude other diseases that cause similar symptoms before labelling a patient with IBS).

Dietary history

Do you eat a normal diet? Vegetarians may develop anaemia.
How frequently do you eat meat?

Menstrual history

How are your menstrual periods? How long do they last? Are they heavy? Do you see clots?

Drug history

Are you taking NSAID or any other medication?

Family history

Does any other member of your family have similar bowel problems?

Social history

- Are you single or married?
- Recent travel or camping *(Giardiasis)*
- Occupation
- Habits
- Sexual history *(HIV enteropathy)*.

Further information not covered (at end of history taking)

Ask the patient the following question: Is there anything else that you feel important and would like to tell me about?

Step 3: Explaining to the patient the diagnosis and the plan of management

Ms Rahma, after reviewing your history, there are some potential reasons for your anaemia and recurrent stomach pain. You most likely have difficulty with absorbing nutrients from the diet. There are many conditions that can lead to this problem. One of these conditions may be celiac disease. Have you heard of this before?

Well, in celiac disease patients have inflammation or irritation of the small bowel with difficulty in absorbing nutrients from the diet. When food containing a protein called gluten is eaten and arrives in the small bowel, the immune system reacts against it and causes an inflammatory reaction in the wall of the bowel and produces antibodies in the blood. Gluten is the name given to certain types of proteins found in wheat, barley, rye, and related grains. We can do a simple blood test to assess Tissue Transglutaminase Antibodies, which is positive in about 98% of people with celiac disease. To further establish a firm diagnosis of celiac disease, we need to take a small piece of the lining of your small bowel (called a biopsy) using endoscopy. Endoscopy involves the insertion of a thin flexible tube through the mouth into the stomach and small bowel. Samples are taken from the wall of the small bowel and are examined under a microscope to look for changes of celiac disease. Does that make sense to you?

I am going to order some blood tests and arrange an appointment with a colleague of mine who is specialised in the digestive system for his opinion and to perform the endoscopy and biopsy.
Check patient understanding and agreement on plan of management.
Does that make sense to you?

Step 4: Ask and address patient's concerns

Do you have any questions or concerns?
Patient's concern: Previously, I was diagnosed with irritable bowel syndrome. Why did the doctor not make the correct diagnosis before?

Reply: The problem with diagnosing celiac disease and differentiating it from irritable bowel syndrome arises from the fact that the two conditions have very similar symptoms. Up to 16% of people with celiac disease are initially labelled as having irritable bowel syndrome before finally receiving a correct diagnosis of celiac disease.

Patient's concern: Is there any treatment for celiac disease?

Reply: Celiac disease is treated by avoiding all foods that contain gluten. Gluten is what causes inflammation in the small bowel. When this is removed from the diet, the bowel will heal and return to normal. Dieticians with expertise in gluten free diets are essential for educating patients and tailoring diets. Medications are not normally required to treat celiac disease except in occasional patients who do not respond to a gluten free diet. There are many celiac disease support groups available for patients and family members.

After answering the person's concerns confirm the agreement by saying; is that ok or does that sound good for you?

Step 5: Summarise the discussion, confirm patient's understandings, and close the meeting

Ms Rahma, I would like to summarise our discussion to be sure that you understand important information mentioned. The most probable cause for your anaemia and tummy pain is a difficulty of your digestive system to absorb nutrients, and the most likely cause is celiac disease. I am going to order some blood tests and arrange an appointment with a colleague who specialises in the digestive system. I will see you in 3-weeks time to give you further answers. Meanwhile, I am going to provide you with my contact number in case you have any further questions or concerns regarding your condition. Does that sound good to you? You can also get some information from the web regarding celiac disease. Thank you and see you soon.

Discussion

Problem

Anaemia in a patient who was misdiagnosed with irritable bowel syndrome.

Diagnosis

Celiac disease.

Other plausible diagnoses

- Crohn's disease
- Whipple's disease (more in men).

Common causes of iron deficiency anaemia in premenopausal women include

- **Abnormal uterine bleeding:**
  Excessive menstruation is a common cause of iron deficiency anaemia in premenopausal women in developed countries; it can lead to varying degrees of iron deficiency anaemia.
- GI source is the second most common cause in this group of patients (30% of cases of iron deficiency anaemia in this age group). If the gynaecologic history is not suggestive of a uterine source, endoscopy should be performed to exclude a GI cause.

In men and postmenopausal women, GI sources of bleeding should be excluded. Current recommendations support upper and lower GI endoscopy.

Important GI causes of iron deficiency anaemia include

- Long-term use of aspirin or other NSAIDs
- Colon carcinoma
- Angiodysplasia
- Gastric carcinoma
- Peptic ulcer disease
- Celiac disease
- Inflammatory bowel disease.

It is crucial to differentiate irritable bowel syndrome from other organic causes of recurrent abdominal pain. People presenting with irritable bowel syndrome symptoms commonly report incomplete evacuation/rectal hypersensitivity, as well as urgency, which is increased in diarrhoea-predominant irritable bowel syndrome.

Abdominal pain or discomfort in irritable bowel syndrome is typically relieved by defecation and associated with altered bowel frequency or stool form. This is a very important symptom in irritable bowel syndrome. This should be accompanied by at least two of the following four symptoms:

- Altered stool passage (straining, urgency, incomplete evacuation)
- Abdominal bloating (more common in women than men), distension, tension or hardness
- Symptoms made worse by eating
- Passage of mucus.

Symptoms not consistent with irritable bowel syndrome should alert the clinician to the possibility of an organic pathology and include the following:

- Onset in middle or older age
- Acute symptoms (irritable bowel syndrome is defined by chronicity)
- Progressive symptoms
- Nocturnal symptoms such as diarrhoea awaking patient from sleep (points to organic cause)
- Anorexia or weight loss
- Fever
- Rectal bleeding
- Painless diarrhoea
- Steatorrhoea
- Gluten intolerance.

Celiac disease or gluten-sensitive enteropathy is an autoimmune condition with an estimated prevalence of 1% in the United States. The initial presentation can be similar to irritable bowel syndrome making the two conditions difficult to distinguish clinically. This can lead to mislabelling, and concern that some patients, in whom irritable bowel syndrome has been diagnosed, may in fact have celiac disease. Multiple clinical guidelines advise routine serologic screening for celiac disease in patients presenting with irritable bowel syndrome-type symptoms. Patients with celiac disease who do not adhere to the gluten-free diet usually continue to suffer from symptoms such as abdominal pain, bloating, gas, diarrhoea, and malabsorption. In addition, these patients are at higher risk for developing complications of celiac disease such as cancer of the small bowel, lymphoma, oesophageal carcinoma, and strictures in the bowel due to inflammation.

Further reading

Loftus C, Murray J. The American College of Gastroenterology. Celiac disease. [online] Available from http://s3.gi.org/patients/gihealth/pdf/celiac.pdf. [Last accessed October, 2019].

Luthra P, Ford AC. Screening for celiac disease in individuals with symptoms suggestive of irritable bowel syndrome: Still a worthwhile exercise. Gastroenterology 2016; 151:368–370.

National Institute for Health and Care Excellence. Irritable bowel syndrome in adults: diagnosis and management. [online] Available from https://www.nice.org.uk/guidance/cg61/chapter/1-Recommendations#diagnosis-of-ibs. [Last accessed October, 2019].

Short MW, Domagalski JE. Iron deficiency anemia: evaluation and management. Am Fam Physician 2013; 87:98–104.

Scenario no. 5

A patient with recurrent arm numbness

Candidate copy

Please read the GP referral letter for Mrs Smith.
The time distribution for this station is as follows:
> You have (---) minutes to take a history from the patient.
> You have (---) minutes to collect your thoughts.
> You have (---) minutes for discussion with the examiners.

Please do not examine the patient

Dear Doctor,

Thank you for seeing Mrs Smith, a 30-year-old who has been complaining of recurrent episodes of numbness in the right arm and sometimes in the left arm over the last few weeks. Her blood count, urea and electrolytes and liver function were all normal.

Yours faithfully,

Please interview the patient and based on the history construct a differential diagnosis and plan of investigation. Provide an explanation to the patient and answer any question she may have.

Surrogate copy

Chief complaint and HPI

- You feel attacks of numbness and tingling in your right arm and sometimes in your left arm for the past 8 weeks.
- The attacks last for a few minutes and then go away.
- On one occasion, you also felt weakness in your right hand but that was only for 1 minute.
- Six months ago, you had a *sudden loss of vision* that lasted for 2–3 minutes. It did not bother you as it did not come back again.
- You do not have numbness elsewhere in your body.
- You never lost consciousness.
- You never lost control of your urine or bowel.
- You never had jerky movement.

Review of systems

Over the past 6 months, you have felt, on occasions, your *heart beats very fast and it was not regular*. This comes and goes but has been increasing in frequency over the past 2 months. It seems to happen when you take a drug called *sumatriptan* 50 mg, prescribed for your migraine.

- You do not feel chest pain.
- You do not have neck pain.
- You do not have a weather preference (hot or cold).
- You have not lost weight and you eat a normal diet.

Menstrual history
Normal and regular.

Dietary history
You eat a normal diet.

Past history
- You have been suffering from *migraine for 4 years and you are taking sumatriptan 50 mg.*
- Your migraine attacks are sometimes severe and prevent you from going to work.
- You do not have disc disease in your neck.
- You do not suffer other diagnosis like multiple sclerosis.

Family history
Nothing significant.

Social history
- You do not smoke or drink alcohol.
- You are a school teacher.

- You are happily married with one kid.

Your main questions/concerns:
- What causes my symptoms?

Steps in history taking in a patient with arm numbness/weakness

Step 1: Introduction, greeting, and confirmation of patient identity
- Good morning Mrs Smith (shakehands with the patient), pleased to meet you.
- I am Dr X working in the medical outpatient clinic.
- Can I confirm that I am talking to Mrs Smith?
- I have just read the referral letter from your GP who states that you complain of arm numbness.
- Can you tell me more about that?
- Allow the patient to speak.
- Avoid interruptions.
- Avoid medical jargon [e.g. transient ischaemic attack (TIA), multiple sclerosis, etc.]
- *Use open ended questions such as:* What else?

Step 2: Elaborating important points in the history

History of presenting illness
- Where did you feel the numbness?
- When did you feel the numbness?
- Did you feel it in any other place?
- Was it sudden or gradual?
- How long did the attack last?
- How many times have you felt it?
- Was it associated with weakness of the arms or legs?
- Was it associated with trouble in speaking or a heavy tongue?
- Did you feel dizziness with the attack?
- Did you lose consciousness?
- Were there any abnormal/involuntary movements in your body?
- Did you feel an increase in your heart rate with the attack?
- Did you lose control of your bowel or bladder?
- How was the attack terminated?
- Did you feel any change or imbalance of your gait?

Review of systems

- Cardiac symptoms: *Palpitations, breathlessness, chest pain (may indicate AF and TIA)*
- Neck pain *(cervical myelopathy is a cause of arm numbness)*
- Blurring or loss of vision *(TIA, multiple sclerosis).*

Past history

- Similar illness in the past
- History of stroke
- History of multiple sclerosis (May cause numbness)
- History of migraine (Migraine aura/ hemiplegic migraine)
- History of epilepsy (Todd's paralysis)
- History of heart disease
- History of HTN
- History of DM
- History of deep vein thrombosis (DVT), thrombophilia
- History of joint pain or connective tissue disease.

Menstrual history

- Have you had recurrent abortions in the past (anti-phospholipid).
- Pregnancy may cause leg oedema.
- Use of oral contraceptive pills (OCPs) (Very important to ask about OCPs in any female with neurologic or thrombosis symptoms or signs as they are thrombogenic).

Family history

- Family history of stroke.
- Family history of heart disease.
- Family history of thrombosis/clots.
- Family history of migraine.

Drug history

- Use of oral contraceptive.
- Use of regular medications or over the counter medication.

Social history

- History of smoking.
- History of alcohol use.
- History of drug abuse (cocaine may cause vasospasm).

Further information not covered (at end of history taking)

Ask the patient the following question: Is there anything else that you feel important and would like to tell me about?

Step 3: Explaining to the patient the diagnosis and the plan of management

Mrs Smith, after reviewing your history, there are some possible reasons for your repeated arm numbness and the previous loss of vision. People who have migraine can get similar symptoms. Now, I do not want you to be alarmed, but these problems may also be caused by a condition that mimics stroke but as it is brief and does not result in permanent brain damage, it is called a "Transient ischaemic attack" or TIA. TIA results from a brief interruption of the blood supply to some parts in your brain. You mentioned that your heart sometimes beats in an irregular manner. One condition that may cause an irregular heart beat and lead to a TIA is called "paroxysmal atrial fibrillation". Paroxysmal atrial fibrillation can result in a clot forming in a chamber of the heart and this, in turn, can travel to and temporarily block a blood vessel to the brain causing numbness or weakness. Have you heard of this before? I would also recommend that you stop the sumatriptan you are using for migraine. This medication is not recommended when there is a problem with blood flow to the brain. Mrs Smith, to check the cause for the transient ischemic attacks and prevent further attacks from happening, I suggest that we admit you to the hospital for a few days. We will perform a scan of your heart, blood vessels of your brain and some blood tests. We will also start some medications that help prevent further TIA. What do you think about that? A team of specialised doctors who deal with TIA and stroke will be looking after you while in hospital. I also recommend that you take a tablet of aspirin (I will order it for you now) which will minimise to some extent the risk of a further TIA.

Check patient's understanding and agreement on plan of management.

Does that sound good to you?

Step 4: Ask about and address patient's concerns

Do you have any questions or concerns?

Patient's concern: What causes my symptoms?

Reply: Your irregular heart beat may be because of a condition called paroxysmal atrial fibrillation. This can result in a clot forming in a chamber of the heart and this, in turn, can travel to and temporarily block a blood vessel to the brain causing numbness or weakness.

After answering each concern, confirm the agreement by saying; "is that alright or does that make sense to you?"

Step 5: Summarise the discussion, confirm patient's understandings and close the meeting

Mrs Smith, I would like to summarise our discussion as it is important for me to be sure that you understand important information mentioned. The most probable cause for your numbness is a condition called transient ischemic attack resulting from brief blockage of the blood supply to your brain. This interruption in blood supply may be related to your irregular heartbeats. I am going to arrange a hospital admission for you, where a team of doctors will perform further testing and imaging. Please make sure that you stop sumatriptan. I am also going to prescribe aspirin for you. Does that make sense to you? You can also have some information from the internet regarding transient ischemic attack. Thank you and see you soon.

Discussion

Problem

Recurrent arm numbness in a patient with migraine (on sumatriptan) and episodic palpitations.

Diagnosis

Transient ischemic attack (palpitations may suggest paroxysmal AF).

Other plausible diagnosis

- Migraine auras
- Sumatriptan-induced cerebral vasospasm and arrhythmia
- Multiple sclerosis.

Sumatriptan can cause vasospasm and cerebrovascular events and should be discontinued if there is a suspicion of cerebrovascular events. It is contraindicated in patients with a history of stroke or TIA. Furthermore, life-threatening arrhythmias including ventricular tachycardia and ventricular fibrillation leading to death have been reported within a few hours of taking 5-HT1 agonists. Sumatriptan is contraindicated in patients with Wolff–Parkinson–White syndrome or arrhythmias associated with other cardiac accessory conduction pathway disorders.

It is essential to identify TIAs promptly because of the increased risk of ischemic stroke, requiring urgent investigation and preventive treatment. On the other hand, it is also important to identify TIA 'mimics', to avoid unnecessary and expensive investigations, incorrect diagnostic labelling, and inappropriate long-term prevention treatment.

There are a number of conditions that may mimic a TIA, called 'TIA Mimics':

- Migraine aura
- Seizures
- Metabolic causes such as hypoglycaemia and electrolyte abnormalities.
- Syncope
- Multiple sclerosis
- Cerebral tumours and space-occupying lesions.

Up to about 20% of patients with suspected TIA have migraine aura. This is a very common mimic of TIA. A diagnostic challenge arises, particularly when the aura occurs with minimal or no headache and associated sensory, motor or speech disturbances. In migraine, different modalities may be involved (e.g. visual and somatosensory) but they often occur sequentially, with one resolving as the other begins, rather than simultaneously as in TIAs. Although auras are typically experienced just before or simultaneously with headache, headache onset can be delayed for more than an hour after the end of the aura.

Further reading

Nadarajan V, Perry RJ, Johnson J, et al. Transient ischemic attacks: mimics and chameleons. Pract Neurol 2014; 14:23–31.

Scenario no. 6

A woman with dysphagia

Candidate copy

Please read the GP referral letter for Mrs Aisha.
The time distribution for this station is as follows:

> You have (---) minutes to take a history from the patient.
> You have (---) minutes to collect your thoughts.
> You have (---) minutes for discussion with the examiners.

Please do not examine the patient

Dear Doctor,

Thank you for seeing Mrs Aisha, a 35-year-old lady who has been complaining of difficulty in swallowing over the last 3 months. Her hemoglobin level is 9 g/dL. Kidney function, liver function, and electrolytes are normal.

Yours faithfully,

Please interview the patient and based on the history construct a differential diagnosis and plan of investigation. Provide an explanation to the patient and answer any questions she may have.

Surrogate copy

Chief complaint and HPI

- Your main complaint is difficulty in swallowing or food sticking in your throat for 3 months.
- You feel that the food is sticking in the mid and lower part of your neck.
- You do not feel pain while swallowing.
- You feel difficulty in swallowing with both solid and liquid food.

Review of systems

- You do not have choking or cough.
- You have no weight loss.
- Your appetite is good.
- You have not vomited blood.
- You have felt frequent *heart burn and acidity* for 1 year.
- You have not noticed any change in the colour of your stool.
- You do not have any family history of similar problems or neurologic diseases.
- You do not have neurologic symptoms.

Review of systems

Questions to be answered only if asked by candidates
- Your *hands turn blue and red* when they are exposed to cold.
- You are suffering from *pain and swelling in your hand joints.*
- You feel that your *skin is becoming tight* and you have *difficulty in opening your mouth.*
- You have not observed thickening of the palms and soles.
- You have fatigue but it does not change between day and night time.

Menstrual history

- Your menses are normal.
- No previous abortions.

Dietary history

You are trying to eat soft food and you find difficulty in swallowing.

Past history

- You do not have a history of neurologic disease.
- You have not had a peptic ulcer.

Family history

- No family history of cancer.
- No family history of neurologic diseases.

Social history

- You are a teacher.
- You do not smoke or drink alcohol.
- You are married with one kid.
- You have never travelled to Latin America *(Chagas disease).*

Drug history

You are not on any medication.

Your questions/concerns

Doctor: I am worried that it might be cancer. What are the chances of it being cancer?

Steps in history taking in a patient with dysphagia

Step 1: Introduction, greeting, and confirmation of patient identity

- Good morning Mrs Aisha (shakehands with the patient), pleased to meet you.
- I am Dr X working in the medical outpatient clinic.
- Can I confirm that I am talking to Mrs Aisha?
- I have just read the referral letter from your GP who states that you have had difficulty with swallowing food.
- Can you tell me more about that?
- Allow the patient to speak.
- Avoid interruptions.
- Avoid medical jargon (e.g. dysphagia, CREST syndrome, oesophagus, achalasia, abdomen, etc.)
- *Use open ended questions such as:* What else?

Step 2: Elaborating important points in the history

History of presenting illness

- What do you mean exactly by difficulty in swallowing?
- When you swallow, does the food stick in your throat?
- Do you feel pain when swallowing? *(Odynophagia is painful swallowing which can be due to ulcers, abscess or local throat lesions. It is different from dysphagia)*
- At which level does the food stick in your throat?
- Do you have problems with swallowing solid food, liquids or both?
- Has the difficulty in swallowing improved, remained the same or worsened?
- Do you have choking or a cough while eating? *(Recurrent aspiration from dysphagia is an important complication of dysphagia)*
- Have you had weight loss?
- How is your appetite or desire for food?
- Have you vomited blood?
- Do you feel frequent heart burn or acidity?
- Have you noticed any change in the colour of your stool?

Review of systems

- Do you have weakness in your arms or legs?
- Do you have difficulty in speaking?
- Do you have joint pain or swelling?
- Do you have any pain or change in the colour of your hands when exposed to cold?
- Is your skin becoming tight or do you have difficulty in opening your mouth?
- Have you observed any unusual thickening of your palms and soles? *(Tylosis is associated with oesophageal cancer)*
- Do you feel fatigue or weakness? And does this fatigue differ in the day or night time?

Past history

- Have you suffered any disease of the brain or nerves? *(Bulbar palsy)*
- Have you suffered from a peptic ulcer or acid reflux?
- Have you suffered any disease of your joints or skin?

Family history

- Do any of your close relatives have stomach or oesophageal cancer?
- Do you have any family member with neurologic disease?
- Do you have any family member who is suffering from thick skin over the soles and palms? *(Tylosis is associated with oesophageal carcinoma)*

Social history

- Do you smoke? If yes, ask details
- Do you drink alcohol? If yes, take detailed history of alcohol intake
- What is your job?
- Have you travelled to Latin America? *(Chagas disease)*

Drug history

Are you taking NSAIDs?

Further information not covered (at end of history taking)

Is there anything else that you feel important and would like to tell me about?

Step 3: Explaining to the patient the diagnosis and the plan of management

Mrs Aisha, your main problem is the difficulty in swallowing and you also feel that your fingers turn blue in cold weather and you have joint pain. These symptoms together may fit a diagnosis called 'systemic sclerosis.' Have you heard of this disease before? Well, systemic sclerosis is a rare disease that can involve different organs in the body. One of the organs affected is the food pipe 'the oesophagus,' causing a weakness of its muscles with recurrent acidity and heart burn and difficulty in swallowing. Other organs in the body that are affected are the skin and blood vessels leading to a change in the colour of the fingers when exposed to cold, and a tightening of the skin with joint pains. However, as there are a number of other reasons for difficulty in swallowing, we need to perform some tests to confirm this diagnosis and exclude other causes. I am going to order some blood tests and refer you to a colleague who specialises in the diseases of the oesophagus who will assess the function and structure of your food pipe by passing a camera down your gullet. I will also refer you to another colleague who specialises in systemic sclerosis for further advice on your management. I will see you in 2 weeks when the results of the tests are ready to plan further management.

Check patient understanding and agreement on plan of management.

Does that make sense to you?

Step 4: Ask about and address patient's concerns

Do you have any questions or concerns?

Patient's concern: Doctor, I am worried that it might be cancer. What are the chances of this being cancer?

Reply: Well, it is true that cancer of the oesophagus can cause difficulty in swallowing. However, cancer of the oesophagus usually affects those above the age of 50 years. In addition, the presence of joint pain and the change in finger colour when you are exposed to cold, point to systemic sclerosis. I am, therefore, going to refer you to colleagues who specialise in the diseases of oesophagus and systemic sclerosis.

After answering each concern, confirm the agreement by saying; "Is that alright or does that make sense to you?"

Step 5: Summarise the discussion, confirm patient's understandings, and close the meeting

Mrs Aisha, I would like to summarise our discussion to be sure that you understand important information mentioned. The most likely cause of difficulty in swallowing in your case is a disease called systemic sclerosis. I am going to order some blood tests and refer you to a colleague who specialises in diseases of the oesophagus and another colleague who specialises in systemic sclerosis for further advice about your management. I will see you in 2 weeks when the results of the tests are ready to give you more information on the diagnosis and management.

Meanwhile, I am going to provide you with my contact number in case you have any further questions or concerns regarding your condition. You can also get information from the internet regarding systemic sclerosis. Does that make sense to you? Thank you and see you soon.

Discussion

Problem

Dysphagia to solid and liquid food suggesting a neuromuscular disorder.

Diagnosis

- **Systemic sclerosis versus CREST syndrome:**
  The patient has dysphagia to both solids and liquids which indicates a neuromuscular cause. In the presence of Raynaud's phenomenon and joint pains, systemic sclerosis becomes a high possibility. The age of the patient, the type of dysphagia, and the presence of other symptoms of scleroderma are against GIT malignancies.

Other plausible diagnoses

- **Oesophageal/gastric cancer:**
  If the patient's age is older (>50) with absence of other symptoms of scleroderma, then this scenario would fit into GIT malignancy.

- **Gastroesophageal reflux disease-related reflux oesophagitis/stricture:**
  Patient gave a history of GERD.

- **Achalasia of the cardia:**
  This will also give dysphagia to both solids and liquids.

- **Oesophageal web:**
  As the patient has anaemia, a differential is Plummer–Vinson syndrome, although this usually gives dysphagia to solids.

Impaired swallowing, or dysphagia, may occur due to a wide variety of structural or functional conditions, including stroke and other neuromuscular diseases, cancer, rheumatologic diseases, and GERD. A thorough history is very important in the diagnosis and treatment of swallowing disorders.

Candidates must ask about the consequences of dysphagia such as recurrent aspiration, weight loss, malnutrition, and GIT bleeding.

Dysphagia to solid food usually suggests mechanical obstruction.

Mechanical obstructions

- Oesophageal stricture/peptic strictures/web/diverticulum
- Patients more than 50 years—oesophageal cancer.

Neuromuscular disorders

- Achalasia
- Scleroderma
- Myasthenia gravis
- Motor neurone disease
- Stroke
- Multiple sclerosis
- Diffuse oesophageal spasm.

The level at which dysphagia is felt is also important. Dysphagia at the level of the pharynx (pharyngeal phase) can be caused by a stricture, pharyngeal web, diverticulum or tumour. Patients may retain excessive amounts of food in the pharynx and experience overflow aspiration after swallowing. This can result in coughing or choking with swallowing due to difficulty in initiating swallowing and drooling. Patients typically feel the food sticks in the throat.

Dysphagia at the oesophageal level causes a sensation of food sticking in the chest. It can result from mechanical obstruction by tumour (oesophageal cancer), a motility disorder or oesophageal muscular weakness or impaired opening of the lower oesophageal sphincter (achalasia).

Patients with chronic GERD are at risk for reflux esophagitis. They are also at risk for peptic strictures, which may obstruct the oesophagus and result in dysphagia. The diagnosis of GERD is associated with a 10–15% risk of Barrett's oesophagus, a change of the normal squamous epithelium of the distal oesophagus to a columnar-lined intestinal metaplasia. Risk factors associated with the development of Barrett's oesophagus include long-standing GERD, male gender, central obesity, and age over 50 years, current or past history of smoking, and a confirmed family history of Barrett's oesophagus or oesophageal adenocarcinoma. Barrett's oesophagus carries a risk (0.2–7%) per year of developing oesophageal adenocarcinoma (the risk depends on the degree of dysplasia observed on biopsy).

Risk factors for oesophageal cancer

- *Tylosis*: A rare dominantly inherited disease characterised by thickening on the areas exposed to pressure and/or friction, as seen on the skin of the palms and soles. The condition is strongly associated with oesophageal cancer.
- Barrett's oesophagus
- Smoking
- Alcohol
- Geographic distribution (China and Asia)
- Presence of other GIT or body cancer.

Oesophageal cancer has two main subtypes–oesophageal squamous cell carcinoma and oesophageal adenocarcinoma. Squamous cell carcinoma accounts for ~90% of oesophageal cancers.

Oesophageal carcinoma is rare in young people and increases in incidence with age, peaking in the seventh and eighth decades of life. Adenocarcinoma is three to four times as common in men as it is in women, whereas the sex distribution is more equal for squamous cell carcinoma.

Systemic sclerosis can be diffuse or limited (previously named CREST '*Calcinosis, Raynaud's disease, Oesophageal dysmotility, Sclerodactyly, Telangiectasia*'). Oesophageal symptoms and disease are very common in patients with systemic sclerosis and can precede other symptoms. Heartburn and dysphagia, and objective findings of oesophageal dysfunction have been reported in 50–90% of patients. Thus, the oesophagus is second only to the skin as the most commonly affected organ in systemic sclerosis. Common abnormalities of gastrointestinal function include weak or absent distal oesophageal peristalsis and reduced lower oesophageal sphincter pressure, a pattern often termed scleroderma oesophagus (even in the absence of systemic sclerosis). Gastroparesis can also develop. These functional abnormalities impair oesophageal acid clearance and predispose patients to GERD and its potential complications.

Further reading

Carlson D, Hinchcliff M, Pandolfino JE. Advances in the evaluation and management of esophageal disease of systemic sclerosis. Curr Rheumatol Rep 2015; 17:475.

Lordick F, Mariette C, Haustermans K, et al. Esophageal cancer: ESMO Clinical Practice Guidelines for diagnosis, treatment and follow-up. Ann Oncol 2016; 27:v50–v57.

Palmer J, Drennan J, Baba M. Evaluation and treatment of swallowing impairments. Am Fam Physician. 2000; 61:2453–2462.

Shaheen NJ, Falk GW, Iyer PG, et al. ACG Clinical Guideline: diagnosis and management of Barrett's esophagus. Am J Gastroenterol 2016;111:30–50.

Scenario no. 7

Headache in a woman

Candidate copy

Please read the GP referral letter for Mrs Amal.
The time distribution for this station is as follows:
>   You have (---) minutes to take a history from the patient.
>   You have (---) minutes to collect your thoughts.
>   You have (---) minutes for discussion with the examiners.

Please do not examine the patient

Dear Doctor,

Thank you for seeing Mrs Amal, a 36-year-old who has been complaining of severe headache for the last 2 weeks associated with blurred vision. Her funduscopic examination revealed papilledema. An urgent plain CT scan of her brain was unremarkable apart from empty sella. Her complete blood count, kidney function test, liver function, and electrolytes were all normal.

Yours faithfully,

Please interview the patient and based on the history construct a differential diagnosis and plan of investigation. Provide an explanation to the patient and answer any questions she may have.

Surrogate copy

Chief complaint and HPI

- You complain of headache for the past 2 weeks.
- The headache is dull and all over your head.
- It is 8/10 on a pain scale.
- It started gradually, and is getting worse.
- It is worse in the morning.
- The headache increases on coughing, bending the head forward and sneezing.
- It may occasionally be relieved by rest.
- You also vomit daily, and it is forceful and sudden.
- You did not lose consciousness.
- You did not have jerky movements in your body.
- You did not and no one else has observed any change in your personality.
- You did not feel any limb weakness or numbness.

Review of systems

- After the delivery of your child 2 years ago, you *gained 15 kg in weight* and it increased from 70 kg to 85 kg.
- You did not feel a fast heartbeat, increased sweating, anxiety or nervousness.
- You have not had fever.

Menstrual history

- You are using *birth control pills/oral contraceptive pill*s.
- There is no relationship between the headache and your menstrual cycle.

Past medical history

- You *had sinusitis 2 months* ago for which you received antibiotics.
- You do not suffer hypertension.
- You do not suffer migraine.
- You have not suffered a previous stroke or other brain lesions.
- You have not suffered head trauma.

Family history

- No family history of migraine.
- No family history of cancer.

Drug history

- You are using the oral contraceptive pill.
- You are using *a medication for acne* (Isotretinoin 20 mg twice daily for the last 3 months).

Social history

- You do not smoke.
- You do not drink.
- No change in personality.
- You have not travelled abroad recently.
- You are married and have one child.

Your main concern or question

- What is the cause of my headache?
- Is this condition serious?

Steps in history taking in a patient with headache

Step 1: Introduction, greeting, and confirmation of patient identity

- Good morning Mrs Amal (shakehands with the patient), pleased to meet you.
- I am Dr X working in the medical outpatient clinic.
- Can I confirm that I am talking to Mrs Amal?
- I have just read the referral letter from your GP who states that you have a severe headache.
- Can you tell me more about that?
- Allow the patient to speak.
- Avoid interruptions.
- Avoid medical jargon (e.g. idiopathic hypertension, neoplasm, cerebral venous thrombosis, trigeminal neuralgia, etc.)
- *Use open ended questions such as:* What else?

Step 2: Elaborating important points in the history of headache

History of presenting illness

Headache like any other pain in the body should be analysed using the LIQOR AAA mnemonic.

Review of systems

- Other neurological symptoms.
- *Trigeminal neuralgia in young*: Ask about other symptoms of MS.
- *Symptoms of pheochromocytoma*: Palpitations, sweating, anxiety, and nervousness.

- *Symptoms suggestive of increased ICP*: Projectile vomiting, personality change, and seizure/weakness/numbness.
- *Recent weight gain*: Idiopathic intracranial hypertension.
- Ask about alarm/red flag symptoms of headache (see below).

Menstrual history

- *Relationship of headache to menstrual cycle*: Catamenial migraine
- *Use of oral contraceptive pill*: Cerebral venous sinus thrombosis, migraine, idiopathic intracranial hypertension.

Past medical history

- Ask about history of hypertension
- Ask about history of migraine
- Ask about previous strokes, brain lesions
- Ask about previous head trauma
- Ask about diseases that cause immunosuppression
- *Recurrent sinusitis*: May cause cerebral venous thrombosis, brain abscess, meningitis.

Family history

- Family history of migraine
- Family history of cancer.

Drug history

- *Oral contraceptive pill*: May be associated with cerebral venous thrombosis, migraine, idiopathic intracranial hypertension.
- Drugs for migraine.
- Steroids
- *Other drugs that may cause headache and ICP*: Isotretinoin, tetracyclines, etc.

Social history

- Smoking *(Risk of malignancy)*
- *Alcohol intake*: Subdural haematoma, bleeding
- Change in personality.
- *Travel history*: Malaria, meningitis.
- *Sexual history:* HIV, neurosyphilis.

Further information not covered (at end of history taking)

Is there anything else that you feel important and would like to tell me about?

Step 3: Explaining to the patient the diagnosis and the plan of management

Mrs Amal, your main complaint is of a severe headache for the last 2 weeks. You have also gained weight over the last 2 years and you are using the birth control pill and isotretinoin for acne. Your GP also found swelling of the nerve at the back of your eyes. All these findings point toward a condition called 'idiopathic intracranial hypertension.' In this condition, there is raised pressure within the skull (raised intracranial pressure), which puts pressure on the brain. Idiopathic means that the cause of this raised pressure is unknown. The main symptoms are headache and blurring of vision. It mostly affects women of childbearing age who are overweight or obese. There are certain conditions that increase the risk of developing idiopathic intracranial hypertension. One of these conditions is being overweight and others include use of birth control pills (oral contraceptive pills) and drugs like isotretinoin that you are using for your acne. Therefore, I would suggest that you stop taking isotretinoin and the oral contraceptive pill. You may ask your dermatologist and gynaecologist to prescribe alternatives such as a contraceptive device for contraception and other acne medications that do not cause raised intracranial pressure. Additionally, I am going to refer you to our weight management clinic to help you lose weight. I am going to arrange urgent imaging of your brain called MRI to make sure that there are no other causes of raised intracranial pressure, such as clots in the veins of the brain that can give a similar picture. If the MRI is okay, then I will arrange with my neurology colleagues to perform a procedure called a lumbar puncture. This is a medical procedure where we insert a needle in your back, and it allows us to measure the pressure of your brain fluid as well as draining some of the fluid to lower the pressure. I can discuss with you further about this procedure after the MRI result. Does that sound clear to you? You will be started on a medication called 'acetazolamide' that lowers the brain pressure and I will discuss further about this medication in the next appointment. I will arrange urgent appointments with my colleagues in neurology and ophthalmology and will see you in 3 days to discuss the result of the MRI. Meanwhile, I will prescribe a pain killer that will help reduce your headache.

Does that make sense to you?

Step 4: Ask about and address patient's concerns

Do you have any questions or concerns?

Patient's concern: What is the cause of my headache?

Reply: Answered above.

Patient's concern: Is this condition serious, doctor?

Reply: This is a very important question. If not treated appropriately, the raised pressure within the skull can cause swelling and compression of the nerve at the back of the eye (optic nerve) which is responsible for your eye sight and can lead to blindness due to damage to that nerve. Therefore, idiopathic intracranial hypertension should be taken seriously.

After answering each concern, confirm the agreement by saying; "Is that alright? Or does that sound clear to you?"

Step 5: Summarise the discussion, confirm patient's understandings, and close the meeting

Mrs Amal, I would like to summarise our discussion to be sure that you understand important information about your illness. The most probable cause of your headache is increased pressure within your skull, a condition called 'idiopathic intracranial hypertension.' I am going to order an urgent MRI of your brain to make sure we are not missing anything else and I am going to get urgent opinions from brain and eye specialists. Please make sure that you stop taking the acne tablets and the contraceptive pill and try to reduce your weight. I will see you urgently in 3 days to give you further advice and plan further management. Meanwhile, I am going to provide you with my contact number in case you have any further questions or concerns regarding your condition. Does that make sense to you? You can also have some information from the internet on 'idiopathic intracranial hypertension.' Thank you and see you soon.

Discussion

Problem

Headache in an obese woman who is using oral contraceptive pills and isotretinoin.

Diagnosis

Idiopathic intracranial hypertension (weight gain, oral contraceptive pill, isotretinoin, papilloedema, and presence of empty sella on CT scan).

Other plausible diagnoses

- **Cerebral venous sinus thrombosis**
  Should be excluded in any newly diagnosed papilloedema (oral contraceptive pill and history of sinusitis).

- **Brain tumour.**

Characteristic features of headache from different aetiologies

Migraine headache

- Usually throbbing or pulsatile.
- Commonly on one side.
- Aggravated by menstrual periods, alcohol, lack of sleep, certain foods such as chocolate, cheese, coffee, etc.
- May be preceded by migraine aura such as problems with vision, dizziness, lip, and facial numbness, etc.
- Usually lasts for hours and sometimes for days.
- Associated with nausea and vomiting, photophobia, phonophobia or depression. Relieved by migraine treatment such as triptans and indomethacin.
- Patients prefer resting in a quiet dark room.

Headache due to increased intracranial pressure

- Usually generalised headache.
- Tends to be of maximal intensity in the morning.
- Usually dull and deep.
- Aggravated by coughing, bending forward, sneezing, and valsalva manoeuvre.
- May be relieved by rest.
- Associated with projectile vomiting.
- May be associated with changes in the level of consciousness, seizure, personality change, limb weakness or numbness.

Hypertension headache

- Usually causes throbbing headache.
- The headache is usually occipital.
- Usually more intense on awakening.
- May persist for days.
- May be associated with palpitation, blurring of vision, confusion, seizure or deterioration of level of consciousness.

Cluster headache

- Unilateral, often severe headache.
- Attacks usually come in clusters, i.e. occur daily for some weeks followed by a period of remission.
- *Typical sites include:* Orbital, supraorbital, or temporal regions.
- Typically associated with autonomic symptoms such as ptosis, meiosis, lacrimation, conjunctival injection, rhinorrhoea, and nasal congestion.
- Attacks typically last for minutes to less than 2 hours.

Trigeminal neuralgia

- Recurrent brief episodes of unilateral electric shock-like pains.
- Onset is sudden.
- Duration is very short (seconds), tend to be repetitive.

- *Location:* In the distribution of one or more divisions of the fifth cranial (trigeminal) nerve (most commonly V2 and V3, very rare in V1).
- The pain usually occurs in paroxysms.
- Classically triggered by light touch of the face in V1, V2, V3 areas.
- *Other triggering factors include:* brushing teeth, chewing, talking, grimacing or smiling.
- Trigeminal neuralgia typically occurs over the age of 50.
- If trigeminal neuralgia is diagnosed before the age of 50, a secondary cause has to be excluded such as demyelinating disease (MS) or cerebellopontine angle tumours. An MRI brain should be obtained before labelling the patient with idiopathic trigeminal neuralgia.

Tension headache

- Frequent headache episodes.
- Minutes to days duration.
- Bilateral pain; pressing.
- Tightening (e.g. "band-like").
- Mild-to-moderate intensity.
- No nausea/vomiting.
- No more than one of photophobia or phonophobia.
- Not aggravated by routine activities.
- May or may not be associated with pericranial tenderness on manual palpation.

What are the red flag symptoms/signs of headache?

- New onset severe headache.
- Severe headache (worst headache in patient's life)/thunderclap headache.
- Presence of other symptoms such as fever, weight loss.
- Development of focal neurological signs such as weakness, seizure or confusion.
- Headache in immune-compromised patient/HIV (toxoplasmosis, tumours).
- New headache in a pregnant woman (pre-eclampsia, cerebral venous sinus thrombosis).
- Headache in older age groups (see below).
- Other symptoms of increased ICP such as projectile vomiting, worsening with stooping, cough, exertion, or sexual activity.

Headache in older patients (above age of 50)

- Brain tumour
- Giant cell arteritis
- Trigeminal neuralgia
- Chronic subdural haematoma.

Idiopathic intracranial hypertension

Idiopathic intracranial hypertension is a clinical diagnosis. Diagnostic criteria include; symptoms and signs of increased intracranial pressure such as headache, blurred vision, and papilledema with evidence of elevated CSF pressure ≥ 25 cm H_2O with normal other CSF analysis. The main reason for performing MRI is to exclude secondary causes such as cerebral venous thrombosis and brain tumours. After excluding a structural intracranial lesion, patients require a lumbar puncture to measure the CSF opening pressure. A CSF sample should be sent for microscopy, protein and glucose and sometimes for xanthochromia and culture to identify secondary causes of raised intracranial pressure. Empty sella is seen in up to 80% of cases of idiopathic intracranial hypertension.

Idiopathic intracranial hypertension was previously called 'benign intracranial hypertension.' This name was given to differentiate it from neoplastic causes of elevated intracranial pressure. However, this name is no longer used as the condition can result in permanent vision loss.

Risk factors for idiopathic intracranial hypertension

Although the disease is idiopathic, different risk factors predispose to idiopathic intracranial hypertension:

- Overweight and obesity, particularly recent weight gain.
- Use of the oral contraceptive pill.
- *Medication:* Tetracyclines, isotretinoin, steroids, nitrofurantoin, hypervitaminosis A, growth hormone, and levothyroxine.

A comprehensive drug history is essential as many cases are linked to these drugs and their withdrawal often resolves the problem. Initial management of idiopathic intracranial hypertension includes weight reduction and use of carbonic anhydrase inhibitors such as acetazolamide to reduce CSF production. For patients with progressive visual loss, surgical intervention with optic nerve sheath fenestration and/or a CSF shunting procedure is recommended. Patients require regular follow-up visits with ophthalmology and neurology clinics with repeated examinations of the visual acuity, visual field and optic disc and lumbar puncture.

Further reading

Canadian Chiropractic Association (CCA), Canadian Federation of Chiropractic Regulatory and Education Accrediting Boards (CFCREAB), Clinical Practice Guidelines Project (CPG): Clinical practice guideline for the management of headache disorders in adults (2012). Available online: www.chiropracticcanada.ca Last accessed April 21st, 2018.

Headache Classification Committee of the International Headache Society (IHS). The international classification of headache disorders, 3rd edition (beta version). Cephalalgia 2013; 33:629–808.

Mollan SP, Markey KA, Benzimra JD, et al. A practical approach to, diagnosis, assessment and management of idiopathic intracranial hypertension. Pract Neurol 2014; 14:380–90.

Scenario no. 8

A patient with joint pain

Candidate copy

Please read the GP referral letter for Mr Davidson. The time distribution for this station is as following:

   You have (---) minutes to take a history from the patient.
   You have (---) minutes to collect your thoughts.
   You have (---) minutes for discussion with the examiners.

Please do not examine the patient

> **Dear Doctor,**
> Thank you for seeing Mr Davidson, a 25-year-old journalist who has been complaining of right ankle and toe pain for the last 10 days. Two weeks earlier, he returned from a journey to Tanzania.
> Yours faithfully,

> Please interview the patient and based on the history construct a differential diagnosis and plan of investigation. Provide an explanation to the patient and answer any questions he may have.

Surrogate copy

Chief complaint and HPI

- You have right ankle pain and swelling for the last 10 days. You also feel some pain and swelling in your right toes. The pain is sometimes severe and prevents you from sleeping.
- You noticed your ankle and toes becoming red.
- The pain is constant.
- There is no fever.
- No other joints in the body are affected.
- This started 2 weeks after returning from an assignment in Africa (Tanzania)—you are a journalist.

Review of systems

- *Only if you are asked you mention:*
  - You have *redness and itching in your eyes.*
  - You have *difficulty in passing urine* as it becomes painful and burning.
  - You were in *Africa (Tanzania)* a month ago and you *had diarrhoea* and *stomach pain* for 5 days after eating at a picnic, but the diarrhoea improved after 5 days without medications.
  - You do not have breathing problems or chest pain.

Past history

- You do not suffer any disease in the past.
- You do not have joint disease.
- You do not have kidney disease.

Family history

Your paternal uncle has *gout* and is on dialysis because of *kidney disease.*

Social history

- You have smoked 10 cigarettes per day for 5 years.
- You drink one glass of wine every day and a bottle on the weekends.
- You are single.
- You work as a journalist for a news channel.
- You were in *Africa (Tanzania)* about a month ago.
- You have had *sex with multiple female partners*, but for the last 3 years you have only one female partner.

Your questions and concerns

What causes my ankle pain?

Steps in history taking in a patient with joint pain

Step 1: Introduction, greeting, and confirmation of patient identity

- Good morning Mr Davidson (shakehands with the patient), pleased to meet you.
- I am Dr X working in the medical outpatient clinic.
- Can I confirm that I am talking to Mr Davidson?
- I have just read the referral letter from your GP who states that you have pain in your ankle joint.
- Can you tell me more about that?
- Allow the patient to speak.

- Avoid interruptions.
- Avoid medical jargon (e.g. reactive, SLE, arthropathy, arthritis, crystal arthropathy, etc.)
- *Use open ended questions such as:* What else?

Step 2: Elaborating important points in the history of leg swelling

History of presenting illness

- **What is the duration of joint pain?**
  - *Acute symptoms:* hours to two weeks; *Chronic symptoms:* >2 weeks
  - Septic arthritis usually presents acutely and typically involves a single large joint.
- **Which joints are affected? And how many are affected?**
  The size (small or large) and kind of joints involved provide major diagnostic clues. Spondyloarthropathies typically involve the spine, including sacroiliac joints and medium/large joints, such as the shoulders, hips, knees, and ankles. RA and lupus typically involve smaller joints such as the wrists, fingers, and toes.
  - *Number of joints affected are also important:* pauciarticular pattern (two to four joints) and polyarticular pattern (five or more joints). Spondyloarthropathies are typically pauciarticular, whereas RA is usually polyarticular. Some spondyloarthropathies, such as psoriatic arthritis, may also present in a polyarticular manner.
- **Is it only pain (arthralgia) or are there other signs of inflammation (swelling and redness)?**
  Two broad categories of arthritis are recognized: (1) Inflammatory, and (2) Noninflammatory (degenerative arthritis). The following symptoms usually suggest inflammatory type: presence of joint swelling, erythema, prolonged morning stiffness (more than 1 hour), and pain at rest. Involvement of weight bearing joints and pain that is mainly on movement are suggestive of non-inflammatory type of arthritis, such as osteoarthritis.
- **Is it symmetrical or asymmetrical?**
  A symmetric presentation suggests an underlying inflammatory arthritis.
- **Does it involve the axial joints?**
  - Ankylosing spondylitis
  - Spondyloarthropathies.
- **Is there morning stiffness?**
  If there is morning stiffness, ask about the duration of this stiffness. Noninflammatory arthritis typically causes less than 1 hour of morning stiffness. Prolonged morning stiffness (more than 1 hour), is suggestive of inflammatory conditions.
- **Is it migratory arthritis?**
  In migratory arthritis, symptoms shift from one joint to another and do not stay in one joint for very long.
- **Conditions that tend to cause migratory arthritis include:**
  - Rheumatic fever
  - Systemic lupus erythematosus
  - Infectious arthritis e.g. gonococcal arthritis
  - Whipple's and Lyme disease.
- **Is it aggravated by activity or rest? And does it wake the patient from sleep?**
  Joint pain at rest that wakes patient from sleep usually indicates inflammatory arthritis.

Review of systems

Many of rheumatologic diseases such as rheumatoid arthritis and SLE are multisystem disorders. Hence, candidates should perform a review of all systems with attention to:

- **Presence of extra-articular symptoms (particularly eyes and skin)**
- **Symptoms of uveitis/conjunctivitis (eye redness and pain):**
  - Ankylosing spondylitis
  - Behcet's disease
  - Rheumatoid arthritis
  - Reactive arthritis.

- **Skin rash/nodules:**
  - Psoriatic arthritis
  - Systemic lupus erythematosus
  - Rheumatoid arthritis (nodules)
  - Henoch-Schonlein purpura.

- **GIT symptoms**
- **Diarrhoea:**
  - Reactive arthritis
  - Inflammatory bowel disease
  - Whipple's disease.

- **Mouth ulcers.**
  - *Behcet's disease*
  - *Systemic lupus erythematosus*
  - *Crohn's disease.*

- **Urethral/GUT**
  Symptoms of urethritis may suggest reactive arthritis.

Past medical history
- Previous joint or rheumatologic diseases
- Chronic kidney disease, hypothyroidism
- Gout, pseudogout.

Family history
- Family history of rheumatologic and autoimmune diseases.

Drug history
- Use of steroids and immune-suppressant medications.

Sexual history
- Gonococcal infection
- HIV
- HBV, HCV (ask about previous transfusions and drug abuse)
- *Chlamydia trachomatis:* Reactive arthritis.

Social history
- Candidate should obtain a detailed social history. Alcohol for example can precipitate gouty arthritis. Particular attention should be paid to the effect of patient's symptoms on his/her functional capabilities, job, financial and family status.

Travel history
- Lyme disease (exposure to ticks in endemic areas)
- Reactive arthritis.

Further information not covered (at end of history taking)
Ask the patient the following question: Is there anything else that you feel important and would like to tell me about?

Discussion

Problem
Arthritis in a young man.

Diagnosis

Reactive arthritis (acute arthritis in young man with recent acute diarrheal illness, sexual history, red eyes, and burning micturition).

Other plausible diagnosis

- **Gonococcal infection**
  Patient has positive sexual history.

- **Acute gouty arthritis**
  Family history of gout and the pattern of joint involvement.

- **HIV arthropathy**
  Reactive arthritis may be the initial manifestation in patients with HIV.

Reactive arthritis, also called Reiter's syndrome, is the most common type of inflammatory polyarthritis in young men. It is very important to observe that Reiter's syndrome can sometimes be the initial manifestation of HIV. It may follow enteric infections such a Salmonella or Shigella or genitourinary infections such as Chlamydia trachomatis. The classic triad of arthritis, urethritis, and conjunctivitis *(Cannot see, cannot pee and cannot climb a tree)*. However, this triad does not occur in all patients. The onset typically occurs 1–3 weeks following the infection and may present acutely or insidiously. Urethritis is often symptomatic in male patients and may present with a mucopurulent discharge or gross haematuria secondary to haemorrhagic cystitis. Females may present with nonspecific cervicitis may occur. However, in either sex, urethritis may be asymptomatic. Joint involvement is often asymmetric oligoarthritis with lower extremity predilection. Skin involvement may include keratoderma blennorrhagica or balanitis circinata. Symptomatic treatment is accomplished with high doses of a potent nonsteroidal anti-inflammatory drug, such as indomethacin. Oral corticosteroids are not as effective as intra-articular steroid injections. When chlamydia is the suspected causative agent, patients may be given doxycycline for up to 3 months. Data on the use of antibiotics following enteric infections are not encouraging.

Gonococcal arthritis is characterised by an acute onset of migratory polyarthralgia that settles in one or more joints and is sometimes associated with tenosynovitis in the small joints of the hands. A helpful diagnostic clue to gonococcal arthritis is the presence of a pustule with an erythematous base on the hand or foot. Gouty arthritis often affects older men, typically affecting the 1st metatarsophalangeal joint (podagra) and severe attacks are usually limited to a matter of days.

Gout typically affects young- and middle-age groups with male predominance. It can be a primary disease or secondary to diseases that are associated with hyperuricemia such as renal failure, myeloproliferative disorders, hypertension, and malignancies, etc.

The typical presentation of an acute gout flare up is a monoarticular severe arthritis seen in ~80% of cases. Other joints that can be affected by acute gouty arthritis include ankle, wrist, finger joints, and knee. Factors that may precipitate the attack of gouty arthritis include certain drugs such as diuretics, alcohol consumption, excessive meat or sea food, trauma or surgery. Pseudogout usually affects large joints such as the knee, ankle, elbow, and wrist joints.

Reiter's syndrome and other reactive arthritis may be seen in HIV-infected patients. Psoriatic arthritis and septic arthritis with opportunistic agents, as well as severe articular pain that is severe, acute, and intermittent, may also occur with HIV infection. An arthritis specific for the acquired immunodeficiency syndrome (AIDS) has been described.

Further reading

Barth W, Segal K. Reactive arthritis (Reiter's Syndrome). Am Fam Physician 1999;60:499–503.
Dearborn JT, Jergesen HE. The evaluation and initial management of arthritis. Prim Care 1996; 23:215–240.
Hainer BL, Matheson E, Wilkes RT. Diagnosis, treatment, and prevention of gout. Am Fam Physician 2014; 90:831–836.
Kaye BR. Rheumatologic manifestations of infection with human immunodeficiency virus (HIV). Ann Intern Med 1989; 111:158–167.
Pujalte GG, Albano-Aluquin SA. Differential Diagnosis of Polyarticular Arthritis. Am Fam Physician 2015; 92:35–41.

Scenario no. 9

Sudden loss of vision in an old man

Candidate copy

Please read the GP referral letter for Mr Amer. The time distribution for this station is as follows:

> You have (---) minutes to take a history from the patient.
> You have (---) minutes to collect your thoughts.
> You have (---) minutes for discussion with the examiners.

Please do not examine the patient

> **Dear Doctor,**
> Thank you for seeing Mr Amer, a 70-year-old man who developed a sudden loss of vision in the right eye this morning. He has been feeling unwell for the last 3 months with increasing malaise and headache.
> Yours faithfully,

> Please interview the patient and based on the history construct a differential diagnosis and plan of investigation. Provide an explanation to the patient and answer any questions he may have.

Surrogate copy

Chief complaints and history of present illness

- You had a sudden loss of sight in your right eye this morning.
- This happened after waking up from sleep.
- It is only in the right eye.
- Although your vision improved after 1 hour, it is still not normal.
- This is the first time you have had such a problem.
- There is no associated pain in your eyes.
- You do not have other symptoms such as seeing moving objects, floaters, flashing lights, halos around lights, distorted colour vision, etc.

- No trauma or injury to the eye.
- You did not feel any weakness or numbness in your legs or arms.
- Your hearing and walking are normal.

Review of systems

- **Questions to be answered only if asked:**
  - You frequently feel *jaw pain* and *discomfort after chewing*. This is becoming very troublesome to you as on many occasions you have had to stop eating.
  - You have had attacks of severe headache on the right side of your head for the last 3 months, this was associated with feeling *unwell* and sometimes *feverish* that keeps coming and going. You thought it might be sinusitis, but this did not go with antibiotics (Augmentin).
  - You suffer from severe *aches in your shoulders and hips* which are worse in the morning.
  - You *cannot move your arms above your head*, especially in the morning.
  - You do not have any chest pain, racing heart or difficulty with breathing.
  - You do not have any clotting problems.
  - You have not had strokes or clots.

Past medical history

- You have not had eye surgery or injury.
- No previous strokes.
- You have had hypertension for 7 years and you are taking Perindopril 10 mg daily with which your blood pressure is controlled in the range of 120–130/70–80 mmHg.
- You have never suffered heart disease.
- You have never suffered migraine.

Drug history

- You are on perindopril 10 mg daily.
- You use painkillers (Paracetamol, Ibuprofen and Voltarol gel) regularly for the severe shoulder pain and headache.

Family history

- Family history of migraine.
- Family history of stroke.

Social history

- You do not smoke.
- You do not drink alcohol.
- You are married and have three kids.
- You are a retired police officer.
- You have good care and support from your family.

Your main concerns and questions to the doctor

- What has caused my loss of vision?
- What treatment will you start for me?
- I am worried about starting steroids; can we wait until the results of the biopsy?
- Will my vision recover?
- What is the relationship of my shoulder pains to vision loss?

Steps in history taking in a patient with sudden vision loss

Step 1: Introduction, greeting and confirmation of patient identity

- Good morning, Mr Amer (shakehands with the patient), pleased to meet you.
- I am Dr X working in the medical outpatient clinic.

Can I confirm that I am talking to Mr Amer?
- I have just read the referral letter from your GP who states that you complain of sudden loss of vision in the right eye.
- Can you tell me more about that?
- Allow the patient to speak.
- Avoid interruptions.
- Avoid medical jargon [e.g. giant cell arteritis, polymyalgia rheumatica, jaw claudication, transient ischaemic attack (TIA), etc.]
- *Use open-ended questions such as:* What else?

Step 2: Elaborating important points in the history of sudden loss of vision

History of presenting illness

- **Is the visual loss monocular or binocular?**
  The differential diagnoses of sudden vision loss are vast. In general, monocular vision loss usually indicates an ocular problem. Binocular vision loss is usually of cerebral origin.

- **Is it just a single episode or were there previous episodes?**
  Recurrent episodes of loss of vision may suggest TIA.

- **How is the onset? (Is it acute or chronic?)**

- **What is the duration?**

- **How is the progression?**

- **Is it painful or painless?**

- **Is the pain worsened when you move your eyes?**
  Optic neuritis usually occurs in the setting of multiple sclerosis. Visual loss is associated with pain on eye movement. The most common reason for painless sudden visual loss is ischaemia.

- **Does it involve the entire visual field or a specific part and which part?**

- **Are there any other visual symptoms?**
  Visual symptoms such as floaters, flashing lights, halos around lights, distorted colour vision, and jagged or mosaic patterns (scintillating scotoma).

- **Is there any history of eye trauma?**
  In addition to diabetic retinopathy, vitreous haemorrhage can also be caused by eye trauma.

Review of systems

- Ask about jaw or tongue claudication (Giant cell arteritis).
- Temporal headache (Giant cell arteritis).
- Proximal muscle pain and stiffness (Giant cell arteritis).
- Headaches (Ocular migraine and giant cell arteritis).
- Review the cardiovascular system carefully for palpitations (AF), coronary artery disease (CAD), intermittent claudication and symptoms of peripheral vascular disease.

Past medical history

- Ask about previous eye disorders (e.g. contact lens use, severe myopia, recent eye surgery or injury).
- Ask about previous strokes.

- Ask about diabetes mellitus as it can cause thrombosis/TIA and vitreous haemorrhage leading to sudden visual loss.
- Other risk factors for vascular disease, e.g. hypertension and haematological disorders (sickle cell, polycythaemia, Waldenström macroglobulinaemia or multiple myeloma that can cause a hyperviscosity syndrome).
- Heart disease and atrial fibrillation (AF).

Drug history

- Oral contraceptive pill (*Risk factor for thrombosis)*
- Ergot alkaloids for migraine
- *Anticoagulants/antiplatelets:* Vitreous haemorrhage.

Family history

- Family history of migraine
- Family history of thrombophilia.

Social history

Detailed smoking history.

Further information not covered (at end of history taking)

Ask the patient the following question: Is there anything else that you feel important and would like to tell me about?

Step 3: Explaining to the patient the diagnosis and the plan of management

Mr Amer, you had a sudden loss of vision in your right eye this morning. You also feel shoulder pain, headache and malaise for the last 3 months and pain in the jaw muscles while eating. I think all these symptoms point to a disease called "giant cell arteritis". Have you heard of this before? Well, giant cell arteritis is a disease-causing inflammation of the large blood vessels. It is called "giant cell" because abnormal large cells develop in the wall of the inflamed arteries. The cause of this condition is unknown. Inflammation inside the blood vessels leads to narrowing and blockage of blood flow in these vessels. Common vessels involved are scalp, neck and arm vessels. Common symptoms include headache and pain around the scalp vessels on each side of the head, pain and stiffness of the muscles around the shoulders and upper arms and sometimes around the hips and neck, pain in the jaw muscles while eating or talking and sometimes loss of eyesight.

If there is loss of vision, treatment has to be started immediately to prevent further worsening of eyesight and to try to prevent the disease from affecting the other eye. I would suggest arranging admission for you to the hospital in order to commence the treatment immediately. Cutting a tiny piece from the blood vessel on your scalp to examine it under a microscope will also help to confirm the diagnosis of giant cell arteritis. Some blood tests and an ultrasound of the blood vessels to your brain will also be arranged as they can help in the diagnosis. A colleague who is specialised in eye diseases will also have a look at your eyes to confirm the cause of loss of vision and exclude other causes. Does this sound ok to you?

Step 4: Ask about and address patient's concerns

Do you have any questions or concerns?

> *Patient's concern: What has caused my loss of vision?*
>
> *Reply:* As I have mentioned Mr Amer, giant cell arteritis causes inflammation in the blood vessels and this can cause them to become narrowed impairing blood flow to the tissue. The arteries that travel to the eye are especially vulnerable in patients with giant cell arteritis. When the blood supply of the eyes diminishes, vision can be affected.

What treatment will you start for me doctor?
We are going to start you on steroids to reduce the inflammation in your blood vessels. Have you heard of this medicine before?
Patient's concern: But doctor, this medicine has many side effects. Why don't you wait until the result of the biopsy is out?
Reply: I understand your concern. It is true that steroids have side effects. However, if there is a strong suspicion of giant cell arteritis which affects eyesight then treatment with steroids has to be started immediately in order to reduce worsening of vision in the affected eye and prevent the other eye from being affected leading to permanent loss of eyesight.
Concern: Will my vision recover?
Reply: Giant cell arteritis can cause transient or permanent loss of vision. I will be able to give you further information after the eye specialist has checked your eye.
Concern: What is the relationship of my shoulder pains to the current problem?
Reply: Giant cell arteritis can be associated with another condition that causes pain and stiffness in the shoulder and hip muscles due to inflammation in these muscles; this condition is called "polymyalgia rheumatica."
After answering each concern, confirm the agreement by asking; "Is that alright? Or does that sound clear to you?"

Step 5: Summarise the discussion, confirm patient's understandings and close the meeting.

Mr Amer, I would like to summarise our discussion to be sure that you understand important information about your illness. The most probable cause for the sudden vision loss in your right eye is a condition called "giant cell arteritis". I will arrange admission for you to the hospital to start treatment immediately, order some tests, and invite specialists in giant cell arteritis and eye diseases to see you. I am going to provide you with my contact number in case you have any further questions or concerns regarding your condition. Does that sound good to you? You can also get some information from the internet regarding giant cell arteritis. Thank you and see you soon.

Discussion

Problem
Sudden monocular loss of vision in an elderly man.

Diagnosis
Central retinal artery occlusion secondary to giant cell arteritis.

Other plausible diagnoses
- Transient ischaemic attack
- Retinal detachment
- Retinal vein or artery occlusion.

Conditions that cause sudden visual loss
- **Transient visual loss**
  - Amaurosis fugax (TIA)
  - Migraine
  - Papilloedema.

- **Visual loss of longer duration which may be permanent**
  - Central retinal artery occlusion
  - Central retinal vein occlusion
  - Vitreous haemorrhage
  - Ischaemic optic neuropathy
  - Optic neuritis
  - Retinal detachment.

It is important to establish whether the visual loss is unilateral or bilateral, as bilateral visual disturbance rarely indicates bilateral ocular or optic nerve disease, but more commonly is a sign of disease posterior to the optic chiasm, including the optic tract and cerebral cortex. It may indicate impaired posterior cerebral circulation or even a migraine.

Loss of vision may be associated with migraine auras. Usually, the visual aura of a migraine presents as zigzag lights or shimmering colours and precedes the headache.

Flashes and floaters are characteristic symptoms of a retinal detachment and vitreous haemorrhage. Poorly controlled diabetes is a risk factor for central retinal artery occlusion (CRAO) (transient or permanent), vitreous haemorrhage or retinal vein occlusion and retinal detachment.

The eye is supplied by several branches of the ophthalmic artery, which derives from the internal carotid artery. These branches include the central retinal artery, the short and long posterior ciliary arteries, and the anterior ciliary arteries. The retina is supplied by the central retinal artery and the short posterior ciliary arteries.

Central retinal artery occlusion is most commonly caused by embolism or thrombosis.

Risk factors for CRAO

- Diseases that cause systemic atherosclerosis leading to embolization of a detached atheroma from the internal carotid (e.g. diabetes, hypertension, dyslipidaemia).
- Giant cell arteritis should be considered in any patient above 50 years with sudden painless blindness.
- Heart disease, e.g. AF, valvular heart disease, intracardiac thrombus, congenital anomalies.
- Hypercoagulable states.
- Migraine.

Patients with CRAO secondary to emboli may initially present with a transient loss of vision called "amaurosis fugax" which may precede persistent loss of vision.

Vitreous haemorrhage should be considered as a cause of painless sudden loss of vision in patients with uncontrolled diabetes and severe diabetic retinopathy or hypertension. Symptoms usually include painless sudden loss of vision with associated unilateral floaters, haze, shadows or a red hue and scotomas. Patients often say vision is worse in the morning due to the blood settling on the back of the eye and covering the macula.

Retinal detachment may be rhegmatogenous (secondary to a retinal tear), tractional (involving scar tissue, e.g. with trauma, and in proliferative diabetic retinopathy) or exudative (e.g. with uveitis, tumours and severe hypertension). Signs and symptoms of retinal detachment may include flashing lights and floaters or dancing flies because of the development of posterior vitreous detachment. A "grey curtain" or shadow that comes over the field of vision from the periphery indicates detachment of the retina.

Optic neuritis refers to inflammation of the optic nerve due to demyelination or infective, immune and infiltrative causes. The common causes of optic neuritis are multiple sclerosis, syphilis, human immunodeficiency virus and sarcoidosis. Optic neuritis occurs in 70% of patients with multiple sclerosis and may be the first sign of demyelination. Patients may have pain on eye movement in typical cases.

Giant cell arteritis (temporal arteritis)

The disease of 50 (Age >50 years, ESR >50, Polymyalgia rheumatic seen in 50% of patients, Second eye will be involved in about 50% if first eye not treated, requires high-dose steroid >50 mg).

Giant cell arteritis is a large vessel vasculitis that affects people above the age of 50 years and most affected people are in their 70s. Characteristically, branches of the carotid artery and the vertebral artery are involved in the inflammatory process. The typical symptoms of giant cell arteritis are bitemporal headaches, jaw claudication, scalp tenderness, visual disturbance, and systemic symptoms such as fever, weight loss and polymyalgia. There is often a significant delay in the diagnosis. Head and muscle pain in older patients can be wrongly assessed for weeks and patients are not referred to an ophthalmologist until they have gone blind in one or both eyes. In 40–60% of patients, giant cell arteritis is associated with polymyalgia rheumatica. These two conditions have overlapping symptoms, and both have a marked acute phase reaction which responds well to corticosteroids. Typical features of polymyalgia rheumatica are proximal myalgia and stiffness of the neck, hip and/or shoulder girdle.

The diagnostic criteria for giant cell arteritis include:

- Age over 50 years.
- New onset of localised headache.
- Abnormality of temporal artery (temporal artery tenderness, reduced pulsation).
- Raised erythrocyte sedimentation rate (ESR) (≥50 mm/1st hour).
- Abnormal arterial biopsy (vasculitis with predominantly mononuclear cell infiltration or granulomatous inflammation or evidence of giant cells).

The eye is involved in up to 70% of patients with giant cell arteritis. If left untreated, in up to 60% of patients, the second eye may also go blind within 1–14 days. The most frequent eye manifestation in giant cell arteritis is anterior ischaemic optic neuropathy resulting from inflammatory occlusion of the posterior ciliary arteries. The occlusion manifests as a sudden, painless loss of vision and/or loss of visual field. The affected optic nerve is swollen and pale with a few haemorrhages and "cotton-wool spots". Other eye manifestations include arterial occlusion (occlusion of a central artery, branch artery or cilioretinal vessel) and amaurosis fugax.

Erythrocyte sedimentation rate (ESR) and C-reactive protein (CRP) should be assessed if giant cell arteritis is suspected. The ESR usually exceeds 50 mm/1st hour. If giant cell arteritis is diagnosed, oral prednisone of at least 1 mg/kg is needed and immediate referral required, as the other eye may also become affected if treatment is not started urgently. Temporal artery biopsy to confirm the diagnosis is the gold standard test for diagnosis and is required in almost all cases of suspected giant cell arteritis as the treatment requires long-term steroid therapy. False negative biopsy results can occur due to the segmental nature of the arteritic involvement by giant cell arteritis due to skip lesions. Biopsy can be done shortly after starting steroid therapy as histological resolution of the inflammation in the affected arteries takes time. Colour Doppler ultrasonography of the temporal arteries can be used as an alternative diagnostic tool in the initial evaluation of giant cell arteritis. Steroid therapy should be started as soon as the clinical diagnosis has been made, particularly in patients who present with visual loss and should not be delayed until the diagnosis is confirmed by biopsy or imaging. Some experts recommend an immediate bolus of intravenous methylprednisolone rather than oral prednisolone when vision is affected to further limit vision loss and to protect the fellow eye from being affected.

Further reading

Chan S. Sudden loss of vision. Hong Kong Med J 2010; 16:155.

Dasgupta B, Cimmino MA, Maradit-Kremers H, et al. Provisional classification criteria for polymyalgia rheumatica: A European League Against Rheumatism/American College of Rheumatology collaborative initiative. Ann Rheum Dis 2012; 71:484–492.

Du Toit N. Sudden loss of vision. S Afr Fam Pract. 2013; 55:235–240.

Ness T, Bley TA, Schmidt WA, et al. The diagnosis and treatment of giant cell arteritis. Dtsch Arztebl Int 2013; 110:376–386.

Sharma N, Ooi JL, Sharma D, et al. Sudden loss of vision - a case study. Aust Fam Physician 2013; 42:48–50.

Scenario no. 10

Sudden loss of vision in a diabetic patient

Candidate copy

Please read the GP referral letter for Mr Johnson. The time distribution for this station is as follows:

> You have (---) minutes to take a history from the patient.
> You have (---) minutes to collect your thoughts.
> You have (---) minutes for discussion with the examiners.

Please do not examine the patient

> **Dear Doctor,**
>
> Thank you for seeing Mr Johnson, a 55-year-old man with long-standing poorly controlled diabetes and diabetic retinopathy, essential hypertension and ischaemic heart disease. He developed a sudden loss of vision in the right eye this morning.
>
> Yours faithfully,

> Please interview the patient and based on the history construct a differential diagnosis and plan of investigation. Provide an explanation to the patient and answer any questions he may have.

Surrogate copy

Chief complaints and history of present illness

- You woke up today in the morning and after breakfast you felt like a curtain came down over your vision in the right eye.
- This is the first time you have had such a problem.
- There is no associated pain in your eye.
- You do not have other symptoms such as seeing moving objects, floaters, flashing lights, halos around lights or distorted colour vision.
- No trauma or injury to the eye.
- You did not feel any weakness or numbness in your legs or arms.
- Your hearing and walking are normal.

Review of systems

- **Questions to be answered only if asked:**
  - You do not feel jaw pain or discomfort after chewing.
  - You do not have headache.
  - You do not feel aches or stiffness in your shoulders and hips.
  - You do not have chest pain, racing heart or difficulty with breathing.
  - You do not have any clotting problems.
  - You have never had strokes or clots.

Past medical history

- You have never had eye surgery or injury.

- No previous strokes.
- You have had diabetes for 20 years. Your diabetes is not controlled and your latest glycosylated haemoglobin (HbA1c) is 10%. Your doctor suggested that you should start insulin, but you did not like the idea of that.
- You have had one session of laser photocoagulation in your left eye 3 years ago.
- You also have hypertension for 10 years and your blood pressure is usually ~150/90 mmHg.
- You suffered a heart attack 5 years ago and you had two stents.
- You have never suffered migraine.

Drug history
- You are taking metformin 1000 mg twice daily, sitagliptin 100 mg and gliclazide 120 mg daily.
- You are taking lisinopril 20 mg daily and amlodipine 10 mg daily.
- You are taking atorvastatin 20 mg daily.
- You are taking aspirin 100 mg daily.

Family history
- You do not have a family history of migraine headaches.
- Your father died from stroke.

Social history
- You stopped smoking after you had a heart attack 5 years ago.
- You smoked 20 cigarettes per day for 25 years.
- You do not drink alcohol.
- You are married and have two sons.
- You are working as a sales manager.
- You have good care and support from your family.

Your main concerns and questions to the doctor
What has caused my loss of vision?

Steps in history taking in a patient with loss of vision

Step 1: Introduction, greeting and confirmation of patient identity
- Good morning, Mr Johnson (shakehands with the patient), pleased to meet you.
- I am Dr X working in the medical outpatient clinic.
- Can I confirm that I am talking to Mr Johnson?
- I have just read the referral letter from your GP who states that you developed a haze and then lost vision in your right eye.
- Can you tell me more about that?
- Allow the patient to speak.
- Avoid interruptions.
- Avoid medical jargon (e.g. TIA, vitreous haemorrhage, retinal detachment, etc.)
- *Use open-ended questions such as:* What else?

Step 2: Elaborating important points in the history of a sudden loss of vision

History of presenting illness
- **Is the visual loss monocular or binocular?**
  The differential diagnoses of sudden vision loss are vast. In general, monocular vision loss indicates an ocular problem and binocular vision loss indicates a cerebral origin.

- **Is it just a single episode or were there previous episodes?**
  Recurrent episodes of loss of vision may suggest TIA.

- **Was the onset sudden?**
- **What is the duration?**
- **Did it progress?**
- **Is it painful or painless?**
- **Is it painful when you move your eyes?**
  Optic neuritis usually occurs in the setting of multiple sclerosis and visual loss is associated with pain on eye movement. The most common reason for painless sudden visual loss is ischaemia.
- **Does it involve the entire visual field or a specific part and which part?**
- **Are there any other visual symptoms?**
  Visual symptoms such as floaters, flashing lights, halos around lights, distorted colour vision and jagged or mosaic patterns (scintillating scotoma).
- **Is there any history of eye trauma?**
  In addition to diabetic retinopathy, vitreous haemorrhage can also be caused by eye trauma.

Review of systems

- Ask about jaw or tongue claudication (giant cell arteritis).
- Temporal headache (giant cell arteritis).
- Proximal muscle pain and stiffness (giant cell arteritis).
- Headaches (ocular migraine and giant cell arteritis).
- Review the cardiovascular system carefully for palpitations (AF), CAD, intermittent claudication and symptoms of peripheral vascular disease.

Past medical history

- Ask about previous eye disorders (e.g. contact lens use, severe myopia, recent eye surgery or injury).
- Ask about previous strokes.
- *Ask about diabetes mellitus:* It can cause thrombosis/TIA and vitreous haemorrhage, and both can lead to sudden visual loss.
- *Other risk factors for vascular disease:* For example hypertension and haematologic disorders (sickle cell, polycythaemia, Waldenström macroglobulinaemia or multiple myeloma that can cause a hyperviscosity syndrome).
- Heart disease and AF.

Drug history

- In female patients, ask about use of the oral contraceptive pill (risk factor for clots—not relevant in this scenario, as the patient is male).
- Ergot alkaloids for migraine.
- *Anticoagulant/antiplatelet drugs:* Vitreous haemorrhage.

Family history

- Family history of migraine.
- Family history of thrombophilia.

Social history

Detailed smoking history.

Further information not covered (at the end of history taking)

Ask the patient the following question: Is there anything else that you feel important and would like to tell me about?

Step 3: Explaining to the patient the diagnosis and the plan of management

Mr Johnson, you had a sudden loss of vision in your right eye since this morning. You also have diabetes that is poorly controlled, hypertension and heart disease. I think the cause of loss of vision in your case is a tiny blood clot in a small blood vessel in your eye. The affected part of the eye was without oxygen for just a few minutes, and then recovered. The most common source of these tiny blood clots is the major carotid and vertebral arteries which are the main arteries in the neck and take blood to the brain. Because of long-standing diabetes and high blood pressure, clots get attached to the walls of these large blood vessels. With time, some of these clots may break off and move to the brain or eyes. This condition is called "transient ischaemic attack". Does that sound clear so far?

It is also worth remembering that poorly controlled diabetes can cause bleeding in the back of your eye, a condition called "vitreous haemorrhage" or separation of the lining of the back of the eye which is called retinal detachment. Both these conditions can cause sudden loss of eyesight in diabetic patients. However, as you do not see moving objects or floaters, these two diagnoses are less likely.

I suggest that we admit you in hospital for 1–2 days to arrange some blood tests, imaging of your brain as well as your eyes. I will also request evaluation of your case by colleagues who specialise in brain and eye diseases. Meanwhile, I suggest that you continue taking your aspirin and cholesterol tablet. I will start a tablet called fenofibrate which has been shown to be beneficial in diabetic eye disease. Your blood sugar and blood pressure need to be better controlled to minimise the chances of further clots. Does this sound clear to you?

Step 4: Ask about and address patient's concerns

Do you have any questions or concerns?

    Patient's concern: Doctor, what has caused my loss of vision?

    Reply: See above

    After answering each concern confirm by saying, is that OK?

Step 5: Summarise the discussion, confirm patient's understanding and close the meeting

Mr Johnson, I would like to summarise our discussion to be sure that you understand important information about your illness. The most probable cause of loss of vision in your case is a blood clot in your eye. However, a bleed in the back of your eye or separation of the retina have to be considered. You will be admitted to the hospital and seen immediately by an eye and brain specialist. Your blood sugar and blood pressure need to be better controlled. Please continue taking the aspirin and cholesterol tablet and I am adding another tablet called fenofibrate which has been shown to be of benefit in diabetic eye disease. I am going to provide you with my contact number in case you have any further questions or concerns regarding your condition. Does that make sense to you? You can also get information from the internet on sudden loss of eyesight in diabetic patients. Thank you and see you soon.

Discussion

Problem

Sudden monocular loss of vision in diabetic patient.

Diagnosis

Transient ischaemic attack causing central retinal artery occlusion (amaurosis fugax).

Other plausible diagnosis

- Vitreous haemorrhage
- Retinal detachment
- Central retinal vein/artery occlusion
- Giant cell arteritis.

Most cases of sudden loss of vision are serious, require referral and have an associated underlying systemic disease.

Conditions that cause sudden visual loss

- **Transient visual loss**
    - *Amaurosis fugax (TIA)*
    - *Migraine*
    - *Papilloedema*
- **Visual loss of longer duration which may be permanent**
    - Central retinal artery occlusion
    - Central retinal vein occlusion
    - Vitreous haemorrhage
    - Ischaemic optic neuropathy
    - Optic neuritis
    - Retinal detachment.

It is important to establish whether the visual loss is unilateral or bilateral, as bilateral visual disturbance rarely indicates bilateral ocular or optic nerve disease, but more commonly is a sign of disease posterior to the optic chiasm, including the optic tract and cerebral cortex. It may indicate impaired posterior cerebral circulation or even a migraine.

Loss of vision may be associated with migraine auras. Usually, the visual aura of a migraine presents as zigzag lights or shimmering colours and precedes a headache.

Flashes and floaters are characteristic symptoms of a retinal detachment and vitreous haemorrhage. Poorly controlled patients with diabetes are at risk of CRAO (transient or permanent), vitreous haemorrhage or retinal vein occlusion and retinal detachment.

Vitreous haemorrhage should be considered as a cause of painless sudden loss of vision in patients with uncontrolled diabetes and severe diabetic retinopathy or hypertension. Symptoms usually include painless sudden loss of vision with associated unilateral floaters, haze, shadows or a red hue and scotomas. Patients often say vision is worse in the morning as blood has settled to the back of the eye, covering the macula.

Retinal detachment may be rhegmatogenous (secondary to a retinal tear), tractional (involving scar tissue, e.g. with trauma, and proliferative diabetic retinopathy) or exudative (e.g. with uveitis, tumours and severe hypertension). Signs and symptoms of retinal detachment may include flashing lights and floaters or dancing flies because of the development of posterior vitreous detachment. A "grey curtain" or shadow that comes over the field of vision from the periphery indicates detachment of the retina.

Further reading

Chan S. Sudden loss of vision. Hong Kong Med J 2010; 16:155.
Du Toit N. Sudden loss of vision. S Afr Fam Pract 2013; 55:235–240.
Sharma N, Ooi JL, Sharma D, et al. Sudden loss of vision - a case study. Aust Fam Physician 2013; 42:48–50.

Scenario no. 11

A patient with dyspepsia

Candidate copy

Please read the GP referral letter for Mr Harrison. The time distribution for this station is as follows:

  You have (---) minutes to take a history from the patient.
  You have (---) minutes to collect your thoughts.
  You have (---) minutes for discussion with the examiners.

Please do not examine the patient

> **Dear Doctor,**
>
> Thank you for seeing Mr Harrison, a 62-year-old man who has been complaining of recurrent epigastric pain and nausea after eating for 10 months. He has long-standing GERD. Despite being on lansoprazole 30 mg daily for 3 months, his symptoms are worsening.
>
> Yours faithfully,

> Please interview the patient and, based on history taking, construct a differential diagnosis and plan of investigation. Provide an explanation to the patient and answer any questions he may have.

Surrogate copy

Chief complaints and history of present illness

- You are 62 years old.
- You complain of a 10-month history of indigestion and stomach pain.
- The pain is in the upper part of your stomach.
- It is dull.
- It develops after food (no particular type of food), but also at night.
- The pain is sometimes felt in your back.
- In the beginning, lansoprazole helped, but for the last 1 month, it has not helped.
- You have lost 4 kg in weight over the past 10 months.
- No difficulty with swallowing and no pain when swallowing.
- You have had heartburn for a long time.
- Sometimes you feel bloated.
- No history of nausea or vomiting.
- No stomach distension.
- You have never passed black stool.
- You have never vomited blood or coffee-coloured vomitus.
- You have not had loose motion or constipation.

Review of systems

As above.

Past medical and surgical history

You were admitted to hospital 10 years ago with pancreatitis, due to excess alcohol. You have stopped drinking alcohol. You do not have any other illness.

Family history

- Your father died of colon cancer at the age of 60 years.

Drug history

- Lansoprazole 30 mg daily.

Social history

- You are a retired carpenter.
- You have smoked 40 cigarettes/day for the past 30 years.
- You stopped drinking alcohol after you had pancreatitis 10 years ago. Before that, you used to drink 3 glasses of wine every day.
- You are married and have one son and one daughter.

Your concerns and questions to the doctor

Do you think I may have cancer doctor?

Steps in history taking in a patient with dyspepsia

Step 1: Introduction, greeting and confirmation of patient identity

- Good morning, Mr Harrison (shakehands with the patient), pleased to meet you.
- I am Dr X working in the medical outpatient clinic.
- Can I confirm that I am talking to Mr Harrison?
- I have just read the referral letter from your GP and it states that you have had indigestion and pain in your stomach for 10 months.
- Can you tell me more about that?
- Allow the patient to speak.
- Avoid interruptions.
- Avoid medical jargon [e.g. dyspepsia, achalasia, gastroesophageal reflux disease (GERD), mesenteric ischaemia etc.]
- *Use open-ended questions such as:* What else?

Step 2: Elaborating important points in the history of epigastric pain/dyspepsia

History of presenting illness

- **What does the patient mean exactly by dyspepsia?**
  Although epigastric pain is the predominant symptom of dyspepsia, it may also include the presence of other symptoms such as heartburn, nausea, or bloating.

- **If the main symptom is pain, then analyse the pain using the mnemonic "LIQOR AAA"**

- **Ask about the relation of the symptoms to food and which type of food aggravates the symptoms [gallbladder disease, peptic ulcer disease (PUD), mesenteric ischaemia, chronic pancreatitis, etc.]**

- **The candidate must seek and ask about the presence of important alarm symptoms for dyspepsia which include:**
  - Unintentional weight loss
  - Older age group >60 years
  - Progressive dysphagia/progressive symptoms
  - Odynophagia
  - Unexplained iron deficiency anaemia
  - Persistent vomiting
  - Palpable mass or lymphadenopathy
  - Family history of upper gastrointestinal cancer.

Review of systems

- Ask about dysphagia.
- Symptoms suggestive of GERD (heartburn, acidity, regurgitation).
- Vomiting, haematemesis, melena, change in bowel habit.

Past history

- Past history of PUD, gallbladder disease, pancreatic disease.
- Past history of AF, diabetes mellitus, hypertension, CAD (may point toward chronic mesenteric ischaemia).

Family history

- Family history of gastrointestinal tract (GIT) malignancies or other malignancies.
- Family history of PUD.

Drug history

- Use of non-steroidal anti-inflammatory drugs (NSAIDs)/steroids—*PUD*.
- Use of warfarin—chronic mesenteric ischaemia [ask about proper use of warfarin and international normalised ratio (INR) levels].

Social history

- Smoking history.
- Alcohol use.

Further information not covered (at end of history taking)

Ask the patient the following question: Is there anything else that you feel important and would like to tell me about?

Step 3: Explaining to the patient the diagnosis and the plan of management

Mr Harrison, your main symptoms are indigestion and stomach pain for about 10 months. You also have had heartburn for a long time. Importantly, you have unintentionally lost weight during this time. You smoke and you are 62 years old. Despite having acidity and heartburn for a long time, which can cause the pain, given the additional issues, I think we need to have a look inside your food pipe and stomach to look for cancer. Does that sound clear to you? I am going to request an endoscopy, which allows the doctor to look inside your food pipe and stomach. The scope is a tube that has a tiny camera attached which will be inserted through your mouth. This is a quick procedure which will need some mild sedation and you can go home after the procedure. I am also going to request some blood tests. Because you had pancreatitis in the past, there is a possibility that this could be related to pancreatitis, though it is less likely. I would strongly recommend that you stop smoking as this is a major risk factor for cancers of the stomach and food pipe. You will be seen shortly by a colleague specialised in the digestive system who will perform the endoscopy.

I am going to arrange another appointment with myself soon after your endoscopy to give you more answers.

Check patient's understanding and agreement on plan of management.

Does that make sense to you?

Step 4: Ask about and address patient's concerns

Do you have any questions or concerns?

Patient's concern: Do you think I may have cancer?

Reply: Well, there are many causes of stomach pain that can range from simple gastritis to more serious causes. However, because you have had this tummy pain for

10 months along with the weight loss and history of smoking, I think it is important to exclude cancer.

After answering each concern, confirm agreement by asking; is that alright? Or does that sound clear to you?

Step 5: Summarise the discussion, confirm patient's understandings and close the meeting.

Mr Harrison, I would like to summarise our discussion to be sure that you understand important information about your illness. Based on your symptoms, age and smoking history, we have to exclude cancer of your stomach or food pipe. Besides blood tests, an urgent endoscopy will be arranged. I will see you soon after the endoscopy to discuss the results. Meanwhile, I am going to provide you with my contact number in case you have any further questions or concerns regarding your condition. Does that sound clear to you? Thank you and see you soon.

Discussion

Problem

Chronic epigastric pain and dyspepsia in a patient above the age of 60 years.

Diagnosis

- Oesophageal/stomach cancer
- Patient has alarm symptoms including weight loss and smoking history. Chronic GERD predisposes to Barrett's oesophagus and oesophageal cancer.

Other plausible alternative diagnosis

- Peptic ulcer disease
- Chronic pancreatitis
- Chronic mesenteric ischaemia.

Dyspepsia is defined as predominant epigastric pain lasting at least 1 month that can be associated with other upper gastrointestinal symptom such as epigastric fullness, nausea, vomiting, or heartburn.

Dyspepsia is a common symptom affecting around 20% of people worldwide. There are multiple causes of dyspeptic symptoms.

Diseases that may cause dyspepsia include:

- Peptic ulcer disease
- GIT malignancies (oesophageal and gastric)
- *Helicobacter pylori* infection
- Gallbladder disease
- Celiac disease
- Lactose intolerance
- NSAID-induced gastritis/PUD
- Chronic pancreatitis
- Chronic mesenteric ischaemia
- Abdominal aortic aneurysm
- Functional dyspepsia.

Alarm symptoms/signs that indicate GIT malignancies include:

- Unintentional weight loss
- Older age group >60 years
- Progressive dysphagia
- Odynophagia
- Unexplained iron deficiency anaemia.
- Persistent vomiting
- Palpable mass or lymphadenopathy
- Family history of upper gastrointestinal cancer.

Risk factors for stomach cancer include:

- Family history of stomach cancer.
- Gastric polyps
- High prevalence of stomach cancer in the country of origin (e.g. Japan).
- Previous partial gastrectomy
- *H. pylori*
- Intestinal metaplasia.

Risk factors associated with oesophageal cancer include:

- 50 years or older of age
- Chronic gastroesophageal reflux disease
- Smoking
- Alcohol consumption
- Elevated body mass index.

A patient's age is an important factor in making the correct diagnosis of dyspepsia. Gastrointestinal neoplasia should be considered seriously in patients aged 60 years or older who present with recurrent dyspepsia. These patients should be evaluated with an endoscopy. Younger patients should have a non-invasive test for *H. pylori* as an initial test, and therapy for *H. pylori* infection if positive. About 10–15% of patients with GERD will have Barrett's oesophagus where the normal squamous cells lining the lower oesophagus transform to columnar epithelium. At endoscopy, this can be seen as a salmon-pink coloured lining of the oesophagus. Patients with Barrett's oesophagus have a 30-fold higher risk of developing oesophageal adenocarcinoma compared to those without Barrett's oesophagus.

Further reading

Family Practice Oncology Network. Clinical Practice Guidelines. Upper Gastrointestinal Cancer – Part 1. Vancouver: BC Cancer Agency; 2016.

Moayyedi PM, Lacy BE. Andrews CA, et al. ACG and CAG Clinical Guideline: management of dyspepsia. Am J Gastroenterol 2017; 112:988–1013.

Talley NJ, Vakil NB, Moayyedi P. American Gastroenterological Association technical review on the evaluation of dyspepsia. Gastroenterology 2005; 129:1756–1780.

Scenario no. 12

A patient with recurrent abdominal pain

Candidate copy

Please read the GP referral letter for Mr Williams. The time distribution for this station is as follows:

You have (---) minutes to take a history from the patient.
You have (---) minutes to collect your thoughts.
You have (---) minutes for discussion with the examiners.

Please do not examine the patient

Dear Doctor,

Thank you for seeing Mr Williams, a 70-year-old man who has been complaining of recurrent abdominal pain and weight loss for the last 3 months. His past history is significant for long-standing diabetes, hypertension and CAD with two coronary stents.

Yours faithfully,

Please interview the patient and, based on history taking, construct a differential diagnosis and plan of investigation. Provide explanation to the patient and answer any questions he may have.

Surrogate copy

Chief Complaints and HPI

- You have recurrent stomach pain for 3 months.
- The pain is cramping and severe.
- The pain occurs mainly after eating.
- It is 8/10 by pain scale severity.
- It usually starts within 30 minutes of eating food and disappears after 1–2 hours.
- Because of the pain, you have started to avoid food.
- You have lost 7 kg weight over the last 3 months because you are afraid to eat because of the pain.
- You do not have nausea or vomiting.
- You have not had loose motion or constipation.
- You have good appetite, but you cannot eat because of the pain.
- No difficulty with swallowing.
- No problem with passing urine.

Review of systems

- You get pain in your calves when you walk more than 100 meters.
- You do get intermittent angina.

Past medical history

- You have had diabetes for 30 years, which is not well controlled with an HbA1c of 10%. You were advised to start insulin, but you did not take it as you do not like injections. The diabetes has affected your eyes and you had laser therapy in both eyes 3 years ago. You also have excess protein in your urine because of diabetes. Last year, you had an ulcer in your right foot because of diabetes, which healed.
- You have high blood pressure which is controlled on medication.
- You had two stents for your heart vessels last year.
- You have had high cholesterol for a long time, and you are on cholesterol tablets.
- You have never had a stomach ulcer.

Past surgical history

- You had your gallbladder removed 15 years ago
- You had coronary artery stents last year.

Family history

- No family history of stomach cancer
- Your brother and one sister have heart disease and diabetes.

Drug history

- Aspirin 100 mg daily
- Clopidogrel 75 mg daily
- Rosuvastatin 20 mg daily
- Metformin 1000 mg twice daily
- Sitagliptin 100 mg daily
- Dapagliflozin 10 mg daily
- Perindopril 10 mg daily
- Amlodipine 10 mg daily.

Social history

- You have smoked 20 cigarettes per day for the last 40 years
- You drink two glasses of whisky every day
- You are retired and you worked as a security man in a bar
- Your wife died 5 years ago, and you are living alone
- Your daughter is visiting you daily and she is taking care of your food.

Your concerns or questions to the doctor

Could this be cancer?

Steps in history taking in a patient with abdominal pain

Step 1: Introduction, greeting and confirmation of patient identity

- Good morning, Mr Williams (shakehands with the patient), pleased to meet you.
- I am Dr X working in the medical outpatient clinic.
- Can I confirm that I am talking to Mr Williams?
- I have just read the referral letter from your GP which states that you have had abdominal pain after eating and weight loss over the last 3 months.
- Can you tell me more about that?
- Allow the patient to speak.
- Avoid interruptions.
- Avoid medical jargon (e.g. dyspepsia, achalasia, GERD, mesenteric ischaemia, etc.)
- *Use open-ended questions such as:* What else?

Step 2: Elaborating important points in the history of epigastric pain/ dyspepsia

History of presenting illness

Abdominal pain like any other pain should be analysed using the mnemonic "LIQOR AAA"

It is very crucial that when you ask about aggravating factors, you consider food. Ask about relation of the symptoms to food and which type of food aggravates the symptoms (gallbladder disease, gastritis and gastric ulcer, mesenteric ischaemia, chronic pancreatitis, etc.)

The candidate must ask about the presence of important alarm symptoms for dyspepsia which include

- Unintentional weight loss
- Older age group >60 years
- Progressive dysphagia/progressive symptoms
- Odynophagia
- Unexplained iron deficiency anaemia
- Persistent vomiting
- Palpable mass or lymphadenopathy
- Family history of upper gastrointestinal cancer.

Review of systems

- Ask about dysphagia
- Symptoms suggestive of GERD (heartburn, acidity, regurgitation)
- Vomiting, hematemesis, melena, change in bowel habit.

Past history

- Past history of PUD, gallbladder disease, pancreatic disease
- Past history of AF, diabetes mellitus, hypertension, CAD (which may point toward chronic mesenteric ischaemia).

Family history

- Family history of GIT malignancies or other malignancies
- Family history of PUD.

Drug history

- Use of NSAIDs/steroids—PUD
- Use of warfarin—chronic mesenteric ischaemia (ask about proper use of warfarin and INR levels)

Social history

- Smoking history
- Alcohol use.

Further information not covered (at end of history taking)

Ask the patient the following question: Is there anything else that you feel important and would like to tell me about?

Step 3: Explaining to the patient the diagnosis and the plan of management

Mr Williams, your main symptoms are tummy pain after you eat and weight loss over the last 3 months. You have had diabetes for 30 years that is not well controlled, high blood pressure, and high cholesterol. You have pain in your legs when you walk, and you have had stents in your heart vessels. This suggests that you are suffering from a condition called "atherosclerosis", which is a hardening and narrowing of the blood vessels in the body. I think you could have a similar narrowing of the blood vessels of your bowel leading to a condition called "mesenteric ischaemia", which can lead to tummy pain shortly after eating because the bowel is not able to get as much blood supply as it needs after you eat. Does that sound clear to you? We need to look into this by doing a CT scan of the blood vessels in your bowel. Importantly, you have to control the risk factors for atherosclerosis, which include diabetes, cholesterol, blood pressure and smoking. I am going to request some blood tests and arrange an appointment with a surgeon who specialises in treating people with mesenteric ischaemia and will see you myself soon after the CT scan to give you more answers.

    Check patient understanding and agreement on plan of management.

    Does that sound clear to you?

Step 4: Ask about and address patient's concerns

Do you have any questions or concerns?

    Patient's concern: Could it be cancer, doctor?

    Reply: Well, stomach cancer can also cause tummy pain and weight loss but the pain you described occurring within 30 minutes of eating food and disappearing after 1–2 hours favours the possibility of mesenteric ischaemia. If the CT scan of the blood vessels does not show narrowing, then of course I will arrange for a procedure called endoscopy that allows us to look inside your stomach and bowel.

    After answering each concern, confirm agreement by asking: is that alright? or does that make sense to you?

Step 5: Summarise the discussion, confirm patient's understandings and close the meeting.

Mr Williams, I would like to summarise our discussion to be sure that you understand the important points mentioned. Based on your symptoms, age and risk factors we have to exclude mesenteric ischaemia which may be reducing the blood supply to your gut. I am going to arrange for a CT scan of these blood vessels and an appointment with a surgeon specialised in dealing with mesenteric ischaemia. I will also see you shortly after the scan to give you further answers. Meanwhile, I am going to provide you with my contact number in case you have any further questions or concerns regarding your condition. Does that sound ok? You can also get information from the internet regarding mesenteric ischaemia. Thank you and see you soon.

Discussion

Problem

Recurrent abdominal pain after food with weight loss in a patient with multiple vascular risk factors.

Diagnosis

Chronic mesenteric ischaemia (abdominal angina)

Patient has a typical history with pain occurring within 1 hour of food and relief after 2 hours. He also has multiple vascular risk factors.

Other plausible diagnoses

- GIT malignancy
- Chronic pancreatitis secondary to alcohol and sitagliptin
- Aspirin and clopidogrel-induced gastric ulcer.

Causes of chronic abdominal pain that is aggravated by food:

- Food intolerance such as lactose intolerance and celiac disease
- Gallbladder disease
- Gastritis, stomach cancer and gastric ulcer (duodenal ulcer typically relieved by food)
- Chronic mesenteric ischaemia
- Chronic pancreatitis
- Irritable bowel syndrome.

Chronic mesenteric ischaemia (also called abdominal angina) requires a high index of clinical suspicion. It is characterised by postprandial abdominal pain and it is typically associated with significant weight loss, food fear, nausea, vomiting, or diarrhoea. The abdominal pain classically starts 15–30 minutes after a meal and lasts for 1–2 hours. The most common cause is atherosclerosis due to long-standing smoking, diabetes, hypertension and hypercholesterolaemia. Less common aetiologies include dissection, vasculitis, fibromuscular dysplasia, radiation, and cocaine abuse. The vessels commonly involved are the proximal portions of the celiac, superior mesenteric, or inferior mesenteric artery. CT angiography, MR angiography or catheter angiography is used to confirm the diagnosis. Treatment is necessary to avoid progression to bowel ischaemia and infarction. Treatment options include open surgical revascularisation and endovascular revascularisation.

Further reading

Hohenwalter EJ. Chronic mesenteric ischaemia: diagnosis and treatment. Semin Intervent Radiol 2009; 26: 345–351.
Sreenarasimhaiah J. Chronic mesenteric ischaemia. Best Pract Res Clin Gastroenterol 2005; 19:283–295.

Scenario no. 13

A patient with weight loss

Candidate copy

Please read the GP referral letter for Ms Arwa.
The time distribution for this station is as follows:

You have (---) minutes to take a history from the patient.
You have (---) minutes to collect your thoughts.
You have (---) minutes for discussion with the examiners.

Please do not examine the patient

Dear Doctor,

Thank you for seeing Mrs Arwa, a 28-year-old woman who has been complaining of weight loss over the last 6 months.

Yours faithfully,

Please interview the patient and, based on history taking, construct a differential diagnosis and plan of investigation. Provide explanation to the patient and answer any questions she may have.

Surrogate copy

Chief complaints and history of present illness

- You have lost 15 kg in weight over the last 6 months
- You are not dieting, and the weight loss is not intentional.

If you are asked:
- Your appetite is good, and you are feeling hungry most of the time. You feel that you are eating more since your illness.
- You do not have stomach pain.
- You do not have constipation.
- You have loose motion and you go to the toilet 5 times per day to evacuate your bowel.
- The stool is not bulky and is easy to flush.

Review of systems

If you are asked:
- You feel your heart beating very fast
- You prefer cold weather and cold places
- You feel that you sweat too much
- You do not feel gritty sensation or bulging of your eyes
- You have not noticed swelling in your neck
- You do not have increased urine frequency
- You do not wake at night for urination.

Menstrual history

You feel that your menses are becoming scanty (the amount of blood is becoming less).

Past history

You were diagnosed with anxiety disorder by your psychiatrist 4 months ago and he prescribed escitalopram 10 mg daily.

Family history

Your younger sister has systemic lupus erythematosus and she is on cortisone therapy.

Drug history

You are taking escitalopram 10 mg.

Social history

- You are a housewife
- You are married and have two kids
- You husband feels you have become very anxious
- You do not smoke
- You do not drink alcohol
- You work as secretary in a construction company.

Your concerns/questions to the doctor
I know that cancer can cause weight loss. I am worried that my weight loss is due to cancer somewhere in my body.

Steps in history taking in a patient with weight loss

Step 1: Introduction, greeting and confirmation of patient identity
- Good morning Mrs Arwa (shakehands with the patient), pleased to meet you.
- I am Dr X working in the medical outpatient clinic.
- Can I confirm that I am talking to Mrs Arwa?
- I have just read the referral letter from your GP who states that you have lost 15 kg in weight over the last 6 months.
- Can you tell me more about that?
- Allow the patient to speak.
- Avoid interruptions.
- Avoid medical jargon (e.g. thyrotoxicosis, celiac disease, anorexia, etc.)
- *Use open-ended questions such as:* What else?

Step 2: Elaborating important points in the history of weight loss

History of presenting illness
- **How much weight did the patient lose?**
  See the classification of significant weight loss in **Table 2**.

- **Intentional or unintentional**
  Ask whether weight loss is intentional or unintentional.

- **How is the patient's appetite?**
  Conditions that cause weight loss with increased appetite include
  - Hyperthyroidism
  - Diabetes mellitus
  - Bulimia nervosa
  - Tumours that cause hypoglycaemia.
  - Anxiety or depression.

- **Dietary history**
  Ask details about patient's dietary history.

- **Use of slimming pills**

- **Recent change in psychological status**
  Depression and anxiety may lead to weight loss.

- **Associated symptoms:**
  - How is your appetite?
  - Palpitations, sweating, heat intolerance, eye problems (bulging, gritty sensation, redness), neck swelling—hyperthyroidism

	Significant weight loss %	Severe weight loss %
1 week	1–2%	>2%
1 month	5%	>5%
3 months	7.5%	>7.5%
6 months	10%	>10%

Table 2 Classification of severity of weight loss

–   Review carefully the GIT system
–   Review all the systems with particular attention to the GIT and endocrine systems.

Menstrual history

Thyrotoxicosis may cause oligomenorrhoea or amenorrhoea.

Dietary history

Ask about the patient's diet.

Past history

Ask about thyroid disorders, malignancies, diabetes and psychiatric disorders.

Family history

Family history of malignant disease or autoimmune disorders such as thyrotoxicosis.

Drug history

Use of slimming pills or psychiatric medications.

Social history

- Ask about smoking and alcohol history.
- Ask about the effect of current illness on the family, job and other aspects of the patient's life.

Further information not covered (at end of history taking)

Ask the patient the following question: Is there anything else that you feel important and would like to tell me about?

Step 3: Explaining to the patient the diagnosis and the plan of management

Mrs Arwa, after reviewing your history, it seems you have lost a significant amount of weight over the past 6 months without any intention to lose weight and in fact your appetite has increased. You feel that your heart is beating faster than usual, and you have become more anxious. You have a reduced amount of blood in your menses. All these symptoms could point to a condition called "hyperthyroidism". Have you heard of this before? Hyperthyroidism is a condition that occurs when the thyroid gland, which is found at the front of your neck, produces too much thyroid hormone. When thyroid hormone levels increase above the normal range, they can result in a fast heartbeat, weight loss and anxiety. Does that sound clear to you? I will perform an examination of your thyroid gland and will order blood tests to assess your thyroid function and will then arrange to see you shortly after that to discuss the results. If they are abnormal, then I will arrange an appointment with a colleague who specialises in the management of thyroid disease.

Check patient understanding and agreement on plan of management.

Does that sound good to you?

Step 4: Ask about and address patient's concerns

Do you have any questions or concerns?

Patient's concern: Doctor, I know that cancer can cause weight loss.

Reply: Well, it is true that cancer can cause weight loss; however, you have other symptoms such as fast heartbeat, increased anxiety and good appetite that make hyperthyroidism the most likely diagnosis in your case. Of course, if the thyroid function comes back normal, then I will look for other diseases.

After answering each concern, confirm the agreement by asking; "Is that alright? Or does that make sense to you?"

Step 5: Summarise the discussion, confirm patient's understandings and close the meeting.

Mrs Arwa, I would like to summarise our discussion to be sure that you understand important information about your illness. The most probable cause for your weight loss is hyperthyroidism. I am going to order thyroid function tests, which is a simple blood test, and depending on the result will seek the opinion of a colleague who specialises in the thyroid gland. Meanwhile, I am going to provide you with my contact number in case you have any further questions or concerns regarding your condition. Does that sound clear to you? You can also get more information on the internet on hyperthyroidism. Thank you and see you soon.

Discussion

Problem

Weight loss.

Diagnosis

Thyrotoxicosis.

Other plausible diagnosis

- **Anxiety disorder**
  Anxiety disorders may give symptoms that are indistinguishable from thyrotoxicosis.
- **Diabetes mellitus**
  Type 1 diabetes mellitus (T1DM) can cause weight loss with normal appetite, but the patient should have osmotic symptoms such as nocturia and polyuria. The patient has polyphagia and a family history of autoimmune disease.
- **Malabsorption syndrome (celiac)**
  Patient has loose motion but no symptoms of steatorrhoea.

Effects of thyroid hormone (active form T3) on body tissues

- Increases tissue basal metabolic rate.
- Reduces serum cholesterol and systemic vascular resistance.
- Clinical effects include:
  - Weight loss
  - Osteoporosis
  - Tachycardia
  - Anxiety
  - Atrial fibrillation
  - Muscle weakness
  - Tremor
  - Neuropsychiatric symptoms
  - Rarely cardiovascular collapse and death.

Assessment of any patient with suspected thyrotoxicosis should include a comprehensive history and physical examination with measurement of the pulse rate, blood pressure, respiratory rate, and body weight. A thorough thyroid gland examination should be performed. Examination of cardiovascular and neuromuscular function is important.

The best initial screening test in suspected thyrotoxicosis is serum thyroid stimulating hormone (TSH) measurement as it has high sensitivity and specificity. Diagnostic accuracy improves when a serum TSH, free thyroxine (T4), and total triiodothyronine (T3) are assessed at the initial evaluation.

In overt hyperthyroidism, serum free T_4, T_3, or both are elevated, and serum TSH is subnormal (usually <0.01 mU/L in a third-generation assay). In mild hyperthyroidism, serum T_4 and free T_4 can be normal, only serum T_3 may be elevated, and serum TSH will be low or undetectable.

Further reading

Ross DS, Burch HB, Cooper DS, et al. 2016 American Thyroid Association guidelines for diagnosis and management of hyperthyroidism and other causes of thyrotoxicosis. Thyroid 2016; 26:1343–1421.

Scenario no. 14

A patient with recurrent headache

Candidate copy

Please read the GP referral letter for Mrs Laila.
The time distribution for this station is as follows:
> You have (---) minutes to take a history from the patient.
> You have (---) minutes to collect your thoughts.
> You have (---) minutes for discussion with the examiners.

Please do not examine the patient

> Dear Doctor,
>
> Thank you for seeing Mrs Laila, a 30-year-old woman who has been complaining of recurrent attacks of severe headache for the last 1 year. She was diagnosed with migraine after a normal MRI brain and basic blood tests. Her headache does not seem to respond to migraine therapy.
>
> Yours faithfully,

> Please interview the patient and, based on history taking, construct a differential diagnosis and plan of investigation. Provide explanation to the patient and answer any questions she may have.

Surrogate copy

Chief complaints and history of present illness

- You have recurrent attacks of headache for the last 1 year.
- The attacks are very severe (9/10 on pain severity scale).
- The headache is mainly at the back of the head and sometimes on the sides.
- Occasionally, you have it only on one side.
- It is a throbbing headache.
- When the attacks come, you also feel nausea, blurring of vision, and fear of death.
- Your heart beats very fast during the attack and you sweat too much.
- The attacks usually last 2–5 hours, occasionally they last longer.
- The attacks come every 5–7 days and they get worse during your periods.
- You know the attack is coming as you feel your heart beats faster.
- When you know the attack is coming, you become very anxious.

Review of systems
- You do not have breathing problems or chest pain.
- You do not have a preference for hot or cold weather.
- You have not lost weight.
- Your desire for food is normal.
- You have not noticed any swelling in your neck.
- You do not have kidney disease.
- You do not have problems with passing urine.
- You do not have frothy urine.

Menstrual history
Your menses are regular with a normal amount of blood.

Past history
- You visited your GP 10 months ago who ordered MRI of the brain and some blood tests which were all normal and he told you that you had migraine. You are taking propranolol 20 mg 3 times daily and sumatriptan and indomethacin tablets, when needed. However, you feel that the attacks have become more severe and more frequent
- You have visited the emergency department frequently for pain relief and you feel only morphine works with you headache
- You are very anxious as your blood pressure shoots up during the attacks as high as 215/115 mmHg and, when the attack is over; your blood pressure goes back to normal.

Family history
Your mother has hypertension and is being treated for thyroid cancer and your older sister had thyroid cancer.

Social history
- You are married and have three kids. You work as a schoolteacher. Your social life and work have been affected significantly by your illness and you have had to take multiple absences from work because of attacks of intolerable headache. Your usual care for your kids and husband has also been affected.
- You do not smoke.
- You do not drink alcohol.

Your concerns/questions to the doctor
What is the cause of my headache?

Steps in history taking in a patient with headache

Step 1: Introduction, greeting and confirmation of patient identity
- Good morning, Mrs Laila (shakehands with the patient), pleased to meet you.
- I am Dr X working in the medical outpatient clinic.
- Can I confirm that I am talking to Mrs Laila?
- I have just read the referral letter from your GP who states that you have had a severe intermittent headache for the last year.
- Can you tell me more about that?
- Allow the patient to speak.
- Avoid interruptions.
- Avoid medical jargon (e.g. idiopathic hypertension, neoplasm, cerebral venous sinus thrombosis, trigeminal neuralgia, etc.)
- *Use open-ended questions such as:* What else?

Step 2: Elaborating important points in the history of headache

History of presenting illness

Headache like any other pain should be analysed using the LIQOR AAA.

Review of systems

- Other neurological symptoms
- *Trigeminal neuralgia in the young:* Ask about other symptoms of multiple sclerosis
- *Symptoms of pheochromocytoma:* Palpitation, sweating, anxiety and nervousness
- *Symptoms suggestive of increased intracranial pressure (ICP):* Projectile vomiting, personality change and seizure/weakness/numbness
- Ask about alarm/red flag symptoms of headache.

Menstrual history

- Relationship of headache to menstrual cycle (catamenial migraine)
- Use of oral contraceptive pills.

Past medical history

- Ask about history of hypertension
- Ask about history of migraine
- Ask about previous stroke, brain lesions
- Ask about previous head trauma
- Ask about diseases that cause immunosuppression
- *Recurrent sinusitis:* Cerebral venous sinus thrombosis, brain abscess, meningitis.

Family history

- Family history of migraine, hypertension or pheochromocytoma.
- Family history of cancer.

Drug history

- *Use of oral contraceptive pills:* Cerebral venous sinus thrombosis, migraine
- Drugs for migraine
- Use of steroids
- *Other drugs that may cause increased ICP:* Isoretinoic acid, tetracyclines, steroids, etc.

Social history

- *Smoking:* Risk of malignancy
- *Alcohol intake:* Subdural haematoma, bleeding
- Changes in personality
- *Travel history:* Malaria, meningitis
- *Sexual history:* Human immunodeficiency virus (HIV), neurosyphilis.

Further information not covered (at end of history taking)

Ask the patient the following question: Is there anything else that you feel important and would like to tell me about?

Step 3: Explaining to the patient the diagnosis and the plan of management

Mrs Laila, you have had recurrent and severe headache for the last 1 year. You had a magnetic resonance imaging scan of your brain which was normal, and your symptoms have not improved on migraine treatment. You have mentioned some very important symptoms like feeling a fast heartbeat, excess sweating and high blood pressure during the attacks. Your mother is hypertensive and is being treated for thyroid cancer and your older sister had thyroid cancer. Putting all these together, you need to be investigated for a condition called pheochromocytoma. Have you heard of this before? Pheochromocytoma is a rare, usually benign growth that develops in a gland situated above the kidney called the adrenal gland.

Pheochromocytoma intermittently releases excess amounts of a hormone called adrenaline that causes episodic attacks of high blood pressure, sweating, fast heartbeat, anxiety and panic-like attacks. Because you have a family history of thyroid cancer, pheochromocytoma may also be part of a syndrome called multiple endocrine neoplasia (MEN) that runs in families and can exist together with thyroid cancer.

We need to measure this hormone in your blood and urine. If the hormone level comes back high, then we will proceed with a CT scan of your adrenal glands. Meanwhile, I am also going to seek help from a colleague who specialises in adrenal glands. Does that sound clear to you? Following the results of blood and urine tests, I will see you again in my clinic to give you further answers.

Does that make sense to you?

Step 4: Ask about and address patient's concerns

Do you have any questions or concerns?

> *Patient's concern:* What is the cause of my headache?

> *Reply*: Answered above.

After answering each concern, confirm the agreement by asking; "Is that alright or does that sound clear to you?"

Step 5: Summarise the discussion, confirm patient's understandings and close the meeting.

Mrs Laila, I would like to summarise our discussion to be sure you understand important information about your illness. The episodes of symptoms you have with the raised blood pressure and your family history may suggest that you have a condition called 'pheochromocytoma'. I will order some blood and urine tests to measure the hormone levels. I will see you after the test results to give you more answers. I am going to provide you with my contact number in case you have any further questions or concerns regarding your condition. Does that sound clear to you? You can get information from the internet regarding pheochromocytoma. Thank you and see you soon.

Discussion

Problem

Recurrent attacks of headache, anxiety, and palpitations.

Diagnosis

Pheochromocytoma (possibly MEN 2A or MEN 2B, but should also have mucosal neuroma and marfanoid body habitus).

(Typical symptoms, episodes of high blood pressure and family history of thyroid cancer).

Other plausible diagnosis

- **Panic attacks**
  Acute panic attacks are an important differential diagnosis of pheochromocytoma.
- **Hyperthyroidism**
- **Migraine**
  Migraine attacks are an important differential diagnosis of pheochromocytoma.
- **Insulinoma**
  Hypoglycaemia may lead to symptoms that are indistinguishable from pheochromocytoma.

Characteristics of headache in certain conditions

Migraine headache
- Usually throbbing or pulsatile
- Commonly on one side
- Aggravated by menstrual periods, alcohol, lack of sleep, certain foods such as chocolate, cheese, coffee, etc.
- May be preceded by migraine aura such as problems with vision, dizziness, lip and facial numbness, etc.
- Usually lasts for hours and sometimes for days
- Associated with nausea and vomiting, photophobia, phonophobia
- Relieved by migraine treatment such as triptans and indomethacin
- In addition, patients tend to prefer resting in a quiet and dark room.

Headache due to increased intracranial pressure
- Usually generalised headache
- Tends to be of maximal intensity in the morning
- Usually dull and deep
- Aggravated by coughing, bending the head forward, sneezing and valsalva manoeuvre
- May be relieved by rest
- Associated with projectile vomiting
- May be associated with changes in the level of consciousness, seizure, personality change, limb weakness or numbness.

Hypertension headache
- Usually cause a throbbing headache
- The headache is usually occipital
- Usually more intense on awakening
- May persist for days
- May be associated with palpitations, blurring of vision, confusion, seizure or deterioration of level of consciousness.

Cluster headache
- Unilateral, often severe headache
- Attacks usually come in clusters, i.e. occur daily for some weeks followed by a period of remission.
- *Typical sites include:* Orbital, supraorbital, or temporal regions
- Typically associated with autonomic symptoms such as ptosis, meiosis, lacrimation, conjunctival injection, rhinorrhoea, and nasal congestion
- Attacks typically last for minutes to less than 2 hours.

Trigeminal neuralgia
- Recurrent brief episodes of unilateral electric shock-like pains
- Onset is sudden
- Duration is very short (seconds), tend to be repetitive
- *Location:* In the distribution of one or more divisions of the fifth cranial (trigeminal) nerve (most commonly V2 and V3, very rare in V1)
- The pain usually occurs in paroxysms
- Pain is classically triggered by light touch of the face in V1, V2, V3 areas
- *Other triggering factors include:* Brushing teeth, chewing, talking, grimacing or smiling
- Trigeminal neuralgia typically occurs over the age of 50 years
- If trigeminal neuralgia is diagnosed before the age of 50 years, a secondary cause has to be excluded such as demyelinating disease (MS) or a cerebellopontine angle tumour. An MRI brain should be obtained before labelling the patient with idiopathic trigeminal neuralgia.

Tension headache
- Frequent headache
- Minutes to days duration
- Bilateral pain, pressing
- Tightening, e.g. 'band-like'
- Mild-to-moderate intensity
- No nausea/vomiting
- No more than one of photophobia or phonophobia

- Not aggravated by routine activities
- May or may not be associated with

pericranial tenderness on manual palpation.

Headache due to pheochromocytoma
- Sudden onset
- Short duration
- Bilateral affecting any part of the head. Occipital, nuchal-occipital, and frontal-occipital regions are the predominant locations
- Throbbing, pulsating
- Frequently associated with palpitations and perspiration
- Other features include apprehension and/or anxiety, often with a sense of impending death, tremor
- Measurement of blood pressure before and after the onset of headache reveals a sudden increase in both systolic and diastolic blood pressure.

What are the red flag symptoms/signs of headache?
- New onset headache
- Severe headache (worst headache in patient's life)/thunderclap headache
- Presence of other serious symptoms such as fever, weight loss
- Development of focal neurological signs such as weakness, seizure or confusion
- Headache in immunocompromised patient/HIV (toxoplasmosis, tumours)
- New headache in pregnant woman (pre-eclampsia, cerebral venous sinus thrombosis)
- Headache in older age groups (as mentioned below)
- Other symptoms of increased ICP such as projectile vomiting, worsening with stooping, cough, exertion, or sexual activity.

Headache in older patients (above age of 50 years)
- Brain tumours
- Giant cell arteritis
- Trigeminal neuralgia
- Chronic subdural haematoma.

Pheochromocytoma

Pheochromocytoma is the 'great mimic'. This is because the symptoms and signs produced by catecholamine excess in this condition can be produced by numerous other clinical conditions. Physicians, therefore, should keep a high index of suspicion for this condition in patients with recurrent headaches, palpitations, diaphoresis, anxiety and episodic attacks of elevated blood pressure. The classic triad of diaphoresis, palpitations and headache has a reported sensitivity of 89% and specificity of 67% for pheochromocytoma and, in the presence of hypertension; it has 91% sensitivity and 94% specificity.

Other important conditions that can mimic pheochromocytoma include
- Anxiety disorders and panic attacks
- Drug withdrawal from benzodiazepines or neuropsychiatric drugs.
- Migraine
- Hyperthyroidism
- Hypoglycaemia, e.g. insulinoma
- Paroxysmal supraventricular tachycardia
- Essential hypertension
- Carcinoid tumours.

Patients with a confirmed diagnosis of pheochromocytoma should be investigated for certain genetic syndromes that may be associated with increased risk for pheochromocytoma, including:
- von Hippel–Lindau (VHL) syndrome
- Multiple endocrine neoplasia type 2
- Neurofibromatosis type 1.

Multiple endocrine neoplasia type 2 is a rare hereditary disorder characterised by the presence of medullary thyroid carcinoma, unilateral or bilateral pheochromocytomas and other hyperplasia and/or neoplasia of different endocrine tissues. The two different forms of MEN 2 are sporadic and familial.

A 24-hour urinary measurement for catecholamines, total and fractionated metanephrines, and vanillylmandelic acid (VMA) have been used to screen patients for pheochromocytoma. Currently, the diagnosis is established by elevated plasma fractionated metanephrines or elevated 24-hour urinary fractionated metanephrines.

Computed tomography is suggested for initial imaging and localization of the tumour, but magnetic resonance imaging is a better option in patients with metastatic disease or when radiation exposure must be limited.

Preoperative alpha-blockade is essential to prevent intraoperative haemodynamic instability during resection of a pheochromocytoma. β-adrenoceptor blockers should never be employed without first blocking α-adrenoceptor mediated vasoconstriction. Adrenalectomy is the mainstay of treatment for pheochromocytoma.

Further reading

Canadian Chiropractic Association (CCA), Canadian Federation of Chiropractic Regulatory and Education Accrediting Boards (CFCREAB), Clinical Practice Guidelines Project (CPG). (2012). Clinical practice guideline for the management of headache disorders in adults. [online]. Available from https://www.researchgate.net/publication/262636337_Clinical_Practice_Guideline_for_the_Management_of_Headache_Disorders_in_Adults. [Last accessed October, 2019].

Chen H, Sippel RS, O'Dorisio MS, et al. North American Neuroendocrine Tumor Society (NANETS). The North American Neuroendocrine Tumor Society consensus guideline for the diagnosis and management of neuroendocrine tumors: pheochromocytoma, paraganglioma, and medullary thyroid cancer. Pancreas 2010; 39:775–783.

Farrugia FA, Martikos G, Tzanetis P, et al. Pheochromocytoma, diagnosis and treatment: Review of the literature. Endocr Regul 2017; 51:168–181.

Headache Classification Committee of the International Headache Society (IHS). The International Classification of Headache Disorders, 3rd edition (beta version). Cephalalgia 2013; 33:629–808.

Watanabe M. Headache in pheochromocytoma. In: Martin JF (Ed). Pheochromocytoma – A new view of the old problem. London: IntechOpen Limited; 2011. pp. 103–110.

Scenario no. 15

A patient with acute kidney injury

Candidate copy

Please read the orthopaedic referral letter for Mr Peterson.
The time distribution for this station is as follows:

You have (---) minutes to take a history from the patient.
You have (---) minutes to collect your thoughts.
You have (---) minutes for discussion with the examiners.

Please do not examine the patient

> Dear Doctor,
>
> Thank you for seeing Mr Peterson, a 34-year-old man who was found to have abnormal kidney function during his preoperative check-up for disc prolapse surgery. His serum creatinine is 260 μmol/L, BUN 14 mmol/L, sodium 145 mmol/L, potassium 5.0 mmol/L and bicarbonate 23 mmol/L. His blood pressure was also high 160/90.
>
> Yours faithfully,

Please interview the patient and, based on history taking, construct a differential diagnosis and plan of investigation. Provide explanation to the patient and answer any questions he may have.

Surrogate copy

Chief complaints and history of present illness

You have been referred by your orthopaedic (bone) doctor because of abnormal kidney function and high blood pressure. You are very surprised because 6 months ago your kidney function and blood pressure were normal. You do not have any symptom apart from back pain which has been there for the last 6 months. You had magnetic resonance imaging of your spine and your orthopaedic doctor informed you that a disc prolapse was causing the pain. This had occurred when you lifted a heavy bag on a holiday 6 months ago. After lifting the bag, you felt a sudden severe pain in the lower back that has worsened over time. Your orthopaedic doctor decided that you need surgery to correct the disc and this was planned for the next month. However, your doctor is now saying that you have problems with your kidneys.

Review of systems
- You do not feel malaise or fatigue
- You did not vomit, and you did not have diarrhoea
- The colour of your urine is normal, and it is not frothy
- You have not noticed any swelling in your legs or below your eyes.

Past history
- Two weeks ago, you had a sore throat and pain with fever. You visited your GP who diagnosed you with acute tonsillitis and you received augmentin 625 mg three times daily for 7 days.
- You do not have any history of kidney disease
- Your kidney function 6 months ago was normal
- You do not suffer high blood pressure, diabetes or any other disease.

Drug history

Only if you are asked, mention you have been taking different painkillers for the past 6 months such as ibuprofen 400 mg three times a day. Last week you visited the emergency department for your back pain, and you received voltaren (diclofenac sodium) injection 100 mg in your muscle.

Social history
- You do not smoke
- You do not drink alcohol
- You work as a computer engineer in a company
- You are happily married and have two kids.

Your questions to the doctor and concerns

My blood pressure was found to be high; could this be the reason for my abnormal kidney function?

Steps in history taking in a patient with acute kidney injury

Step 1: Introduction, greeting and confirmation of patient identity

- Good morning Mr Peterson (shakehands with the patient), pleased to meet you.
- I am Dr X working in the medical outpatient clinic.
- Can I confirm that I am talking to Mr Peterson?
- I have just read the referral letter from your orthopaedic doctor who states that your kidney function is not normal, and your blood pressure is high.
- Can you tell me more?
- Allow the patient to speak.
- Avoid interruptions.
- Avoid medical jargon (e.g. acute kidney injury, analgesia, renal, periorbital, etc.)
- *Use open-ended questions such as:* What else?

Step 2: Elaborating important points in the history of back pain and abnormal kidney function

History of presenting illness

Ask about symptoms suggestive of kidney disease

- Malaise
- Fatigue
- Nausea and vomiting
- Weight loss
- Abdominal pain
- Pruritus

Take details of urinary symptoms including

- *Change in amount:* Oliguria may suggest acute kidney injury (AKI) and anuria may suggest obstruction or acute tubular necrosis (ATN) or severely impaired kidney function.
- Change in colour.
- Foamy or frothy urine suggestive of proteinuria.
- *Symptoms of obstruction/prostatism:* Urgency, hesitancy or dribbling?

Ask about symptoms that suggest the presence of nephrotic syndrome:

- Leg swelling
- Periorbital swelling
- Abdominal distention.

History of recent upper respiratory tract infection

- This is very important as some kidney diseases tend to occur following an upper respiratory tract infection.

Review of systems

- *Cardiac symptoms:* Dyspnoea, paroxysmal nocturnal dyspnoea, orthopnoea, chest pain
- *Renal symptoms:* Frothy urine, reduced urine output, change in urine colour
- *GIT symptoms:* Diarrhoea, vomiting and GIT bleeding (causing hypovolaemia)
- *Musculoskeletal:* Joint pain or swelling which may suggest connective tissue disease
- History of recent upper respiratory tract infection, tonsillitis or viral illness.

Past history

- History of chronic kidney disease
- History of hypertension
- History of diabetes mellitus
- History of hepatitis C and B
- History of rheumatologic disorders.

Family history

Family history of kidney disease (Alport's disease, autosomal dominant polycystic kidney disease).

Drug history

Ask about the use of nephrotoxic drugs including over-the-counter medications such NSAIDs and angiotensin-converting enzyme (ACE) inhibitors or antibiotics.

Social history

- History of smoking.
- History of alcohol use.

- History of drug abuse (hepatitis).
- Sexual history.

Further information not covered (at end of history taking)

Ask the patient the following question: Is there anything else that you feel important and would like to tell me about?

Step 3: Explaining to the patient the diagnosis and the plan of management

Mr Peterson, you have been referred by your orthopaedic doctor because of abnormal kidney function and high blood pressure. You have had back pain for 6 months for which you are taking painkillers. Importantly, you had a recent sore throat with fever for which you received Augmentin tablets. I think there are a number of possible causes for the abnormal kidney function in your case. Most important are the medications you are taking. Painkillers are well-known to affect kidney function by various mechanisms and the antibiotic Augmentin can also affect the kidneys. I strongly suggest that you stop taking ibuprofen and Voltaren immediately. For your back pain, you may use other painkillers that do not have major effects on the kidneys. Another possible reason of your abnormal kidney function is that certain bacteria called *Streptococcus* can cause throat infection and, indirectly, a kidney disease called post-streptococcal glomerulonephritis. Sometimes kidney disease can also happen after viral infection. Does that make sense to you?

I will order some urine and blood tests for you and an ultrasound scan of your kidneys to look for the cause of your abnormal kidney function. Meanwhile, please stop taking the painkillers and drink plenty of water to help increase the blood flow to your kidneys. I will also prescribe a tablet to help control your blood pressure. A colleague who specialises in kidney diseases will see you shortly. In case your kidney function does not get better. We may need to take a tiny piece from your kidney to examine it under the microscope and identify the exact cause of kidney damage. I will see you again in one week to reassess your kidney function and discuss the results of the tests.

Check patient understanding and agreement on plan of management.

Does that make sense to you?

Step 4: Ask about and address patient's concerns

Do you have any questions or concerns?

Patient's concern: My blood pressure was also found to be high although I did not have high blood pressure before. Could this be the reason for my abnormal kidney function?

Reply: Well, it is true that high blood pressure can cause abnormal kidney function. However, high blood pressure could also result from the abnormal kidney function. Since you did not have high blood pressure before, this is unlikely to be the cause of your kidney damage. In either case, blood pressure has to be controlled as it can cause further kidney damage.

After answering each concern, confirm agreement by asking; is that alright? Or does that make sense to you?

Step 5: Summarise the discussion, confirm patient's understandings and close the meeting.

Mr Peterson, I would like to summarise our discussion to be sure you understand important information about your illness. The most probable cause of your abnormal kidney function is the painkiller drugs. I would suggest that you stop these drugs immediately. I am going to prescribe an alternative medication for your back pain that does not affect your kidney function. Given your throat infection 2 weeks ago, it is important to exclude post-streptococcal glomerulonephritis. I will arrange for some blood and urine tests and will see you in 1 week to give you further answers. Meanwhile, I am going to provide you with my contact number in case you have any further questions or concerns regarding your condition. Does that sound clear to you? You can also get more information from the internet on abnormal kidney function caused by painkillers. Thank you and see you soon.

Discussion

Problem

Acute kidney injury.

Diagnosis

Drug-induced (NSAIDs, Augmentin) AKI.

Other plausible diagnosis

- Post-streptococcal glomerulonephritis
- Immunoglobulin A (IgA) nephropathy
- Hypertensive nephropathy.

Definition of acute kidney injury

Acute kidney injury is defined as any of the following
- Increase in serum creatinine by 0.3 mg/dL (26.5 µmol/L) or more within 48 hours.
- Increase in serum creatinine to 1.5 times above baseline within the prior 7 days.
- Decrease in urine volume of 0.5 mL/kg/hour or less over 6 hours.

Chronic kidney disease is defined as glomerular filtration rate <60 mL/minute/1.73 m^2 for 3 months or more.

Causes of acute kidney injury

Prerenal
- Decrease intake
- *Volume loss:* Bleeding, diarrhoea, vomiting, sweating, third space loss, diuretics, hypercalcaemia
- Renal vasoconstriction
- NSAID, ACE inhibitors, angiotensin receptor blockers
- Hepatorenal syndrome
- Sepsis.

Intrinsic renal

- *Glomerular*
  - Post-infectious such as post-streptococcal glomerulonephritis and other glomerulonephritides.
  - Connective tissue diseases.
- *Interstitial*
  - *Medications:* Penicillins, cephalosporins, sulphonamides, fluoroquinolones, NSAIDs, etc.
  - Infections (e.g. direct infection of renal parenchyma or systemic infections)
  - *Viruses:* Epstein–Barr virus, cytomegalovirus, human immunodeficiency virus
  - *Bacteria: Streptococcus* species, *Legionella* species

- Fungi: Candidiasis, histoplasmosis
- *Systemic disease:* Sarcoidosis, lupus.
- *Tubular*
  - Acute tubular necrosis from prolonged ischaemia/hypoperfusion.
  - *Drugs:* Aminoglycosides and amphotericin B.
  - *Toxins:* Ethylene glycol, contrast nephropathy, venoms
  - Rhabdomyolysis
  - Tumour lysis.
- *Vascular*
  - Renal vein thrombosis, malignant hypertension, scleroderma renal crisis, renal atheroembolic disease and renal infarction.

Postrenal
- *Obstruction*: Prostatic hypertrophy, tumours, stones, retroperitoneal fibrosis, etc.

Kidney diseases following upper respiratory tract infection

- Post-streptococcal
- IgA nephropathy
- Sometimes, connective tissue diseases such as SLE.

The period from the onset of upper respiratory infection to the detection of haematuria is important to predict the cause of abnormal kidney function. This period is usually between 1 week and 3 weeks with beta-haemolytic streptococcal pharyngitis (longer for streptococcal skin infection) compared with less than 5 days in IgA nephropathy.

Nonsteroidal anti-inflammatory drugs inhibit cyclooxygenase (COX) enzymes which lead to reduction in prostaglandin synthesis. Prostaglandins are vasodilator. Inhibition of prostaglandin synthesis will cause vasoconstriction of the renal vasculature and reversible renal ischaemia with reduced GFR.

Risk factors for NSAID-induced kidney injury

- Hypovolaemia (such as diarrhoea, vomiting, bleeding)
- Use of diuretics
- Use of ACE inhibitors
- Old age
- Presence of chronic kidney disease.

Renal effects of NSAIDs

- Acute renal failure
- Acute interstitial nephritis
- Acute papillary necrosis.

The most common cause of acute interstitial nephritis is drugs. Other causes include infections and autoimmune disorders. Drug-induced acute interstitial nephritis can be asymptomatic and is not dose or time dependent and can occur at any dose and up to several weeks after exposure to the offending drug. Acute interstitial nephritis may present with abnormal kidney function. Less common presentation may include fever, rash and eosinophilia. Laboratory tests typically show eosinophilia and eosinophiluria. The urine sediment usually reveals white cells and white cell casts.

Further reading

Kellum JA, Lameire N, Aspelin P, et al. Kidney Disease: Improving Global Outcomes (KDIGO) Acute Kidney Injury Work Group. KDIGO clinical practice guideline for acute kidney injury. Kidney Int Suppl 2012; 2:1–138.

Praga M, González E. Acute interstitial nephritis. Kidney Int 2010; 77:956–961.

Rahman M, Shad F, Smith MC. Acute kidney injury: a guide to diagnosis and management. Am Fam Physician 2012; 86:631–639.

Whelton A. Nephrotoxicity of nonsteroidal anti-inflammatory drugs: physiologic foundations and clinical implications. Am J Med 1999; 106:13S–24S.

Scenario no. 16

Dizziness in a patient with type 1 diabetes mellitus

Candidate copy

Please read the GP referral letter for Mr. Donald.
The time distribution for this station is as follows:
 You have (---) minutes to take a history from the patient.
 You have (---) minutes to collect your thoughts.
 You have (---) minutes for discussion with the examiners.

Please do not examine the patient

> **Dear Doctor,**
>
> Thank you for seeing Mr Donald, a 28-year-old with type 1 diabetes mellitus (T1DM) who has been complaining of increasing dizziness over the last few weeks. His supine blood pressure is 120/70 and on standing it is 85/50. He frequently feels nausea and abdominal pain.
>
> Yours faithfully,

> Please interview the patient and, based on history taking, construct a differential diagnosis and plan of investigation. Provide explanation to the patient and answer any questions he may have.

Surrogate copy

Chief complaint and HPI

You have felt dizziness and tiredness over the past 8 weeks. You cannot perform your usual work as a pharmaceutical representative. Your dizziness often forces you to sit or lie down. It particularly happens when you stand up from a sitting or lying position. You have fallen over when getting up from sleep to walk to the bathroom. This has worsened over the last week.

 You have recurrent tummy pain and occasional loose motions. The pain is dull, comes and goes and is not related to food. You also have nausea and increasing fatigue.

Review of systems

- You do not feel chest pain
- You do not feel a racing heart beat
- You do not have a hearing problem
- You do not feel numbness or tingling in your hands or feet
- You do not feel weakness in your legs or arms
- You do not see double images.

If asked only: You feel that your skin is becoming darker and your appendectomy scar is getting darker and darker.

Dietary history

You are eating a healthy diabetic diet.

Past history and drug history

You have had type 1 diabetes mellitus since the age of 16 years, and you are taking glargine 20 units in the evening and aspart insulin 10 units before breakfast, lunch, and dinner. Your blood sugar is well-controlled with a haemoglobin A1C of 7.0%. However, over the last 1 month you have noticed your sugar readings have been lower and your GP has reduced your glargine to 15 units and aspart to 8 units. You regularly see your doctor for your diabetes and your annual retinal screening and urine protein test were normal. You do not suffer any other illness.

Family history

Your sister had hyperthyroidism for which she received radioactive iodine.

Drug history

Other than insulin, you are not on any other medication.

Social history

- You work as a representative for a pharmaceutical company.
- You do not smoke.
- You do not drink alcohol.
- Your dizziness has severely affected your capability to perform your job.
- You are not married.

Your questions to the doctors and concerns

Can diabetes be the cause of my dizziness?

Steps in history taking in a patient with dizziness

Step 1: Introduction, greeting, and confirmation of patient identity

- Good morning Mr Donald (shakehands with the patient), pleased to meet you.
- I am Dr X working in the medical outpatient clinic.
- Can I confirm that I am talking to Mr Donald?
- I have just read the referral letter from your GP who states that you have had severe dizziness over the last 8 weeks, especially when you stand up from lying down or sitting.
- Can you tell me more about that?
- Allow the patient to speak.
- Avoid interruptions.
- Avoid medical jargon (e.g. addison, adrenal, celiac, vertigo, etc.)
- *Use open ended questions such as:* What else?

Step 2: Elaborating important points in the history of dizziness/vertigo

History of presenting illness

- **What does the patient exactly mean by dizziness?**
  Patients may use the term dizziness to describe a range of sensations such as vertigo, presyncope, disequilibrium/unsteadiness or light-headedness.
- **Was the onset sudden or gradual?**
- **How long does the dizziness last?**

- **How severe is the dizziness?**
- **What triggers the dizziness?**
    - *Head movement:* Inner ear disease such as benign positional vertigo or vestibular disorders.
    - *Standing or sitting from recumbent position:* Postural hypotension.
    - *Fasting:* Hypoglycaemia.
- **Important associated symptoms:**
    - *Vertigo*: A false sense that you or your surroundings are spinning or moving is called vertigo.
    - *Palpitations or chest pain*: May suggest a cardiac cause such as ischemia or arrhythmia.
    - *Bleeding*: Particularly GIT bleeding.
    - *Increased skin pigmentation and GIT symptoms*: Adrenal insufficiency
    - *Sweating, nervousness, palpitations, and presyncope*: Hypoglycaemia
    - *Limb weakness, numbness, diplopia, imbalance, facial deviation or swallowing difficulties*: Posterior circulation stroke, intracranial haemorrhage
    - *Peripheral numbness and burning*: Autonomic neuropathy
    - *Nausea and vomiting*: Peripheral or central vertigo or adrenal insufficiency
    - *Ear symptoms such as hearing loss and tinnitus*: Hearing loss may suggest Meniere disease, vestibular neuritis.

Review of systems

Candidate should pay particular attention to CNS, CVS, GIT, and endocrine systems. Ask about increased skin pigmentation for adrenal insufficiency.

Menstrual history

- Menorrhagia.

Dietary history

- Vegetarians may develop B12 deficiency.
- Poor food intake may lead to anaemia and dizziness.

Past history

- History of diabetes.
- History of HTN.
- History of heart disease.
- History of CNS diseases such as stroke.
- History of GIT or other bleeding diseases.
- Recent surgery.

Drug history

Medications are implicated in about a third of causes of dizziness. It is very important to enquire about drugs taken by the patient particularly over-the-counter medications. Ask in particular about the use of NSAIDs that can cause GIT bleeding.

Family history

Family history of autoimmune diseases.

Social history

- Effects of dizziness at work and other aspects of patient's life.
- Smoking history
- Alcohol history
- *Occupation:* Such as exposure to sun.

Further information not covered (at end of history taking):

Ask the patient the following question: Is there anything else that you feel is important and would like to tell me about?

Step 3: Explaining to the patient the diagnosis and the plan of management

Mr Donald, you have T1DM and your main complaint is dizziness that occurs on standing. Your doctor found a difference in your blood pressure when you were standing and when lying. You have also had tummy pain and occasional loose motion and your skin is becoming darker. You have also observed that your blood sugar readings are becoming lower than normal. Putting all this together points to a problem in the glands that lie above your kidneys and it could be a condition called 'Addison's disease.' Have you heard of this disease before? People with T1DM have an increased chance of developing autoimmune diseases where the body's own immune defence system turns against different organs in the body. If these antibodies attack the gland that lies above your kidneys (called the adrenal gland), then it will reduce or stop secreting a hormone called cortisol. Lack of cortisol in the body may lead to fatigue, dizziness, and low blood pressure. It also may cause the body colour to darken. Does that make sense to you? I will arrange an urgent blood test called a short synacthen to be done today. In this test, we measure your cortisol level after giving you an injection to stimulate cortisol release. If this is Addison's disease, then we will treat it by replacing the hormones that the adrenal glands are no longer making. A synthetic cortisol called hydrocortisone is taken once or twice a day to replace cortisol. I would suggest that you start taking hydrocortisone immediately after performing the blood test today. This is because if not treated quickly, Addison's disease can lead to a severe illness called adrenal crisis in which the blood pressure may drop suddenly, and serious consequences may result. A colleague who specialises in adrenal glands will also see you shortly. I will see you again after the test results and provide further information on Addison's disease and the medications used to treat it.

Check patient's understanding and agreement on plan of management.

Does that sound clear to you?

Step 4: Ask about and address patient's concerns

Do you have any questions or concerns?

Patient's concern: Can diabetes be the cause of my dizziness?

Reply: Yes, diabetes can cause dizziness for a number of reasons. It can cause a drop in the blood pressure when standing if it affects the autonomic nerves that helps to maintain our blood pressure. Low blood sugar readings associated with insulin can also cause dizziness. However, in the presence of the other symptoms you have mentioned such as tummy pain, loose motion, and darkening of the skin, it is important to look for Addison's disease.

After answering each concern confirm agreement by saying: 'is that okay or does that make sense to you?'

Step 5: Summarise the discussion, confirm patient's understandings, and close the meeting

Mr Donald, I would like to summarise our discussion to be sure that you understand important information about your illness. The most probable cause for your dizziness and low blood pressure when you stand up is Addison's disease. I am going to order the special blood tests to look for this and I will also prescribe cortisol tablets which you need to take immediately after performing the test. I will see you shortly to inform you about the test results and plan further treatment. A colleague who specialises in adrenal glands will see you soon. Meanwhile, I am going to provide you with my contact number in case you have any further questions or concerns regarding your condition. Does that make sense to you? You can also get information from the internet on Addison's disease. Thank you and see you soon.

Discussion

Problem

Dizziness, postural hypotension, new onset hypoglycaemic episodes, abdominal pain, and loose motion.

Diagnosis

Adrenal insufficiency.

Other plausible diagnosis

- **Diabetic autonomic neuropathy**
  The patient has no other complications like retinopathy and nephropathy, so this is highly unlikely.
- **Celiac disease**
  Patient's age is against this and he does not have other symptoms.
- **Inflammatory bowel disease**

Causes of new onset hypoglycaemic episodes in patients with type 1 diabetes mellitus whose sugar was controlled

- Aggressive insulin therapy
- Excessive physical activity
- Significant reduction of carbohydrate intake
- Development of Addison's disease
- Development of Celiac disease
- Development of acute or chronic kidney disease
- Liver disease
- Alcohol abuse
- Development of non-neutralizing insulin-binding antibodies induced by exogenous insulin.

The typical clinical presentation of primary adrenal insufficiency includes weight loss, orthostatic hypotension due to dehydration, hyponatremia, hyperkalemia, changes in blood count (anaemia, eosinophilia, lymphocytosis), and hypoglycaemia. Hyperpigmentation of the skin and mucous membranes results from excess ACTH and other pro-opiomelanocortin peptides. Due to nonspecific presentation, the diagnosis is frequently delayed, resulting in a clinical presentation with an acute life-threatening adrenal crisis. Some relatively frequent conditions predisposing patients to primary adrenal insufficiency include certain autoimmune disorders (e.g., T1DM, autoimmune gastritis/pernicious anaemia, and vitiligo) as well as infectious diseases (tuberculosis, HIV, cytomegalovirus, candidiasis, histoplasmosis). Addison's disease may constitute a diagnostic challenge in patients with T1DM. It should be a diagnostic consideration in patients with T1DM who present with unexplained orthostatic hypotension/persistent hypotension or abrupt recurrent hypoglycaemia in patients with previously controlled DM. The corticotropin stimulation test (short Synacthen test) is the diagnostic 'gold standard' for the diagnosis of primary adrenal insufficiency. Treatment with hydrocortisone (15–25 mg) or cortisone acetate (20–35 mg) in two or three divided oral doses per day is recommended as soon as diagnosis is made. Patients with confirmed aldosterone deficiency should receive mineralocorticoid replacement with fludrocortisone (starting dose, 50–100 µg in adults) and not restrict their salt intake. Patients with suspected adrenal crisis should be treated with an immediate parenteral injection of 100 mg hydrocortisone, followed by appropriate fluid resuscitation and 200 mg of hydrocortisone/24 hours (via continuous IV therapy or 6 hourly injections).

Prevention of adrenal crisis in patients with primary adrenal insufficiency

- Adrenal crisis in patients with known primary adrenal insufficiency is best prevented by patient education.
- Increase the glucocorticoid dosage in situations of stressors known to increase cortisol requirements (such as infections, anaesthesia, medications that induce the drug-metabolizing enzyme CYP3A4, surgery and trauma).
- Parenteral self- or lay-administration of emergency glucocorticoids (patients should be provided with a glucocorticoid injection kit for emergency use).
- Provide patients with a steroid emergency card and medical alert identification.

Further reading

Bornstein SR, Allolio B, Arlt W, et al. Diagnosis and Treatment of Primary Adrenal Insufficiency: An Endocrine Society Clinical Practice Guideline. J Clin Endocrinol Metab 2016; 101:364–389.

Muncie HL, Sirmans SM, James E. Dizziness: Approach to evaluation and management. Am Fam Physician 2017; 95:154–162.

Passanisi S, Timpanaro T, Lo Presti D, et al. Recurrent hypoglycaemia in type-1 diabetes mellitus may unravel the association with Addison's disease: a case report. BMC Research Notes 2014; 7:634.

Scenario no. 17

A patient with cough and breathlessness

Candidate copy

Please read the GP referral letter for Mr Jamil.
The time distribution for this station is as follows:

    You have (---) minutes to take a history from the patient.
    You have (---) minutes to collect your thoughts.
    You have (---) minutes for discussion with the examiners.

Please do not examine the patient

Dear Doctor,

Thank you for seeing Mr Jamil, a 60-year-old with a history of hypertension and coronary artery stenting. He has been complaining of cough and exertional breathlessness for 3 months. His ramipril was changed to Irbesartan since the start of his symptoms, but this did not seem to relieve his symptoms which are getting worse. His echocardiography showed an EF of 58%.

Yours faithfully,

Please interview the patient and, based on history taking, construct a differential diagnosis and plan of investigation. Provide explanation to the patient and answer any questions he may have.

Surrogate copy

Chief complaint and HPI

- You complain from a dry cough for the past 3 months.
- You have had similar episodes of cough in the past for short periods of time.
- You have started feeling breathless when going up one flight of stairs for the last 2 months.
- The breathlessness gets better when you rest or sleep.
- You do not wake up at night with breathlessness.
- You do not feel chest pain.
- You have not observed any swelling in your legs.
- You are sleeping on one pillow.

Review of systems

- You do not have any problems with your urine.
- You do not have symptoms of recurrent sneezing, itchy nose, or throat clearing sensation.
- You do not have recurrent heart burn.
- Your urine is not frothy.
- You have not noticed any swelling in your tummy.
- You do not have kidney disease.

Past history and drug history

- You have had high blood pressure for 10 years.
- You were on ramipril 5 mg for 10 years, but your GP changed that to Irbesartan 150 mg since the start of your cough as he thought that ramipril was the cause of the cough.
- You had a stent of your largest coronary artery 5 years ago.
- A recent echocardiograph was normal.

Social history

- You have never smoked.
- You do not drink alcohol.

Questions you answer only if you are asked

- You have worked as a technician in a glass factory (manufacturing glass) for 20 years.
- You *keep pigeons* at home and clean their cages daily.
- You are happily married with two kids.
- Your questions to the doctor and concerns.

Could the cause of cough and breathlessness be related to my heart?

Steps in history taking in a patient with cough and breathlessness

Step 1: Introduction, greeting, and confirmation of patient identity

- Good morning Mr Jamil (shakehands with the patient), pleased to meet you.
- I am Dr X working in the medical outpatient clinic.
- Can I confirm that I am talking to Mr Jamil?
- I have just read the referral letter from your GP who states that you have a dry cough and difficulty with breathing.
- Can you tell me more about that?
- Allow the patient to speak.
- Avoid interruptions.
- Avoid medical jargon (e.g. oedema, cardiac, haemoptysis, etc.)
- *Use open ended questions such as:* What else?

Step 2: Elaborating important points in the history of cough and breathlessness

History of presenting illness

- How long have you had the cough?
- Is it dry or with phlegm, if so what colour?
- History of wheezing.
- History of dyspnoea, orthopnoea or paroxysmal nocturnal dyspnoea (PND).
- Hoarse voice.
- Did you ever cough blood up?
- Have you had any leg swelling?
- Do you suffer nasal or throat symptoms such as itchy nose, frequent sneezing, itchy throat or desire to clear the throat? (Upper airway diseases such as allergic rhinitis and post nasal drip are the most common causes of chronic cough).
- Do you have acidity or heart burn? [Gastroesophageal reflux disease (GERD) is a cause of chronic cough).
- *Diurnal variation of cough:* GERD/asthma.
- Seasonal variation of cough (exposure to different allergens such as pollens during spring).

Review of systems

- *Cardiac symptoms*: Dyspnoea, PND, orthopnoea, chest pain, leg swelling
- *Respiratory*: Wheeze, sputum
- *GIT symptoms*: GERD, dysphagia
- *General*: Fever, weight loss.

Past history

- *History of pulmonary disease:* Chronic obstructive pulmonary disease (COPD), asthma, interstitial lung disease (ILD), etc.
- History of heart disease.
- History of hypertension (HTN).
- History of diabetes mellitus (DM).
- Previous hospital admissions and vaccination.

Menstrual history in females

Not applicable.

Family history

- Family history of asthma or allergic rhinitis.
- Family history of communicable diseases.

Drug history

- Use of angiotensin-converting-enzyme (ACE) inhibitor or sitagliptin
- Hydralazine
- Alpha-blockers
- Nonsteroidal anti-inflammatory drugs
- Pioglitazone.

Social history

- History of smoking.
- History of alcohol use.
- *Recent and past occupation:* Exposure to chemicals or pollution causing lung diseases, asbestos exposure.
- Keeping pets or birds.

(Respiratory history is never complete without asking about details of occupation and keeping pets or birds)

Further information not covered (at end of history taking)

Ask the patient the following question: Is there anything else that you feel important and would like to tell me about?

Step 3: Explaining to the patient the diagnosis and the plan of management

Mr Jamil, you appear to have had a cough for 3 months and breathlessness for 2 months. You have hypertension, which is controlled, you had a stent of one of your heart vessels 5 years ago and your recent echocardiography is normal. Of relevance, you keep pigeons and clean their cages and you work as a technician, manufacturing glass. An important cause of your cough to be considered is the pigeons. Bird antigens present in the feathers and droppings can cause repeated inflammation in the lungs of people who keep birds resulting in a condition called 'hypersensitivity pneumonitis.' Repeated attacks of hypersensitivity pneumonitis can cause scarring and damage of the lungs. It is, therefore, important that you either remove the pigeons or stop contact with them to stop further damage to your lungs. In addition, as you have been working as a technician manufacturing glass, you are at risk of breathing silica dust present in the sand material used to make glass, which can cause scarring of the lungs, a disease called 'silicosis.' I will order a chest X-ray, lung function test, and some blood tests (to detect immune response to the bird antigens) as initial investigations. Based on these tests, we will see if further imaging (high resolution CT scan) or testing will be needed. A colleague who specialises in lung diseases will see you shortly.

I am also going to arrange another appointment with myself in a weeks time to see the results of the chest X-ray and lung function.

Check patient understanding and agreement on plan of management.

Does that sound clear to you?

Step 4: Ask about and address patient's concerns

Do you have any questions or concerns?

Patient's concern: Could the cause of cough and breathlessness be related to my heart?

Reply: Well, the echocardiography done recently showed normal heart contraction which makes it less likely that the problem is related to your heart. However, as you have had long-standing hypertension, it can affect how well your heart relaxes and that can give you breathlessness.

After answering each concern confirm agreement by asking; 'is that alright? Or does that sound clear to you?'

Step 5: Summarise the discussion, confirm patient's understandings, and close the meeting

Mr Jamil, I would like to summarise our discussion to be sure that you understand important information about your illness. The most probable cause for your cough and breathlessness is hypersensitivity pneumonitis caused by the pigeons. The second possibility is silicosis due to the possibility of inhaling silica dust during glass manufacturing. I am going to order a chest X-ray, blood tests as well as lung function test and will see you with the results in a weeks time. I will also arrange for you to see a lung specialist. Meanwhile, I am going to provide you with my contact number in case you have any further questions or concerns regarding your condition. Does that make sense to you? You can get more information from the internet on hypersensitivity pneumonitis and silicosis. Thank you and see you soon.

Discussion

Problem

Chronic cough and breathlessness on exertion.

Diagnosis

Hypersensitivity pneumonitis (extrinsic allergic alveolitis) due to birds.

Plausible differential diagnoses

- Silicosis (working with glass)
- Heart failure with preserved ejection fraction.

Hypersensitivity pneumonitis is a complex syndrome resulting from repeated exposure to a variety of organic particles. Hypersensitivity pneumonitis may present as acute, subacute, or chronic clinical forms but with frequent overlap of these various forms. There are many allergens that can cause the disease. Bird breeder's or pigeon fancier's disease is caused by avian droppings, feathers, serum. It can occur with exposure to parakeets, budgerigars, pigeons, chickens, and turkeys.

Farmer's lung is caused by *Saccharopolyspora rectivirgula* which is present in mouldy hay, grain, and silage. The acute form of hypersensitivity pneumonitis can be indistinguishable from an acute respiratory infection caused by viral or mycoplasma agents and is characterised by an influenza-like syndrome occurring a few hours after substantial exposure. Symptoms gradually decrease over hours/days but often recur with re-exposure. Subacute hypersensitivity pneumonitis may result from repeated low-level exposure to inhaled antigens. It is characterised by an insidious onset of dyspnoea, fatigue, and cough that develops over weeks to a few months. The chronic form is characterised by progressive dyspnoea, cough, fatigue, malaise, and weight loss. Digital clubbing may be present and predicts clinical deterioration. Often, these patients develop progressive fibrosis, and in advanced forms the disease may mimic idiopathic pulmonary fibrosis (IPF). Investigations include chest radiograph and HRCT chest that shows ground glass opacities in the acute form and fibrosis in the chronic form. Bronchoalveolar lavage (BAL) shows an elevated lymphocyte count (>15%). (BAL lymphocyte count >50% is very suggestive of HP); serologic testing for antibodies against different antigens causing HP and lung biopsy may be required. Lung function is important to detect the degree of impairment. The mainstay treatment of hypersensitivity pneumonitis is to avoid the predisposing factors (birds, farming, etc.). Corticosteroids may be used.

Silicosis is caused by the inhalation of crystalline silicon dioxide or silica which comes from chipping, cutting, drilling, or grinding soil, sand, granite, or other minerals. Any occupation where the earth's crust is disturbed can cause silicosis. Chronic silicosis is the most common form of the disease and usually develops after 10 years or more of exposure at low concentrations. Radiologically, it may cause nodules, fibrosis, and egg-shell calcifications of the hilar lymph nodes. Silicosis can predispose to many diseases such as tuberculosis, chronic obstructive pulmonary disease, autoimmune diseases such as scleroderma and rheumatoid arthritis and lung cancer.

Further reading

Leung CC, Yu IT, Chen W. Silicosis. Lancet 2012; 379:2008–2018.

Meyer KC, Raghu G, Baughman RP, et al. An official American Thoracic Society clinical practice guideline: the clinical utility of bronchoalveolar lavage cellular analysis in interstitial lung disease. Am J Respir Crit Care Med 2012; 185:1004–1014.

Selman M, Pardo A, King TE Jr. Hypersensitivity pneumonitis; insights in diagnosis and pathobiology. Am J Respir Crit Care Med 2012; 186:314–324.

Scenario no. 18

A patient with persistent diarrhoea

Candidate copy

Please read the GP referral letter for Mrs Cooper.
The time distribution for this station is as follows:

You have (---) minutes to take a history from the patient.
You have (---) minutes to collect your thoughts.
You have (---) minutes for discussion with the examiners.

Please do not examine the patient

Dear Doctor,

Thank you for seeing Mrs Cooper, a 40-year-old lady who has been complaining of diarrhoea over the last 3 weeks. Her diarrhoea seems to be worsening despite being treated with loperamide. Please do the needful.

Yours faithfully,

Please interview the patient and based on history taking, construct a differential diagnosis and plan of investigation. Provide explanation to the patient and answer any questions she may have.

Surrogate Copy

Chief complaint and HPI

- Your main complaint is loose motion (diarrhoea) for the past 3 weeks.
- In the first week, you went to the toilet 5 times per day, but this increased over the following 2 weeks to 10 times per day.
- You also wake up at night to pass stool.
- The stool is watery.
- You have also noticed mucus in the stool.
- There is no blood in the stool.
- You feel campy pain all over your tummy.
- You feel nausea but you have not vomited.
- You have lost 3 kg of your weight during this time.
- The diarrhoea is not related to any specific type of food.
- The stool is not oily and is easily flushed by water.

Review of systems

- No history of fever
- No racing heart beat
- You do not have preference for hot or cold weather.

Past history and drug history

Only if asked: You had a urinary infection more than a month ago for which you received an antibiotic called ciprofloxacin, which you took for 10 days. The diarrhoea started on the last day of the antibiotic.

Family history

There is no member of your family who suffers diarrhoea.

Social history

- You do not smoke.
- You do not drink alcohol.
- You are a social worker.
- You are happily married with two kids.
- *Only if asked:* You returned 2 months ago from a holiday to Egypt where you visited the pyramids and camped in the desert. You ate from local restaurants in Egypt.
- You have recently got two new puppies at home.

Your questions to the doctors and concerns

What is the cause of my diarrhoea?

Steps in history taking in a patient with diarrhoea

Step 1: Introduction, greeting, and confirmation of patient identity

- Good morning Mrs Cooper (shakehands with the patient), pleased to meet you.
- I am Dr X working in the medical outpatient clinic.
- Can I confirm that I am talking to Mrs Cooper?
- I have just read the referral letter from your GP which states that you complain of loose motion.
- Can you tell me more about that?
- Allow the patient to speak.
- Avoid interruptions.
- Avoid medical jargon (e.g. malabsorption, cardiac, colitis, pseudomembranous, etc.)
- *Use open ended questions such as:* What else?

Step 2: Elaborating important points in the history of diarrhoea

History of presenting illness

- How long have you had the diarrhoea?
- What is the appearance of the stool?
- How often do you pass stool per day?
- Do you wake up at night with the urge to pass stool?
    - Gluten in celiac disease
    - Milk or milk products in lactose intolerance.
- Is there any blood in the stool?
- Is there any mucus or pus in the stool?
- Is it associated with flushing of the face or neck? *(Carcinoid syndrome)*
- Is it related to certain types of food?
- Are there any symptoms suggestive of malabsorption (steatorrhoea, weight loss, flatulence, and abdominal distension)?
  Steatorrhoea is the result of fat malabsorption and typically manifests with passage of pale, bulky, and offensive stools. Due to the presence of fat, stools often float on top of the toilet water and are difficult to flush. Patients may also be able to observe oil droplets in the toilet after defecation.

- Is it associated with heat intolerance, palpitations or other symptoms of thyrotoxicosis?
  - Has the patient received any antibiotics prior to the onset of diarrhoea?
    - Drug-induced diarrhoea and clostridium difficile infection
- **Is there any recent history of camping or travel?**
  People who go for camping are at risk of exposure to water sources contaminated with *Giardia* organisms. Bacteria are the most common cause of traveller's diarrhoea. Overall, the most common pathogen is enterotoxigenic *Escherichia coli*, followed by *Campylobacter jejuni*, *Shigella* species, and *Salmonella* species. Other bacteria include *Aeromonas* spp. Viral causes of traveller's diarrhoea include: norovirus, rotavirus, and astrovirus. Protozoal causes include *Giardia* and *Entamoeba*.
- **How long after return from travel did the diarrhoea begin?**
  - Bacterial toxins generally cause symptoms within a few hours.
  - Bacterial and viral pathogens have an incubation period of 6–72 hours.
  - Protozoal pathogens generally have an incubation period of 1–2 weeks and rarely present in the first few days of travel.
- Enquire about history of contact with sick people.
- Enquire about history of contact with animals.
  - Exposure to young dogs or cats is associated with *Campylobacter* organisms.
  - Exposure to turtles is associated with *Salmonella* organisms.
- Ingestion of contaminated/rotten food.

Review of systems
- Enquire about symptoms of malabsorption.
- Enquire about symptoms of thyrotoxicosis.
- Enquire about symptoms of carcinoid.

Past medical and surgical history
- Similar diarrhoeal illness previously
- History of colonic disease/malabsorption syndrome/food intolerance.
- Past history of thyroid disease.
- Past history of diabetes.
- *Past surgery for the colon:* Blind loop syndrome and bacterial overgrowth.
- Organ transplant.

Family history
Similar illness in the family or in contacts.

Drug history
Enquire carefully about recent use of antibiotics/laxatives.

Social history
- Recent travel
- Recent camping
- Eating habits
- Sick contacts
- *Alcohol:* Chronic pancreatitis
- *Sexual history:* HIV enteropathy.

Further information not covered (at end of history taking):
Ask the patient the following question: Is there anything else that you feel important and would like to tell me about?

Step 3: Explaining to the patient the diagnosis and the plan of management
Mrs Cooper, after reviewing your history, your main complaint is loose motion or diarrhoea that has worsened with time. The loose motion started while you were taking ciprofloxacin for a urinary infection. You have also recently travelled to Egypt for a

holiday where you went camping in the desert and you recently got 2 puppies at home. I think the most likely cause of your loose motion is the recent use of the ciprofloxacin. Prolonged use of antibiotics can kill not only the bacteria causing the urinary infection, but also bacteria in the intestines allowing other bacteria called *Clostridium difficile* to overgrow. Overgrowth of *Clostridium difficile* can cause inflammation of the colon, a condition called 'pseudomembranous colitis.' Symptoms of pseudomembranous colitis can begin as soon as 1–2 days after you start taking an antibiotic or can come on several weeks after you finish taking the antibiotic. However, I am going to order some stool tests to check for bacterial toxin and other bacteria or parasites in the stool. Because you were recently camping in Egypt, you could have also ingested parasites like *Giardia* and Amoeba that can cause loose motion. Therefore, I will order a stool test to check for such parasites. I will also prescribe another antibiotic called metronidazole, which specifically kills the *Clostridium* and other possible parasites such as Giardia and Amoeba. You need to take it for 10 days. Meanwhile, I strongly recommend that you take plenty of fluids to compensate for the water you are losing through the stool and prevent dehydration. I will also notify the infection control staff in the hospital to prevent other people from getting the infection.

I will see you next week to discuss the results of the stool tests and see how your symptoms respond to treatment with metronidazole.

Check patient understanding and agreement on plan of management.

Does that make sense to you?

Step 4: Ask about and address patient's concerns

Do you have any questions or concerns?

Patient's concern: What causes my loose stool?

Reply: Answered.

After answering each concern, confirm the agreement by saying; "is that okay or does that sound good for you?"

Step 5: Summarise the discussion, confirm patient's understandings, and close the meeting

Mrs Cooper, I would like to summarise our discussion to be sure that you understand important information about your illness. The most probable cause for your loose motion is a condition called pseudomembranous colitis caused by the antibiotic ciprofloxacin. I will request some stool tests and prescribe metronidazole. I would suggest that you drink plenty of water and fluids. I will see you next week to give you more answers about your illness. Meanwhile, I am going to provide you with my contact number in case you have any further questions or concerns regarding your condition. Does that sound clear to you? You can also get information from the internet on pseudomembranous colitis. Thank you and see you soon.

Discussion

Problem

Persistent diarrhoea.

Diagnosis

Pseudomembranous colitis (patient received ciprofloxacin for UTI, and the diarrhoea started on day 10 of the antibiotic).

Other plausible diagnosis

- **Giardiasis**
  She recently went camping in Egypt.

- **Campylobacter infection**
  She recently got two puppies.

Clostridium difficile is a Gram-positive, spore-forming bacterium usually spread by the feco-oral route. It is noninvasive and produces toxins A and B that cause the disease. Most patients present with mild to moderate watery diarrhoea. Bloody diarrhoea is rare, occurring in less than a quarter of patients. Other symptoms include cramping abdominal pain, anorexia, malaise and fever, especially in more severe cases.

Risk factors for *clostridium difficile* infection (CDI)

The two major risk factors are:
1. Exposure to antibiotics.
2. Exposure to the organism.

Others risk factors include

- Chemotherapeutic agents
- Prolonged hospitalisation or residence in nursing homes
- Old age
- Use of proton pump inhibitors
- Ulcerative colitis or Crohn's disease.

All patients with inflammatory bowel disease hospitalised with a disease flare should undergo testing for *C. difficile*. Only stool from patients with diarrhoea should be tested for *C. difficile*. Previously, toxin A + B enzyme-linked immunoassays were the most widely used diagnostic tests because of ease of use and objective interpretation. Nucleic acid amplification tests for *C. difficile* toxin genes such as PCR are superior to toxins A + B enzyme immunoassay as a standard diagnostic test for CDI.

Management of suspected CDI

- Empiric therapy for CDI should be considered if clinically suspected regardless of the laboratory testing.
- Any inciting antimicrobial agent(s) should be discontinued, if possible.
- Either vancomycin or fidaxomicin is recommended over metronidazole for an initial episode of CDI.
- The dosage of vancomycin 125 mg orally 4 times per day or fidaxomicin 200 mg twice daily for 10 days.
- If vancomycin or fidaxomicin are not available, Metronidazole can be used for an initial episode of non-severe CDI only.
- For fulminant CDI, vancomycin administered orally is the regimen of choice. The dosage is 500 mg orally 4 times per day and 500 mg in approximately 100 mL normal saline per rectum every 6 hours as a retention enema. Intravenously administered Metronidazole should be administered together with oral or rectal vancomycin, particularly if ileus is present.
- The use of antiperistaltic agents to control diarrhoea from confirmed or suspected CDI should be limited or avoided, as they may obscure symptoms and precipitate complicated disease. Use of antiperistaltic agents in the setting of CDI must always be accompanied by medical therapy for CDI.
- Supportive care should be delivered to all patients with CDI and includes fluid resuscitation and electrolyte replacement.
- In the absence of ileus or significant abdominal distention, oral or enteral feeding should be continued.

Complications of pseudomembranous colitis include

- Volume and electrolyte loss
- Toxic megacolon
- Sepsis
- Bowel perforation.

Giardiasis is a ubiquitous parasitic infection. The infection produces classic steatorrhoea and malabsorption associated with bloating, nausea, and emesis. The disease is often difficult to differentiate from inflammatory bowel disease. *Giardia* may be transmitted via contaminated food, water or direct person-person contact (faecal oral spread common in day care centres and residential institutions). Giardiasis comprises an appreciable percentage of travel-associated infection mediated persistent/chronic diarrhoea. The diagnosis is best rendered with a stool ELISA measuring the *Giardia* antigen. Treatment is affected with a 7–10 days course of metronidazole. *Campylobacter* organisms can also be an important cause of traveller's diarrhoea. Infected animals and their products are the major source of infection. Transmission to humans may occur through consumption of infected animal products such as unpasteurised animal milk and milk products, undercooked poultry, and through contaminated drinking water. Recent contact with pets, especially puppies, has been identified as an important source of the infection. Most colonised animals develop a lifelong carrier state.

Further reading

Duplessis CA, Gutierrez RL, Porter CK. Chronic and persistent diarrhoea with a focus in the returning traveller. Trop Dis Travel Med Vaccines 2017; 3:9.

Gutierrez RL, Goldberg M, Young P, et al. Management of service members presenting with persistent and chronic diarrhoea, during or upon returning from deployment. Mil Med 2012; 177:627–634.

McDonald LC, Gerding DN, Johnson S, et al. Clinical practice guidelines for Clostridium difficile infection in adults and children: 2017 update by the Infectious Diseases Society of America (IDSA) and Society for Healthcare Epidemiology of America. Clin Infect Dis 2018; 66:e1–e48.

Sarkar SR, Hossain MA, Paul SK, et al. Campylobacteriosis: an overview. Mymensingh Med J 2014; 23:173–180.

Surawicz CM, Brandt LJ, Binion DG, et al. Guidelines for diagnosis, treatment, and prevention of Clostridium difficile infections. Am J Gastroenterol 2013; 108:478–498.

Scenario no. 19

A young woman with chest pain

Candidate copy

Please read the emergency room doctor referral letter for Ms Halpern.
The time distribution for this station is as follows:

>   You have (---) minutes to take a history from the patient.
>   You have (---) minutes to collect your thoughts.
>   You have (---) minutes for discussion with the examiners.

Please do not examine the patient

> **Dear Doctor,**
>
> Thank you for seeing Ms Halpern. She is a 33-year-old woman who had recurrent episodes of retrosternal chest pain while sleeping last night. The pain is radiating to the left shoulder. Her ECG done after sublingual nitroglycerine was unremarkable and her serum troponins were normal.
>
> Yours faithfully,

> Please interview the patient and based on history taking construct a differential diagnosis and plan of investigation. Provide explanation to the patient and answer any questions she may have.

Surrogate Copy

Chief complaint and HPI

- You came to the emergency room because of severe retrosternal chest pain.
- The pain is squeezing in nature.
- It started late in the night the previous day and lasted for 1 hour.
- It was relieved by a nitroglycerine tablet that was given to you by the emergency room doctor.
- You have had similar episodes of pain over the last 6 months and you have visited emergency room 3 times in the last month.
- The pain is not related to exercise but rather you feel it comes on more at rest, particularly at night.
- It is not related to eating.
- There is no difficulty in breathing.
- There is associated sweating during the attack of pain and a feeling of dizziness.
- You have had multiple ECGs in emergency room during your previous visits. Apart from one ECG that showed a little elevation in the chest leads, all the other ECGs were normal.
- Your GP told you it might all be psychological.

Review of systems

- You do not have stomach or acid problems.
- You do not have breathlessness.
- Although you feel some dizziness during the attacks of pain, you have never lost consciousness.

Past history and drug history

- You have been suffering from migraine for the past 3 years, which affects one side of your head and you are taking sumatriptan 100 mg for the acute attacks and propranolol 40 mg three times daily regularly.
- You have not had heart disease or clots in your legs.

Menstrual history

- Your periods are normal and regular
- You are using the contraceptive pill.

Family history

Your sister had a clot in her leg late during her pregnancy. She took treatment for 3 months.

Social history

- You do not smoke.
- You *drink alcohol* 3–4 glasses of whisky every week.
- You work as a waitress in a hotel.
- You sniff cocaine almost daily.
- You are single.
- You had a boyfriend.

Your questions to the doctors and concerns

I know a friend of mine who had chest pain and turned out to have clot in her lung? Is my condition serious?

Steps in history taking in a patient with chest pain

Step 1: Introduction, greeting, and confirmation of patient identity

- Good morning Ms Halpern (shakehands with the patient), pleased to meet you.
- I am Dr X working in the medical department.
- Can I confirm that I am talking to Ms Halpern?
- The emergency room doctor requested my opinion regarding your chest pain.
- Can you tell me more about that?
- Allow the patient to speak.
- Avoid interruptions.
- Avoid medical jargon (e.g. myocardial infarction, manometry, coronary, etc.)
- *Use open ended questions such as:* What else?

Step 2: Elaborating important points in the history of chest pain

History of presenting illness

- Chest pain should be analysed with LIQOR AAA
- Enquire about associated symptoms:
  - *Dyspnoea, PND, orthopnoea:* Cardiac cause
  - *Palpitations:* Pulmonary embolism
  - Syncope
  - Dizziness
  - *GIT symptoms:* Heart burn/acidity.

Review of systems

Review carefully the cardiovascular, respiratory, and GIT systems.

Menstrual history

- History of recurrent abortions (pulmonary embolism/antiphospholipid).
- Use of oral contraceptive pills (pulmonary embolism).

Past medical history

- Heart disease
- *Coronary risk factors:* Diabetes, hypertension, dyslipidaemia
- Previous pulmonary embolism or deep vein thrombosis (DVT)
- History of GERD, oesophageal disease or peptic ulcer.

Family history

- Heart disease
- Pulmonary embolism/DVT.

Drug history

- *Migraine tablets:* Triptans and ergot alkaloids may cause coronary vasospasm (Prinzmetal angina).
- Use of cardiac medications or other medications.

Social history

- Smoking
- Alcohol
- *Drugs abuse:* Cocaine (may cause spasm), use of NSAIDs
- Occupation
- *How pain has affected the patient's life:* Job, finance, family, daily activity, and sexual life.

Further information not covered (at end of history taking)

Ask the patient the following question: Is there anything else that you feel important and would like to tell me about?

Step 3: Explaining to the patient the diagnosis and the plan of management

Ms Halpern it seems you have been getting recurrent attacks of a squeezing chest pain that usually comes on at night and is not related to activity. You have migraine and you are taking sumatriptan during the attack and propranolol on a daily basis. You also sniff cocaine almost every day. I think the most probable cause of your chest pain is spasm of one of the vessels that supply your heart muscles with blood. This condition is called 'Prinzmetal angina.' it decreases the width of the coronary artery and deprives the heart muscles of blood and oxygen, triggering chest discomfort. There are also some other conditions that can precipitate the spasm in the heart arteries. These include migraine tablets, cocaine, and beta-blockers drugs like propranolol. Does this make sense to you?

I understand that my colleagues in emergency room have undertaken a tracing of electrical activity of your heart (ECG) and taken some blood tests, which were all normal. Unfortunately, these tests can be normal particularly if you take nitroglycerine before they are done. I am going to ask one of my cardiology colleagues to have a look at you and perform coronary angiogram where he will visualise your heart vessels using a contrast material. Meanwhile, I am going to request some blood tests to exclude other causes of chest pain such as clots in the lungs. I will also prescribe for you some medications to relax your artery muscles and help reduce the spasm. These medications are called calcium channel blockers. It is very important that you quit cocaine as it can precipitate coronary artery spasm. If you agree, I will also seek the opinion of my colleagues who specialise in treating addiction. In addition, you also need to discuss with your migraine doctor about changing your sumatriptan and propranolol for an alternative medication like naproxen.

Check patient understanding and agreement on plan of management.

Does that make sense to you?

Step 4: Ask about and address patient's concerns

Do you have any questions or concerns?

Patient's concern: One of my friends had chest pain and she turned out to have a clot in her lung?

Reply: Clots in the lungs can also cause chest pain, but the pain due to clots is typically sharp or knife-like and worsens when you take a big breath in. Of course, it is important to exclude such clots, keeping in mind that your sister had a clot in her leg, and you are on the contraceptive pill. Therefore, I am going to order a blood test called D-dimer to help exclude a clot in the lungs.

Patient's concern: Is my condition serious?

Reply: Prinzmetal angina, if prolonged and not treated appropriately, can cause death of heart muscle and can precipitate an abnormal heart rhythm leading to sudden death.

After answering each concern confirm agreement by saying, 'is that okay or does that make sense to you?'

Step 5: Summarise the discussion, confirm patient's understandings, and close the meeting

Ms Halpern, I would like to summarise our discussion to be sure you understand important information about your illness. The most probable cause for your chest pain is repeated spasm in the arteries supplying blood to your heart. A colleague who specialises in heart disease will see you and undertake imaging of the heart arteries. Meanwhile, it is very important that you quit cocaine and you change your current migraine treatment. I will prescribe some medications that help to reduce the spasm of the coronary arteries. Meanwhile, I am going to provide you with my contact number in case you have any further questions or concerns regarding your condition. Does that sound good to you? You can also get information from the internet on Prinzmetal angina. Thank you and see you soon.

Discussion

Problem

Chest pain.

Diagnosis

Prinzmetal angina precipitated by cocaine and migraine treatment.

Other plausible diagnosis

- Pulmonary embolism
- Unstable angina.

Differentiating the cause of chest pain

Anginal pain

- Usually central/retrosternal
- Burning, tightening, or heaviness
- Radiates to left shoulder, arm and jaw
- Aggravated by exertion and emotional stress (sometimes meals)
- Relieved by sublingual nitroglycerine/ rest
- Angina lasts up to 10 or 20 minutes
- May be associated with dyspnoea, nausea, vomiting, dizziness.

Myocardial infarction pain:

- Crushing type
- Lasts >20 minutes
- Not relieved by rest
- Associated with dyspnoea, nausea, vomiting, dizziness.

Prinzmetal angina (variant angina/angina inversa)

- Caused by coronary vasospasm rather than atherosclerosis.
- The pain is similar to angina pain.
- But it comes at rest and very rarely on exertion.
- It is usually episodic.
- Usually occurs while resting and during the night or early morning hours.
- Usually severe.
- Can be relieved by nitroglycerine.
- Associated with ST elevation but normal troponins.
- *Risk factors include:* Heavy cigarette smoking, use of cocaine, use of migraine medication such as triptans and exposure to severe cold weather.

Pulmonary embolism/pleuritic pain

- Usually
- Sharp/stabbing
- Aggravated by deep breathing
- Associated with palpitations
- Lasts for days.

Acute aortic dissection

- Tearing pain
- Sudden onset
- Radiates to the back
- Very severe
- Persistent
- Associated with high blood pressure
- May lead to stroke, paraplegia.

Oesophageal spasm

- Retrosternal
- Usually squeezing

- May radiate to the back.
- Aggravated by swallowing food
- There may be a long history of GERD.
- May be relieved by sublingual nitroglycerine.

Gastroesophageal reflux

- Burning
- Retrosternal and epigastric
- Aggravated by certain types of food (spicy, sour), lying supine
- Relieved by antacids, proton pump inhibitors (PPIs).

Vasospastic angina, variant angina, or prinzmetal angina is a clinical entity which is characterised by chest pain at rest with transient ischemic electrocardiographic changes in the ST segment, with prompt response to nitrates. These symptoms are attributed to coronary artery spasm. There are multiple triggers for vasospastic angina including drugs such as ephedrine and sumatriptan which can cause coronary artery spasm. Recreational substances like cocaine, amphetamines, alcohol, and marijuana are also possible precipitating factors. Exposure to cold weather or bathing with very cold water can also cause spasm in the coronaries. The chest pain caused by coronary spasm is typically at rest, occurs between midnight and early morning and responds to nitroglycerine but is not related to exertion. The diagnostic criteria of Prinzmetal angina include clinical response to nitrates during a spontaneous angina episode, transient ischemic electrocardiographic changes and evidence of coronary vasospasm during angiography. The diagnosis is established by visualisation of coronary spasm during cardiac catheterisation that is seen spontaneously or under induction using ergonovine or acetylcholine. An ambulatory electrocardiogram can be used to record transient electrocardiographic changes during acute spontaneous events. Calcium antagonists are the first-line treatment due to their vasodilation effect in the coronary vasculature. They alleviate symptoms in 90% of patients and prevent myocardial infarction. A high dose of long-acting calcium antagonists like diltiazem, amlodipine, nifedipine, or verapamil are recommended.

Further reading

JCS Joint Working Group. Guidelines for diagnosis and treatment of patients with vasospastic angina (Coronary Spastic Angina) (JCS 2013). Circ J 2014; 78:2779–2801.

Rodriguez Ziccardi M, Gossman WG. Angina, Prinz metal. In: StatPearls. Treasure Island (FL): StatPearls Publishing; 2018-2017.

Scenario no. 20

A patient with chest pain

Candidate copy

Please read the GP referral letter for Mrs Amal.
The time distribution for this station is as follows:

 You have (---) minutes to take a history from the patient.
 You have (---) minutes to collect your thoughts.
 You have (---) minutes for discussion with the examiners.

Please do not examine the patient

Dear Doctor,

Thank you for seeing Mrs Amal, a 55-year-old with a history of mixed connective tissue disease and hypertension. She is on oral corticosteroids and methotrexate. She complains of retrosternal squeezing chest pain that radiates to the back for the last 2 weeks and is relieved by sublingual nitroglycerin. Her ECG and cardiac troponins were unremarkable.

Yours faithfully,

Please interview the patient and based on history taking construct a differential diagnosis and plan of investigation. Provide explanation to the patient and answer any questions she may have.

Surrogate Copy

Chief complaint and HPI

- You suffer from pain in the centre of your chest.
- The pain comes and goes.
- Each episode of pain lasts for 1–2 hours.
- The pain is squeezing.
- The pain is sometimes so severe that it prevents you from sleeping.
- It is not related to exercise and can come on at rest.
- The pain is also felt in your back but does not go to your shoulders, arms or neck.
- It usually gets worse after eating particularly after dinner when you go to sleep.
- There is no difficulty in breathing.
- There is no sweating during the attack of pain.
- Your GP prescribed a nitroglycerine tablet that you put under the tongue and it relieves the pain.
- *Only when asked:*
  - There is difficulty in swallowing food and water and sometimes the food sticks in your throat.
  - You have suffered acidity and heart burn for a long time.
  - You also suffer regurgitation of food.

Review of systems

- You do not have joint pain.
- You have not had hair loss.
- You do not have mouth ulcers or skin rash.
- You do not have any problems with your urine.
- You have not noticed any swelling in your abdomen.
- You do not have kidney disease.
- Your urine is not frothy.

Past history and drug history

You have had mixed connective tissue disease since the age of 35. It started with pain in your hand and knee joints with fatigue and muscle weakness. You had multiple blood tests and your doctor who specialises in joints told you it was a mixed connective tissue disease. You are taking prednisolone 10 mg daily and methotrexate 10 mg weekly. You also have severe osteoporosis and you are taking vitamin D 50,000 units and alendronate (Fosamax) 70 mg weekly.

The mixed connective tissue disease is well controlled, and it has not affected your kidneys or lungs.

Menstrual history

Your periods stopped 4 years ago.

Social history

- You do not smoke.
- You do not drink alcohol.
- You work as a school teacher.
- You are married with two children.

Your questions to the doctors and concerns

Could the pain be coming from my heart?

Steps in history taking in a patient with chest pain

Step 1: Introduction, greeting, and confirmation of patient identity

- Good morning Mrs Amal (shakehands with the patient), pleased to meet you.
- I am Dr X working in the medical outpatient clinic.
- Can I confirm that I am talking to Mrs Amal?
- I have just read the referral letter from your GP who states that you have chest pain.
- Can you tell me more about that?
- Allow the patient to speak.
- Avoid interruptions.
- Avoid medical jargon (e.g. angina, myocardial infarction, manometry, coronary, etc.)
- *Use open ended questions such as:* What else?

Step 2: Elaborating important points in the history of chest pain

History of presenting illness

- Chest pain should be analysed with LIQOR AAA.
- Enquire about associated symptoms:
  - Dyspnoea, PND, orthopnoea (cardiac cause)
  - Palpitations (pulmonary embolism)
  - Syncope
  - Dizziness
  - Heart burn/acidity.

Review of systems

Review carefully the cardiovascular, respiratory, and GIT systems.

Menstrual history

- History of recurrent abortions (pulmonary embolism/antiphospholipid).
- Use of oral contraceptive pill (pulmonary embolism).

Past medical history:

- Heart disease
- *Coronary risk factors:* Diabetes, hypertension, dyslipidaemia
- Previous pulmonary embolism or DVT
- History of GERD, oesophageal disease or peptic ulcer.

Family history

- Heart disease
- Pulmonary embolism/DVT

Drug history
- *Migraine tablets*: Triptans and ergot alkaloids may cause coronary vasospasm.
- Use of cardiac medications or other medications.

Social history
- Smoking
- Alcohol
- *Drug abuse*: Cocaine (may cause spasm), NSAIDs
- Occupation
- *How has pain affected the patient's life*: Job, finance, family, daily activity, and sexual life.

Further information not covered (at end of history taking)
Ask the patient the following question: Is there anything else that you feel important and would like to tell me about?

Step 3: Explaining to the patient the diagnosis and the plan of management
Mrs Amal, you have been getting recurrent attacks of chest pain that are squeezing in nature and get worse after food. You also suffer with difficulty in swallowing and heart burn. You are currently being treated for mixed connective tissue disease and osteoporosis. Your GP has done an ECG and some blood tests, and they are both normal. The most likely cause of your chest pain is a problem with your food pipe or oesophagus. Up to 80% of people who suffer scleroderma, a component of mixed connective tissue disease, can develop abnormal function of their oesophagus. This can take the form of abnormal movement of the muscles of the oesophagus called 'motility disorder,' regurgitation of stomach acid into the oesophagus leading to inflammation and irritation of the esophagus 'called GERD' or development of narrowed segments of the oesophagus called a 'stricture.' All these, particularly the motility disorder can cause chest pain difficulty in swallowing and regurgitation of food. Another potentially important contributor is the alendronate tablet for osteoporosis as it can cause inflammation in the oesophagus and may cause heart burn or chest pain. I assume that you have already been told to take this tablet in the morning before food with plenty of water and to stay upright for at least 30 minutes after swallowing the tablet, to reduce the chances of inflaming the oesophagus. Finally, steroids and methotrexate can increase your risk of fungal infection in the oesophagus. I am going to order a test called manometry to measure the function of the muscles of the oesophagus. I am also going to refer you to my colleague who specialises in diseases of the oesophagus to pass a special camera into your oesophagus to look for inflammation, infection or narrowing. Meanwhile, I will prescribe some tablets to reduce the production of the acids in your stomach, which will help to relieve your symptoms.

I am going to arrange another appointment with myself in 1 week, to see the effect on your symptoms and to discuss the results of your investigations.

Check patient understanding and agreement on plan of management.

Does that make sense to you?

Step 4: Ask about and address patient's concerns
Do you have any questions or concerns?

Patient's concern: Could this pain be due to angina?

Reply: Well, angina does give chest pain, but this is usually related to activity or exercise and relieved by rest. In addition, you have other symptoms like the difficulty in swallowing and heart burn which can occur in mixed connective tissue disease.

The normal ECG and heart blood tests point to an oesophageal origin of your pain.

After answering each concern confirm agreement by saying, 'is that ok or does that make sense to you?'

Step 5: Summarise the discussion, confirm patient's understandings, and close the meeting

Mrs Amal, I would like to summarise our discussion to be sure you understand important information about your illness. The most probable origin for your chest pain is your oesophagus because of the scleroderma component of your mixed connective tissue disease, which may have been worsened by the alendronate. In addition, steroids and methotrexate can also lead to fungal infection in the oesophagus. I am going to arrange for oesophageal manometry and will refer you to a colleague who will pass a camera into your oesophagus and see if there are any problems there. Meanwhile, I will prescribe some medication to relieve your symptoms and will see you in a week time to give you further answers. Meanwhile, I am going to provide you with my contact number in case you have any further questions or concerns regarding your condition. Does that sound good to you? You can also get information from the internet on oesophageal diseases in scleroderma. Thank you and see you soon.

Discussion

Problem

Chest pain.

Diagnosis

Scleroderma-related oesophageal spasm, GERD or stricture.

Other plausible diagnosis

- Candida esophagitis
- Alendronate-induced esophagitis.

Differentiating the cause of chest pain

Anginal pain

- Usually central/retrosternal
- Burning, tightening or heaviness
- Radiates to left shoulder, arm, and jaw
- Aggravated by exertion and emotional stress (sometimes meals)
- Relieved by sublingual nitroglycerine/rest
- Angina lasts up to 10–20 minutes
- May be associated with dyspnoea, nausea, vomiting, dizziness.

Myocardial infarction pain

- Crushing type
- Lasts >20 minutes
- Not relieved by rest
- Associated with dyspnoea, nausea, vomiting, dizziness.

Pulmonary embolism/pleuritic pain

- Sharp/stabbing
- Aggravated by deep breathing
- Associated with palpitations
- Lasts for days.

Acute aortic dissection

- Tearing pain
- Sudden onset
- Radiates to the back
- Very severe
- Persistent
- Associated with high blood pressure
- May lead to stroke, paraplegia.

Oesophageal spasm

- Retrosternal
- Usually squeezing
- May radiate to the back
- Aggravated by swallowing food
- There may be a long history of GERD.
- May be relieved by sublingual nitroglycerine.

Gastroesophageal reflux

- Burning
- Retrosternal and epigastric
- Aggravated by certain types of food (spicy, sour), lying supine
- Relieved by antacids, PPI.

Oesophageal involvement in systemic sclerosis is common, occurring in up to 80% of patients. It carries significant morbidity and mortality, which can be improved by early diagnosis and treatment. Patients with systemic sclerosis and oesophageal involvement usually report two types of symptoms: GERD due to heartburn and regurgitation, and/or oesophageal dysmotility leading to chest pain or dysphagia. Dysphagia may not only represent a symptom of dysmotility but could also be the result of Candida esophagitis or a peptic stricture due to complicated GERD. High-resolution manometry is the gold standard method to identify systemic sclerosis patients with oesophageal motility disorders. It uses multiple closely spaced pressure sensors that allow an assessment of the whole oesophagus and especially of the lower oesophageal sphincter. Treatment for systemic sclerosis-related esophageal disorders includes use of PPIs, prokinetics, and endoscopic interventions. Buspirone, a 5-HT1A receptor agonist has shown a significant benefit on both manometric and clinical parameters in systemic sclerosis patients with oesophageal involvement.

Further reading

Denaxas K, Ladas SD, Karamanolis GP. Evaluation and management of esophageal manifestations in systemic sclerosis. Ann Gastroenterol 2018; 31:165–170.

Scenario no. 21

A patient with breakthrough seizure

Candidate copy

Please read the GP referral letter for Mrs Bolton.
The time distribution for this station is as follows:
    You have (---) minutes to take a history from the patient.
    You have (---) minutes to collect your thoughts.
    You have (---) minutes for discussion with the examiners.

Please do not examine the patient

> **Dear Doctor,**
>
> Thank you for seeing Mrs Bolton, a 35-year-old who was diagnosed with epilepsy 2 years ago. Her epilepsy was well-controlled on sodium valproate 500 mg twice daily as she has been seizure-free for 12 months. However, over the past week, she has experienced breakthrough seizures despite taking her valproic acid regularly.
>
> Yours faithfully,

Please interview the patient and based on history taking construct a differential diagnosis and plan of investigation. Provide explanation to the patient and answer any questions she may have.

Surrogate copy

Chief complaint and HPI

You were diagnosed with epilepsy at the age of 33 and you are taking sodium valproate tablets 500 mg twice daily. Your epilepsy has been well-controlled on this medication and for the last 12 months, you have not had any seizures. However, over the last week you have had 1–2 seizures daily. During the attack, your husband states that your arms and legs start shaking and you have bit your tongue and lost consciousness. On two occasions, you found that you had wet yourself. These attacks usually last a few minutes. You see zigzag lines before each attack.

Review of systems

- You do not have a fever.
- You have suffered from a headache when you fell 2 weeks ago after having getting drunk. You had a minor head injury and have some bruises on the right side of your head.
- The headache is a mild ache, mainly on the right side and gets better with paracetamol.

Menstrual history

Normal.

Family history

Normal.

Past history

You have had recurrent urinary tract infections since the age of 3 years. The last infection was 3 weeks ago with antibiotic-resistant bacteria.

Drug history

You are taking valproic acid 500 mg twice daily for 2 years and you take your medication regularly and you have never stopped it. You are taking paracetamol for your recent headache after the fall. You have been taking Orlistat 120 mg three times daily to reduce weight over the last 2 months and you have lost 3 kg. You recently completed a course of intravenous Ertapenem for a urinary tract infection.

Social history

- You smoke 5 cigarettes every day for the last 5 years.
- You are married but you do not have children.
- You have drunk two glasses of whisky every day since the age of 25. However, after the death of your father last month, you have been drinking 1 bottle of whisky every day.
- You work as a supervisor in a construction company.

Your questions to the doctors and concerns

What has caused my seizures to come back?

Steps in history taking in a patient with uncontrolled seizure

Step 1: Introduction, greeting, and confirmation of patient identity

- Good morning Mrs Bolton (shakehands with the patient), pleased to meet you.
- I am Dr X working in the medical outpatient clinic.
- Can I confirm that I am talking to Mrs Bolton?
- I have just read the referral letter from your GP who states that your epilepsy has no longer been controlled over the last week.
- Can you tell me more about that?
- Allow the patient to speak.
- Avoid interruptions.
- Avoid medical jargon (e.g. coma, status epilepticus, etc.)
- Use open ended questions such as: What else?

Step 2: Elaborating important points in the history of uncontrolled seizure

History of presenting illness

- Was it witnessed by someone else?
- Was it sudden?
- What were the circumstances before the episode?
- What was the patient doing when the seizure occurred?
- Did the patient become unaware of the surrounding?
- Was the attack preceded by an aura?
- Was the attack preceded by headache?
- How many times did it happen?
- How long did the attack last?
- Did the patient sustain any head trauma before the attack?
- Did the patient bite his/her tongue/injure him/herself during the attack?
- Did the patient lose sphincter control during the attack?
- Were there any jerky movements with the attack? If yes, where did they start and how did they proceed?
- Was the attack associated with weakness, tingling/numbness, headache, double vision?
- How did the attack end?
- Did it end spontaneously or with the administration of glucose or benzodiazepines?
- What happened after the attack?
- Did the patient experience any confusion or weakness?
- Was any blood test done before or during the attack, e.g. blood sugar and electrolytes and what was the result?

Review of systems

- Ask about other neurological symptoms in detail.
- Ask about palpitations and chest pain (arrhythmia can lead to a loss of consciousness).
- Review other systems.

Past history

- Past history of similar episodes.
- Past history of epilepsy.
- Past history of diabetes (if yes enquire about details of glycaemic control and hypoglycaemia).
- Past history of neurological, cardiac, renal disease.
- Past history of depression or psychiatric diseases (drugs/suicide).
- Previous accidents or head trauma.

Family history

- Family history of epilepsy.
- Family history of arrhythmias.

Drug history

- Drug history must be checked very carefully, particularly in the elderly.
- Ask about adherence and use of antiepileptic medications. Make sure that the patient is taking the correct dose in a regular manner and the right antiepileptic medication.
- Name the drugs you were taking before the incident.
- What over the counter medications were you taking?
- Ask about any withdrawal or sudden discontinuation of any medication (such as benzodiazepines and neuropsychiatric medications) before the incident. Drug withdrawal is an important cause for the loss of consciousness, seizure, and confusion. Check drug interaction with antiepileptic medications.

Social history

- Details of alcohol intake (excessive alcohol consumption may lead to poor epilepsy control/withdrawal/head injury, etc.)
- Drug abuse
- Living conditions
- Recent travel.

Further information not covered (at end of history taking)

Ask the patient the following question: Is there anything else that you feel important and would like to tell me about?

Step 3: Explaining to the patient the diagnosis and the plan of management

Mrs Bolton, it seems your main complaint is the recent return of epileptic seizures over the last week following a 12-month period of controlled epilepsy on valproate tablets. You have had a fall and head injury after excessive alcohol consumption 2 weeks ago. You also received a course of Ertapenem for a urinary infection shortly before this problem and you are taking Orlistat to lose weight for about 2 months. There are some potential reasons why you have had a worsening of your epilepsy. Firstly, both Ertapenem and Orlistat can interfere with the action of valproic acid by decreasing the blood concentration of valproic acid and reduce its effect. Increased alcohol consumption can also lead to increased seizures. Head injury can lead to the collection of blood under the skull and trigger seizures. We need to urgently undertake a CT scan of your brain to exclude a blood collection. I also strongly recommend that you gradually reduce your alcohol consumption as this will help to reduce the seizure activity. I also recommend that you stop taking Orlistat which can interfere with the action of valproate. You can ask your obesity doctor to change it to an alternative medication for obesity. Please always alert your doctors about your antiepileptic medication so that they do not prescribe other medications that interfere with its action.

I am going to arrange an immediate CT scan of your brain to exclude a blood collection in the head and I will see you shortly to be able to give you further answers. A colleague who specialises in epilepsy will also see you soon. I assume your epilepsy doctor has already informed you about driving, contraception, and pregnancy while having epilepsy.

Check patient understanding and agreement on plan of management.

Does that sound good to you?

Step 4: Ask about and address patient's concerns

Do you have any questions or concerns?

> *Patient's concern*: What caused my seizures to come back?

> *Reply*: Answered

> After answering each concern, confirm agreement by saying, 'is that ok or does that sound good for you?'

Step 5: Summarise the discussion, confirm patient's understanding, and close the meeting

Mrs Bolton, I would like to summarise our discussion to be sure you understand important information about your illness. The possible causes for loss of control of your epilepsy are the use of Ertapenem and Orlistat, the recent head injury, and the increase in alcohol consumption. I am going to arrange an urgent CT scan of your head to exclude a blood collection and I strongly recommend that you gradually reduce your alcohol consumption and stop Orlistat. A colleague who specialises in epilepsy will see you very soon. Meanwhile, I am going to provide you with my contact number in case you have any further questions or concerns regarding your condition. Does that sound good to you? You can also get some information from the internet regarding epilepsy. Thank you and see you soon.

Discussion

Problem

Uncontrolled epilepsy with breakthrough seizure.

Diagnosis

- *Drug interaction with antiepileptic medication*
  - Ertapenem and Orlistat.
- *Head injury*
  - Concussion/subdural haematoma.
- *Excessive alcohol consumption.*

Other plausible diagnosis

- Poor adherence to antiepileptic medication.
- Improper treatment of epilepsy/inadequate dosage.

Breakthrough seizures

When a patient with a sustained period free from seizures (seizure control) suddenly experiences a seizure, such an event is commonly referred to as a breakthrough seizure.

Causes of a breakthrough seizure

- Poor compliance with antiepileptic medication.
- Persistent epileptic focus
- Recent neurologic insult (stroke, haemorrhage)
- Use of medications that interact with antiepileptic drugs.
- Excessive alcohol consumption
- Sleep deprivation
- Excessive TV/game watching
- Exertion and emotional stress
- Ongoing infections
- Metabolic events (such as a decrease in sodium or glucose levels).

Further reading

Bonnett LJ, Powell GA, Tudur Smith C, et al. Breakthrough seizures—further analysis of the Standard versus New Antiepileptic Drugs (SANAD) study. PLoS ONE 2017; 12:e0190035.

Ettinger AB, Adiga RK. Breakthrough Seizures—Approach to prevention and diagnosis. US Neurology 2008; 4:40–42.

Kaddumukasa M, Kaddumukasa M, Matovu S, et al. The frequency and precipitating factors for breakthrough seizures among patients with epilepsy in Uganda. BMC Neurol 2013; 13:182.

Kumar S. Factors precipitating breakthrough seizures in well-controlled epilepsy. Indian Pediatr 2005; 42:182–183.

Scenario no. 22

A patient with facial pain

Candidate copy

Please read the referral letter for Ms Ruby from her dentist.
The time distribution for this station is as follows:

> You have (---) minutes to take a history from the patient.
> You have (---) minutes to collect your thoughts.
> You have (---) minutes for discussion with the examiners.

Please do not examine the patient

Dear Doctor,

Thank you for seeing Ms Ruby, a 25-year-old who has been complaining of recurrent severe right facial pain over the last 3 months. The pain is becoming very severe and not responding to NSAIDs. Her dental examination was unremarkable.

Yours faithfully,

Please interview the patient and based on history taking construct a differential diagnosis and plan of investigation. Provide explanation to the patient and answer any questions she may have.

Surrogate copy

Chief complaint and HPI

- You have been referred from your dentist as you complain of severe pain in the right side of your face for the past 3 months.
- In the beginning, you thought this may be caused by problems with your teeth as your pain was sometimes triggered by chewing. However, your dentist reassured you that your teeth are fine.
- The pain comes in attacks and suddenly without warning.
- In the beginning, the pain only lasted for a few seconds but for the last month it tends to stay for a few minutes.

- The pain is often electric, shock-like, and sometimes stabbing.
- It is now becoming very severe and occurs every 3–4 hours.
- The pain may be triggered by chewing food, brushing your teeth, and touching the right side of your face.
- There is nothing that reduces the pain and it usually goes by itself.
- You have tried different pain killers such as paracetamol, ibuprofen but they did not work.
- No hearing problems.
- *If asked:*

You have felt repeated numbness and tingling in your feet for the last 4 months. The numbness usually lasts for a few days and then comes again after a few days.

Six months ago, you suddenly lost vision in your right eye for one day, but it improved by itself.

Review of systems

- No weakness in your arms or legs.
- No problems with speech.
- No difficulty in walking.
- No loss of consciousness or abnormal movement.
- No vomiting.

Menstrual history

- Your menses are regular and normal.
- You do not feel that the pain is related to your menses.
- You are not using the oral contraceptive pill.

Past history and drug history

- You have not suffered any chronic illness.
- No past history of migraine.
- You are not taking any medication apart from pain killers.

Social history

- You do not smoke**.**
- You do not drink alcohol.
- You work as a school teacher.
- You are single.

Your questions to the doctors and concerns

Is there any treatment that can relieve my pain?

Steps in history taking in a patient with facial pain

Step 1: Introduction, greeting, and confirmation of patient identity

- Good morning Ms Ruby (shakehands with the patient), pleased to meet you.
- I am Dr X working in the medical outpatient clinic.
- Can I confirm that I am talking to Ms Ruby?
- I have just read the referral letter from your dentist regarding the pain in your face.
- Can you tell me more about that?
- Allow the patient to speak.
- Avoid interruptions.
- Avoid medical jargon (e.g. neuralgia, hemifacial, trigeminal, etc.)
- *Use open ended questions such as:* What else?

Step 2: Elaborating important points in the history of facial pain/headache

History of presenting illness

Headache/facial pain, like any other pain in the body, should be analysed using the LIQOR AAA mnemonic.

Review of systems

- Other neurological symptoms.
- *Trigeminal neuralgia in young*: Ask about other symptoms of multiple sclerosis.
- *Symptoms of pheochromocytoma*: Palpitations, sweating, anxiety, and nervousness
- *Symptoms suggestive of increased ICP*: Projectile vomiting, personality change, and seizure/weakness/numbness
- *Recent weight gain*: Idiopathic intracranial hypertension
- Ask about alarm/red flag symptoms of headache.

Menstrual history

- *Relationship of headache to menstrual cycle*: Catamenial migraine
- *Use of oral contraceptive pill*: Cerebral venous sinus thrombosis, migraine, idiopathic intracranial hypertension.

Past medical history

- Ask about history of hypertension.
- Ask about history of migraine.
- Ask about previous strokes, brain lesions.
- Ask about previous head trauma.
- Ask about diseases that cause immunosuppression.
- *Recurrent sinusitis:* Cerebral venous sinus thrombosis, brain abscess, meningitis.

Family history

- Family history of migraine.
- Family history of cancer.
- Family history of other neurologic disorders.

Drug history

- *Oral contraceptive pill use*: Cerebral venous sinus thrombosis, migraine, idiopathic intracranial hypertension
- Drugs for migraine
- Use of steroids
- *Other drugs that may cause ICP*: Isotretinoin, tetracyclines, etc.

Social history

- Smoking *(risk of malignancy)*
- *Alcohol intake*: Subdural haematoma
- Change in personality
- *Travel history*: Malaria, meningitis
- *Sexual history*: HIV, neurosyphilis.

Further information not covered (at end of history taking)

Ask the patient the following question: Is there anything else that you feel important and would like to tell me about?

Step 3: Explaining to the patient the diagnosis and the plan of management

Ms Ruby, you have had a pain along the right side of your face over the past 3 months. The pain is electric, shock-like, and sometimes triggered by chewing and touching the area. You have also had recurrent numbness in your feet over the past 4 months and on one occasion you temporarily lost vision in your right eye. Putting all these together, the most likely cause of your pain is a condition called 'Trigeminal neuralgia'. Have you heard of this before? Trigeminal neuralgia is a disorder of the trigeminal nerve that provides sensation to the face. The exact cause of this disorder is not fully understood.

However, it can be caused by a blood vessel pressing on the trigeminal nerve. It can also occur in people with multiple sclerosis. Very rarely, trigeminal neuralgia can be caused by nerve compression from a tumour. The condition causes extreme, sporadic, sudden burning or shock-like facial pain in the area of the face where the branches of the nerve are distributed. Trigeminal neuralgia typically occurs in people above the age of 50. When it occurs in people who are younger than this age (as in your case), we should exclude other underlying diseases that can cause trigeminal neuralgia, especially a condition called 'multiple sclerosis.' Have you heard of this term before? Multiple sclerosis is a disorder of the immune system in which there is damage to the nerve. It can result in different symptoms. One such symptom is trigeminal neuralgia in young people. Therefore, I think it is very important that you undergo an MRI scan of your brain and spinal cord to look for multiple sclerosis. I am also going to write an urgent referral to one of my colleagues who specialise in neurology to have his input. Does that make sense to you?

Step 4: Ask about and address patient's concerns

Do you have any questions or concerns?

> *Patient's concern*: Is there any treatment that can relieve my pain? I have tried many pain killers, but they did not work.
>
> *Reply*: Simple pain killer do not work very well in trigeminal neuralgia. The drug that gives good results in trigeminal neuralgia is called carbamazepine. I am going to prescribe this medication to you and will shortly explain to you its dose and side effects.
>
> After answering each concern, confirm agreement by saying, 'is that okay or does that sound good for you?'

Step 5: Summarise the discussion, confirm patient's understanding, and close the meeting

Ms Ruby, I would like to summarise our discussion to be sure you understand important information about your illness. The most likely cause of your facial pain is trigeminal neuralgia. Because of your age and history of numbness in your feet and temporary loss of eye sight, you must undergo MRI of the brain and spinal cord to exclude multiple sclerosis. I am going to prescribe a drug called carbamazepine to help relieve the pain and I will write an urgent referral to a neurologist. I will see you in 2 weeks to give you further answers. Meanwhile, I am going to provide you with my contact number in case you have any further questions or concerns regarding your condition. Is that okay? You can get more information from the internet on trigeminal neuralgia. Thank you and see you soon.

Discussion

Problem

Recurrent facial pain in a young woman.

Diagnosis

Trigeminal neuralgia in a young woman most likely secondary to multiple sclerosis.

Other plausible diagnosis:

- Cluster headache
- Migraine.

The idiopathic form of trigeminal neuralgia occurs typically after the age of 50. Females are more affected than males. Trigeminal neuralgia in young people should raise the suspicion of an underlying disease, most commonly multiple sclerosis or a tumour along the trigeminal nerve. MRI brain should be obtained to exclude multiple sclerosis or a cerebellopontine angle tumour.

Characteristics of pain from trigeminal neuralgia

- Recurrent brief episodes of unilateral electric shock-like pain.
- Onset is sudden.
- Duration is very short (seconds) tend to be repetitive.
- *Location:* In the distribution of one or more divisions of the fifth cranial (trigeminal) nerve (most commonly V2 and V3, very rare in V1 distribution).
- The pain usually occurs in paroxysms.
- Trigeminal neuralgia pain is classically triggered by light touch of the face in V1, V2, V3 areas.
- *Other triggering factors include:* Brushing teeth, chewing, talking, grimacing or smiling.

The pain of trigeminal neuralgia is often mistakenly attributed to a tooth problem owing to its presentation in the two lower branches of the trigeminal nerve. Patients may undergo unnecessary and sometimes irreversible dental treatment before the condition is recognised.

Red flags signs that may point to secondary causes of trigeminal neuralgia

- Presence of other sensory symptoms in the body (multiple sclerosis).
- Deafness or other ear problems (underlying tumours).
- Difficulty achieving pain control and poor response to carbamazepine.
- History of any skin lesions (herpes).
- Pain along the ophthalmic division only or bilateral (malignancy or multiple sclerosis).
- Age of onset under 40 years, optic neuritis, family history of multiple sclerosis.

The drug of choice in the treatment of trigeminal neuralgia is carbamazepine. The second drug of choice is oxcarbazepine, a keto derivative of carbamazepine that has shown similar efficacy to carbamazepine but increased tolerability and fewer drug interactions. Surgical options include microvascular decompression to decompress the trigeminal nerve and palliative destructive procedures damaging the trigeminal nerve root to relieve pain.

Further reading

Zakrzewska JM, Linskey ME. Trigeminal neuralgia. BMJ 2014; 348:g474.

Scenario no. 23

A patient with abnormal liver function

Candidate copy

Please read the general surgery referral letter for Mrs Salma.
The time distribution for this station is as follows:
  You have (---) minutes to take a history from the patient.
  You have (---) minutes to collect your thoughts.
  You have (---) minutes for discussion with the examiners.

Please do not examine the patient

Dear Doctor,

Thank you for seeing Mrs Salma, a 48-year-old who is awaiting a right inguinal hernia repair. She was found to have abnormal liver function tests on the routine preoperative checkup. Her ALT is 100 U/L (0–40), AST 90 U/L (0–37), ALP 49 U/L (20–140), and total bilirubin is 16 µmol/L (1.7–20).

Yours faithfully,

Please interview the patient and based on history taking construct a differential diagnosis and plan of investigation. Provide explanation to the patient and answer any questions she may have.

Surrogate copy

Chief complaint and HPI

You had a routine blood check-up before surgery for an inguinal hernia and you were found to have abnormal liver function tests.

Review of systems

- You have had fatigue and easy tiredness over the last 1 year, during the day and night.
- *If asked only:* You have had joint pain in the right index and middle finger for 1 year.
- You have not noticed any yellowish discoloration of the eyes or skin.
- You have not noticed any change in the colour of your urine or stool.
- You have not felt any tummy pain.
- You do not have liver disease.

Menstrual history

Your periods stopped 3 months ago, but you thought it may be because you are 48-years old.

Past history and drug history

- You have a hernia and you are being considered for surgery.
- You have high blood lipids and you are following dietary restrictions for that.
- You are overweight and you are under follow-up of the obesity specialist, who has advised diet and exercise.

Family history

- Your younger sister has been diagnosed recently with systemic lupus erythematosus and she is on cortisone.
- You had a road traffic accident 15 years ago for which you required a blood transfusion.

Drug history

None.

Social history

- You do not smoke.
- You do not drink alcohol.
- You work as a school teacher.
- You are happily married with two kids.
- You do not have extramarital sexual relations.

Your questions to the doctors and concerns

Is this condition risky?

Is there any treatment for this condition?

Steps in history taking in a patient with abnormal liver function/jaundice

Step 1: Introduction, greeting, and confirmation of patient identity

- Good morning Mrs Salma (shakehands with the patient), pleased to meet you.
- I am Dr X working in the medical outpatient clinic.
- Can I confirm that I am talking to Mrs Salma?
- I have just read the referral letter from your surgeon about your abnormal liver function tests.
- Can you tell me more about that?
- Allow the patient to speak.
- Avoid interruptions.
- Avoid medical jargon (e.g. jaundice, cholestasis, hepatic, etc.)
- *Use open ended questions such as:* What else?

Step 2: Elaborating important points in the history of abnormal liver function/jaundice

History of presenting illness/analysis of jaundice

- Onset of jaundice (sudden/gradual)
- Duration of jaundice
- *Progression*: Progressive/improvement/same status
- Was it observed by patient/colleague/family or diagnosed by a doctor?
- Does the yellow discoloration involve only eyes or both skin and eyes?
- Is there any skin itching (obstructive jaundice)?
- Is there any fever (cholangitis/cholelithiasis with bile duct stone)?
- What is the colour of your stool and urine? (dark urine or pale stool indicate obstructive jaundice)
- Is there any change in your appetite or weight loss (hepatobiliary malignancy)?
- Do you feel nausea/vomiting? (acute hepatitis)
- Do you have any abdominal pain (painless cholestatic jaundice suggests underlying malignancy)?
- Do you feel abdominal distension? (ascites/malignancy)
- Any vomiting of blood or dark tarry stool?

Review of systems

- Ask about fatigue (primary biliary cirrhosis/chronic liver disease/anaemia).
- Ask about fever.
- *Rheumatologic system:* Joint pains/body pains (autoimmune hepatitis/haemolytic anaemia)
- *Joint pains involving metacarpophalangeal joints*: Haemochromatosis
- *Increased skin pigmentation:* Haemochromatosis.

Past history

- Past history of liver disease/stones.
- Past history of jaundice.
- History of gallbladder stones.
- History of cancer.
- Past history of blood transfusions.

- Autoimmune diseases (autoimmune hepatitis)
- Haemolytic anaemia
- *Obesity and over weight*: Nonalcoholic fatty liver disease (NAFLD).

Menstrual history

- Amenorrhoea (autoimmune hepatitis/primary biliary cirrhosis)
- Use of oral contraceptive pill (may predispose to cholestasis and liver tumours).
- *Decreased libido and infertility:* Haemochromatosis.

Family history

- *Family history or contact with other people with jaundice or liver disease*: Hepatitis A, E
- Family history of liver disease/GIT malignancy.
- Family history of autoimmune diseases (autoimmune hepatitis)
- Family history of haemolytic anaemia.

Drug history

- Inquire about use of anabolic steroids in young men/bodybuilders.
- Take a detailed drug history including over the counter medications.

Social history

- Details of alcohol intake
- Smoking
- *Drug abuse particularly intravenous drug abuse*: Risk of hepatitis/HIV
- *Travel history*: Hepatitis A, E, other infections and infestations causing hepatitis
- *Details of sexual history*: Hepatitis/HIV.

Further information not covered (at end of history taking)

- *Ask the patient the following question:* Is there anything else that you feel important and would like to tell me about?

Step 3: Explaining to the patient the diagnosis and the plan of management

Mrs Salma, you have abnormal liver function tests which were found incidentally. You do complain of fatigue which does not seem to bother you too much. You are overweight and you are following a weight reduction diet. You have not had your menses for the last 3 months and you have had some joint pains of the index and middle finger. There are several reasons why you might have abnormal liver function tests. In relation to your weight, you might have a condition called 'NAFLD' which occurs due to an accumulation of excess fat in the liver. However, given the history of joint pain in the fingers, the family history of systemic lupus erythematosus (SLE) and the loss of menstrual cycles, other conditions such as haemochromatosis where there is an excess accumulation of iron in the body and autoimmune hepatitis, which causes liver inflammation, should be excluded. I am going to order some blood and an ultrasound of your liver to look for these other causes. Does this make sense to you so far?

Patient: Is this condition risky?

Although having fat in the liver is not normal, by itself it probably does not damage the liver. A small group of people with NAFLD may develop a more serious condition called nonalcoholic steatohepatitis (NASH), where the fat accumulation is associated with liver cell inflammation and scarring. Cirrhosis can occur when the liver sustains substantial damage, and the liver cells are gradually replaced by scar tissue, resulting in the inability of the liver to work properly. Some patients who develop cirrhosis may eventually require a liver transplant to remove the damaged liver and replace it with a 'new' liver.

Doctor: Is there any treatment for this condition?

Yes, the most important recommendation for people with fatty liver is to lose weight. This can be achieved by diet, exercise, medications, and/or surgery. Avoiding alcohol and medications that affect liver function is also very important. As you have high lipids, lipid lowering medications can be beneficial in reducing fat accumulation in the liver. Other medications that can be used include insulin sensitisers and antioxidants that can decrease liver inflammation.

I will send you for some blood tests to exclude other less likely causes of abnormal liver function and confirm the diagnosis of NAFLD by a liver ultrasound. I will also prescribe you a lipid lowering drug to reduce your blood lipids and fat in the liver. A colleague of mine who specialises in liver diseases will also see you in few days.

I am going to arrange another appointment with myself in 2 weeks to see the results of blood tests and liver ultrasound and I hope by that time I will be able to give you more answers.

Check patient understanding and agreement on plan of management.

Does that sound okay?

Step 4: Ask about and address patient's concerns

Do you have any questions or concerns?

Already answered

Step 5: Summarise the discussion, confirm patient's understandings, and close the meeting

Mrs Salma, I would like to summarise our discussion to be sure you understand important information about your illness. The most probable cause for your abnormal liver function is a condition called NAFLD for which I am going to arrange some blood tests and a liver ultrasound. You will also receive an appointment with a liver specialist, and I will prescribe a lipid lowering drug. I will see you again in 2 weeks.

Meanwhile, I am going to provide you with my contact number in case you have any further questions or concerns regarding your condition. Does that sound good to you? You can get more information on NAFLD from the internet. Thank you and see you soon.

Discussion

Problem

Incidentally discovered abnormal liver function with mildly elevated ALT and AST.

Diagnosis

Nonalcoholic fatty liver disease.

Other plausible diagnosis

- *Autoimmune hepatitis*
  - Amenorrhoea, family history of autoimmune disease.
- *Haemochromatosis*
  - History of recurrent joint pain (small hand joints).
- *Hepatitis B/C viral infection*
  - Past history of blood transfusion.

Nonalcoholic fatty liver disease is a highly prevalent condition characterised by the presence of hepatic fat accumulation. NAFLD manifests as nonalcoholic fatty liver (NAFL) or NASH. In NAFL, hepatic steatosis is present without evidence of significant inflammation, whereas in NASH, hepatic steatosis is associated with hepatic inflammation. NAFL tends to be benign and nonprogressive while NASH can progress to cirrhosis, which in rare cases gives rise to hepatocellular carcinoma. The diagnosis of NAFLD is based on: (1) a history of no or limited daily alcohol intake (<20 g for women and <30 g for men); (2) presence of hepatic steatosis by imaging or by histology; and (3) exclusion of other liver diseases. The differentiation of NAFL from NASH requires a liver biopsy. NAFLD is considered a part of metabolic syndrome and commonly coexists with central obesity, insulin resistance, type 2 diabetes mellitus, and dyslipidaemia. Most patients with NAFLD are asymptomatic and commonly diagnosed incidentally when elevated liver aminotransferases are found, or fatty liver is found on ultrasound imaging. The elevation of ALT and AST is usually mild and the AST to ALT ratio is less than one (alcoholic fatty liver disease typically has a ratio >2). Other causes of elevated ALT and ALT should be excluded. Blood should be sent for viral hepatitis serology, iron profile (to exclude haemochromatosis), ANA, AMA, and anti-LKM antibodies and serum gamma globulin levels to exclude autoimmune hepatitis. Ultrasonography often reveals a hyperechoic and bright liver due to diffuse fatty infiltration. Patients with simple steatosis on biopsy are at low risk for developing significant fibrosis, whereas those with NASH are at higher risk. The risk increases when transaminases are >2 times the upper limit of normal in patients with a high BMI. Poor outcomes are more frequent in patients in whom biopsies show ballooning degeneration and Mallory hyaline or fibrosis. The most important step in the management of NAFLD is weight loss for patients who are overweight or obese. Other treatments include thiazolidinediones, orlistat, statins, Pentoxifylline, and antioxidant therapy such as vitamin E.

Further reading

Hashimoto E, Tokushige K, Ludwig J. Diagnosis and classification of non-alcoholic fatty liver disease and non-alcoholic steatohepatitis: Current concepts and remaining challenges. Hepatol Res 2015; 45:20–28.

Matteoni CA, Younossi ZM, Gramlich T, et al. Nonalcoholic fatty liver disease: a spectrum of clinical and pathological severity. Gastroenterology 1999; 116:1413–1419.

Patient Education & Resource Center. American College of Gastroenterology. Non-alcoholic Fatty Liver Disease (NAFLD). [online] Available at http://patients.gi.org/topics/fatty-liver-disease-nafld/. [Last accessed October, 2019.

Scenario no. 24

An elderly man with recurrent falls

Candidate copy

Please read the GP referral letter for Mr Johnson
The time distribution for this station is as follows:
   You have (---) minutes to take a history from the patient.
   You have (---) minutes to collect your thoughts.
   You have (---) minutes for discussion with the examiners.

Please do not examine the patient

Dear Doctor,

Mr Galston is a 78-year-old man who has had recurrent falls at home. He is living alone in his house after the recent death of his wife. His daughter feels that this may be due to depression following the death of his wife. Mr Galston and his daughter are very concerned about his recurrent falls.

Yours sincerely,

Please interview the patient and based on history taking construct a differential diagnosis and plan of investigation. Provide an explanation to the patient and answer any questions she may have.

Surrogate copy

Chief complaints and history of present illness

- You are 78-years-old.
- You experienced recurrent falls (5 times) at your home.
- You have fallen three times while going to bathroom.
- Twice while walking to the kitchen.
- Falls did not happen after standing or sitting from a lying position.
- In your last fall, you sustained small bruises on your face.
- You did not lose consciousness when you fell down.
- You did not have any jerky movement in your limbs.
- You did not have any limb weakness.
- You have full control of your bladder and bowel habits.
- You did not miss any meals.

Questions to be answered only if asked:

- You felt some dizziness and light-headedness just before the fall, which comes on suddenly.
- On multiple occasions, you have felt that your heart beats fast.
- The fast heartbeats are irregular.

Review of systems

You feel significant numbness and tingling in your feet particularly at night. Your doctor said that this is because of diabetes.

Past history

- You have had high blood pressure for the last 10 years, but this is well controlled.
- You have had diabetes for the last 15 years.
- You had a heart attack 5 years ago and a stent was placed in one of your heart vessels.

Drug history

- Aspirin
- Atorvastatin
- Gliclazide
- Atenolol
- Quetiapine
- Indapamide

Social history

- You are a retired police officer.
- You are living alone after the recent death of your wife.
- Your daughter visits you daily and helps with shopping and washing.
- Your GP has recently prescribed quetiapine tablet for you to help your depression after the death of your wife.

Patient's concern

- What has caused my falls?
- Is there any treatment for it?

Steps in history taking in an elderly patient with recurrent falls

Step 1: Introduction, greeting and confirmation of patient identity

- Good morning, Mr Galston (shakehands with the patient), glad to meet you. I am Dr X working here in the medical outpatient clinic. Can I confirm that I am talking to Mr Galston?
- The referral letter from your GP states that you have had recurrent falls, recently. Can you tell me more about that?
- Allow the patient to speak fully.
- Avoid interruptions.
- Avoid medical jargon (e.g. palpitations, cardiac, neurogenic, cerebrovascular accident, etc.)
- *Use open-ended questions repeatedly such as:* OK, what else?

Step 2: Elaborating important points in the history

After open-ended question, use the following closed-ended questions.

History of presenting illness

- How did the fall happen?
- What were you doing when you fell down?
- When was the fall (night/daytime)?
- Did you trip over anything?
- Where did you fell down? House, office, outdoor, etc.
- Did you feel any dizziness/spinning before you fell down?
- Did you feel a racing heartbeat before you fell down?
- Did the fall happen after standing or sitting from a lying/sitting position?
- Did you lose consciousness at the time of your fall?
- Do you have any visual blurring when you stand up from a lying/sitting position?
- Did anyone witness your fall?
- Was there any witnessed jerking movement of your limbs or tongue biting? (seizure)
- Do you have any weakness or confusion after the fall? (postictal)
- Do you have shaking or jerky movement of your hands and legs? (Parkinson's disease)
- Do you have difficulty standing from a sitting position? (proximal muscle weakness)
- Do you have any problems with the sensation in your legs? (peripheral neuropathy)

Review of systems

- *Neurological system:* Visual problem, dizziness, vertigo, weakness, peripheral neuropathy symptoms
- *Cardiovascular system:* Palpitations, chest pain, breathlessness
- *Locomotor:* Joint problems, walking aids, muscle weakness
- *Respiratory:* Symptoms of sleep apnoea such as witnessed nighttime snoring/abnormal breathing during sleep (apnoeic episodes), daytime sleepiness and fatigue.

Past history

- *History of diabetes mellitus (DM):* If yes, details of level of glucose control and hypoglycaemia, complications (particularly neuropathy)
- History of hypertension and the level of control.
- History of heart disease.
- History of stroke.

Family history
- Family history of any chronic diseases of the heart, brain, lung and kidney.
- Family history of sudden death.
- Family history of thrombosis/clots.

Drug history
Particular attention should be paid to the following drugs in the elderly with recurrent falls:
- Neuro-psychiatric drugs such as sedatives/anxiolytics/antidepressant medications: these medications have multiple neurologic and cardiac side effects, particularly in the elderly.
- Diuretics, especially thiazide diuretics, can cause postural hypotension and electrolyte abnormalities.
- Antihypertensive medications and cardiac medications.
- Diabetic medications can cause hypoglycaemia.

Social history
- Details of alcohol history
- Smoking history
- Do you live alone? (pay attention to social support)
- *Housing condition:* Which floor is your bedroom in? Are there mechanical obstructions?
- Ask about depression?
- Occupation or work?
- Effects of falls on different aspects of patient's life.

Further information not covered (at end of history taking)
Is there anything you feel is important to you and you would like to discuss?

Step 3: Explaining to the patient the diagnosis and the plan of management
Mr Galston, your main complaint is recurrent falls over the past 2 months. You have felt dizziness and light-headedness just before the fall on two occasions and on multiple occasions, you have felt irregular heartbeats. You suffer from long-standing high blood pressure and diabetes and you have had a previous heart attack for which you are on treatment. You are now living alone and feel depressed after the death of your wife. The most likely underlying reason for your falls is an underlying heart problem, given your heart attack 10 years ago and you have felt some missed heartbeats. I am going to order a trace of your heart rhythm through a simple test called an ECG and will arrange to monitor your heart rhythm through a 24-hour ambulatory ECG. Other possible causes of your recurrent falls, are some of the drugs you are currently taking. The water pill called indapamide can cause an abnormality in the salts in your blood and it may lower your blood pressure which may lead to recurrent falls. The quetiapine pill prescribed for your depression can affect the heart and cause an abnormal heart rhythm as well as other side effects leading to recurrent falls. I suggest that we change these medications to others with fewer side effects. Having diabetes for a long time can also damage the nerves in your legs and this may, in turn, cause recurrent falls. I am going to order a tracing of your nerve activity in your legs.

I am also going to order some blood tests to make sure that your sugar, sodium, potassium and kidney function are normal, and you do not have anaemia.

I would strongly recommend that you avoid suddenly standing from a lying position and you should sit on the bedside for a while before you stand when you wake up from sleep.

Diabetes and the medications for blood pressure can also cause a drop in the blood pressure on standing. I will check your blood pressure when lying and standing to see if there is any evidence of a condition called postural hypotension. A walking frame to help support you while walking may help. I will discuss with our social worker to arrange more frequent visits to your home to take care of your needs. It is important to minimise your falls as they carry a risk of fractures in older people.

I will give you an appointment with me in a week's time to follow up with your results. Is that OK and does that make sense to you?

Step 4: Ask about and address patient's concerns

Do you have any questions or concerns?

Patient: What is the cause of my recurrent falls?

Reply: Answered above

Patient: Is there any treatment for this?

The treatment depends on the cause. If we find that you have an underlying heart rhythm problem, then we can give you medicine to help reduce this or we may have to think about a pacemaker. If it is your medication, then we can stop or change your medication. We will also assess your blood sugar levels using a special wearable sensor to look for episodes of low sugar.

If we find a drop in your blood pressure on standing from a sitting position, then we will give you some medication to improve this condition.

After answering each concern confirm agreement by saying; is that OK or does that sound good to you?

Step 5: Summarise the discussion, confirm patient's understanding and close the meeting

Mr Galston, I would like to summarise our discussion to be sure you understand important information about your illness. The likely cause of your recurrent falls is a problem with your heart rhythm. Other possible causes may be medications such as the water pills and the antidepression pills. I will order a trace of your heart rhythm, some blood tests and trace of your leg nerve activity. I will also arrange for a social worker visit your home and will change some of your medications that may cause recurrent falls to ones with fewer side effects. I will see you in a week's time and will be able to give you further information.

Discussion

Problem

Recurrent falls in the elderly.

Diagnosis

Arrhythmias: Patient has a past history of a heart attack and is feeling recurrent missed beats. This might have been exacerbated by atenolol and quetiapine.

Other plausible diagnosis

- **Diuretics**
  They can induce electrolyte abnormality and cause weakness. Increased urinary frequency can lead to recurrent falls, especially in elderly patients.
- **Quetiapine**
  It can induce recurrent falls in elderly by causing arrhythmia (prolonged QT), dizziness, and other side effects.

- **Diabetic peripheral and autonomic neuropathy**
- **Hypoglycaemic** symptoms may be masked by beta-blockers.

Causes of recurrent falls in the elderly

- **Neurologic diseases**
  - Cerebrovascular accidents/tumours
  - Parkinsonism
  - Peripheral neuropathy.
- **Drugs**
  - Psychiatric medications (antidepressants/sedatives/antipsychotics)
  - Cardiac medications
  - Diabetic medications
  - Alcohol.
- **Postural hypotension** (e.g. from medications)
- **Cardiovascular causes**
  - Cardiac syncope from arrhythmia/aortic stenosis/ischaemia
  - Carotid stenosis.
- **Metabolic causes**
  - Electrolyte abnormalities/hypoglycaemia
  - Renal/liver/thyroid diseases.
- **Cognitive impairment**
- **Mechanical obstacles/visual problems**

What are the risks of falls in elderly?

- Hip fractures with poor healing.
- Prolonged hospitalisation
- One-fourth of elderly persons who sustain a hip fracture after a fall die within 6 months and more than 50% of older patients who survive a hip fracture are discharged to a nursing home, and half of these patients are still in a nursing home 1 year later.

Management of elderly with recurrent falls

- Take a detailed history to identify the cause and treat it
- Physical examination
  - Look for postural hypotension
  - Examine sensation
  - Examine proximal strength (vitamin D deficiency)
  - Examine lower limb joints
  - Examine the heart.
- Eliminate/change culprit medications such as psychiatric medications/sedatives/anti-hypertensives.
- Provide social support and involve the family.
- Remove physical obstacles in the house and install grab bars or raised toilet seats and provide walking frames.

Further reading

Fuller GF. Falls in the elderly. Am Fam Physician 2000; 61:2159–2168.
Rubenstein LZ. Falls. In: Yoshikawa TT, Cobbs EL, Brummel-Smith K (Eds.) Ambulatory Geriatric Care. St. Louis: Mosby; 1993. pp. 296–304.

Scenario no. 25

A patient with cholestatic jaundice

Candidate copy

Please read the GP referral letter for Mr Hamid.
The time distribution for this station is as follows:

    You have (---) minutes to take a history from the patient.
    You have (---) minutes to collect your thoughts.
    You have (---) minutes for discussion with the examiners.

Please do not examine the patient

> **Dear Doctor,**
>
> Thank you for seeing Mr Hamid, a 28-year-old man who has been complaining of yellowish discoloration of his eyes and skin for 1 month. He also noticed some weight loss. Laboratory tests showed AST: 42 U/L (5–45), ALT: 62 U/L (13–45), ALP: 1167 U/L (40–120), total bilirubin: 547.2 µmol/L (0–21) and direct bilirubin: 542.07 µmol/L. Ultrasound of his abdomen did not show evidence of dilated extrahepatic bile ducts or any other obvious pathology.
>
> Yours faithfully,

> Please interview the patient and based on history taking construct a differential diagnosis and plan of investigation. Provide explanation to the patient and answer any questions she may have.

Surrogate copy

Chief complaints and history of present illness

- Your main complaint is of a yellowish discolouration of your skin and eyes over the past month, which was noticed by your friend. This yellow discolouration has been increasing over the last month and now the colour is turning greenish. There is severe itching particularly at night that is disturbing your sleep. You have lost about 15 kg in the last month. Initially, you thought the weight loss was due to excessive exercise and training at the gym as you are a body builder and you are working hard to achieve a good body image to participate in a big competition. However, even after you stopped training at the gym, the weight loss persisted.
- Your appetite is good.
- You do not feel any tummy pain.
- You do not feel nausea.
- You do not vomit.

Only if asked:
- You do not feel fever.
- You noticed that your stool colour is becoming very yellow and pale.
- You noticed your urine is becoming dark yellow to brown.

Review of systems

You have had fatigue and easy tiredness.

Past history

Apart from tonsillitis, you are healthy.

The last attack of tonsillitis was 2 months ago and it resolved with a 7-day course of Augmentin.

Family history

Your grandfather died from pancreatic cancer 20 years ago.

Drug history

- You took Augmentin 2 months ago for tonsillitis.
  Only if asked: For the last 3 months, you have been taking a drug called Anabol (Methandrostenolone) 3 tablets daily for bodybuilding. You bought this medication from a gym mate, who told you that this was going to make you more muscular.

Social history

- You do not smoke.
- You do not drink alcohol.
- You work as a physiotherapist.
- You have been married for 1 year but have no children.
- Over the last 3 months, you have lost the desire for sex and you are not getting normal erections.

Your questions to the doctors and concerns

Could it be cancer?

Is the change in my sex life related to this problem?

Steps in history taking in a patient with jaundice

Step 1: Introduction, greeting and confirmation of patient identity

- Good morning Mr Hamid (shakehands with the patient), pleased to meet you.
- I am Dr X working in the medical outpatient clinic.
- Can I confirm that I am talking to Mr Hamid?
- I have just read the referral letter from your GP about your abnormal liver function tests.
- Can you tell me more about that?
- Allow the patient to speak.
- Avoid interruptions.
- Avoid medical jargon (e.g. jaundice, cholestasis, hepatic, etc.)
- *Use open-ended questions such as:* What else?

Step 2: Elaborating important points in the history of abnormal liver function/ jaundice

History of presenting illness/analysis of jaundice

- Onset of jaundice (sudden/gradual)
- Duration of jaundice
- *Progression:* Progressive/improvement/same status
- Was it observed by patient/colleague/family or diagnosed by a doctor?
- Does the yellow discolouration involve only eyes or both the skin and eyes?
- Is there any skin itching (obstructive jaundice)?
- Is there any associated fever? (cholangitis/cholelithiasis with bile duct stone)

- What is the colour of the stool and urine? (dark urine or pale stool indicate obstructive jaundice)
- Is there any change in your appetite or weight loss (hepatobiliary malignancy)?
- Do you feel nausea/vomiting? (acute hepatitis)
- Do you have any abdominal pain (painless cholestatic jaundice suggests underlying malignancy)?
- Do you feel abdominal distension? (ascites/malignancy)
- Melena/haematemesis.

Review of systems
- Ask about fatigue (primary biliary cirrhosis/chronic liver disease/anaemia).
- Ask about fever.
- *Rheumatologic system:* Joint pains/body pains (autoimmune hepatitis/haemolytic anaemia)
- *Joint pains involving metacarpophalangeal joints:* Haemochromatosis
- *Increase skin pigmentation:* Haemochromatosis.

Past history
- Past history of liver disease/stones.
- Past history of jaundice.
- History of gallbladder stones.
- History of cancer.
- Past history of blood transfusions.
- Autoimmune diseases (autoimmune hepatitis).
- Haemolytic anaemia.
- *Obesity and overweight:* Non-alcoholic fatty liver disease.

Menstrual history
- Amenorrhea (autoimmune hepatitis/primary biliary cirrhosis)
- Use of oral contraceptive pills (may predispose to cholestasis and liver tumours)
- *Decreased libido and infertility:* Haemochromatosis.

Family history
- *Family history or contact with people with jaundice or liver disease:* Hepatitis A, E
- Family history of liver disease/GIT malignancy.
- Family history of autoimmune diseases (autoimmune hepatitis).
- Family history of haemolytic anaemia.

Drug history
- Inquire about use of anabolic steroids in young men/bodybuilders.
- Take detailed drug history including over-the-counter medications.

Social history
- Details of alcohol intake.
- Smoking
- *Drug abuse particularly intravenous drug abuse:* Risk of hepatitis/HIV
- *Travel history:* Hepatitis A, E, other infections and infestations causing hepatitis.
- *Details of sexual history:* Hepatitis/HIV.

Further information not covered (at end of history taking)
Ask the patient the following question: Is there anything else that you feel is important and would like to tell me about?

Step 3: Explaining to the patient the diagnosis and the plan of management
Mr Hamid, your main complaint is the yellow discoloration of your eyes and skin, and weight loss. Apart from tonsillitis for which you took Augmentin 2 months ago and the

Anabol tablet which you started 3 months ago for bodybuilding; you do not take any other medication. Your grandfather died from pancreatic cancer. The most likely reason for your symptoms is the Anabol, which is an anabolic steroid. Anabolic steroids are synthetic substances made from testosterone and are controlled substances. They precipitate and block the small bile ducts in the liver leading to bile substances passing via the blood to the skin leading to a yellow discolouration. I strongly recommend that you immediately stop taking this medication to prevent further damage to your liver. This will improve your symptoms but may take some time. I am also going to prescribe some medications that will help your itching (Ursodeoxycholic acid and antihistamine). Augmentin can also cause similar symptoms, although you took it over a month ago, so it is less likely to be the cause of your symptoms. Meanwhile, I am going to arrange a magnetic resonance imaging scan of your liver to exclude other possible causes since you have a family history of pancreatic cancer. I will also arrange an appointment with a colleague who specialises in liver disease.

Check patient understanding and agreement on plan of management.

Does that make sense to you?

Step 4: Ask about and address patient's concerns

Do you have any questions or concerns?

Patient's concern: Could it be a cancer?

Reply: Cancer of the pancreas and in the bile ducts is one of the causes of yellow discoloration of the body. However, as your ultrasound did not show dilatation of the bile ducts, this diagnosis becomes less likely. Anabolic steroids can also put you at a risk of liver cancer, which is why I am doing the MR scan.

Patient's concern: Is the change in my sexual life related to this problem?

Reply: This is an important question. A major side effect of anabolic steroids is they can cause a loss of sexual desire and failure of erection. In fact, anabolic steroids are among the most common causes of such problems in young men.

Step 5: Summarise the discussion, confirm patient's understandings and close the meeting.

Mr Hamid, I would like to summarise our discussion to be sure you understand important information about your illness. The most probable cause for your symptoms is the anabolic steroid, which you need to stop immediately. I will prescribe some medications to help your itching and arrange a magnetic resonance imaging scan of your liver. I will arrange for you to be seen by a colleague who specialises in liver disease and repeat your liver function in 2 weeks.

Meanwhile, I am going to provide you with my contact number in case you have any further questions or concerns regarding your condition. Does that sound OK? You can get more information from the internet regarding the problems of taking anabolic steroids. Thank you and see you soon.

Discussion

Problem

Painless cholestatic jaundice.

Diagnosis

Anabolic steroid-induced cholestasis.
(This diagnosis should be considered in any young man with unexplained cholestatic jaundice).

Other plausible diagnosis

- **Cholangiocarcinoma/pancreatic head cancer**
  Although the patient presented with cholestatic jaundice and weight loss with a family history of pancreatic cancer, the absence of dilatation of extrahepatic biliary ducts and the temporal association with ingestion of anabolic steroids is against this diagnosis.
- **Augmentin-induced cholestasis**
  Augmentin is probably the most common cause of drug-induced cholestasis. However, the progressive jaundice despite the discontinuation of Augmentin a month ago argues against this diagnosis.

Cholestasis is a defect in bile acid transport from the liver to the intestine. It has two forms; intrahepatic and extrahepatic. In intrahepatic cholestasis, the impairment of bile secretion occurs primarily within the liver. It can result from hepatocellular functional defects or from obstructive lesions of the intrahepatic bile ducts. Extrahepatic causes occur at the level of large bile ducts.

Common causes of extrahepatic cholestasis include:
- Choledocholithiasis (most common cause)
- Obstruction of the biliary tract due to malignancy (pancreas, gallbladder, bile duct cancer, or metastasis to perihilar lymph nodes).
- Primary sclerosing cholangitis
- AIDS cholangiopathy.

Causes of intrahepatic cholestasis include:
- Drugs (e.g. augmentin, anabolic steroids)
- Primary biliary cirrhosis
- Viral hepatitis
- Cholestasis of pregnancy
- Infiltrative diseases (tuberculosis, lymphoma, sarcoidosis)
- Sepsis
- Total parenteral nutrition.

Hepatic imaging (particularly ultrasound) to look for evidence of intra or extrahepatic bile duct dilation is usually the first step in the evaluation of a patient with cholestatic jaundice. A nondilated biliary system suggests that the cause of cholestatic jaundice is intrahepatic. Drug induced liver injury can present in several forms including hepatocellular, cholestatic, or mixed. The pattern of liver injury is classified based on R values [alanine aminotransferase (ALT) value/ALT upper limit of normal divided by the alkaline phosphatase (ALP) value/ALP upper limit of normal]. A case is considered hepatocellular when R is 5 or greater, cholestatic when R is 2 or less, and mixed when the R value is between 2 and 5. Anabolic steroid-induced cholestasis should be considered in any young man who presents with unexplained cholestasis. Patients often tend to hide using anabolic steroids unless asked directly about these medications. Despite being classified as controlled substances in many countries, their use is becoming widespread and no longer limited to bodybuilders or elite athletes. A striking side effect of anabolic androgenic steroids is hepatotoxicity and the 17αalkylated anabolic androgenic steroids (e.g. methandrostenolone and methyltestosterone) that have the greatest potential for liver injury. The use of anabolic androgenic steroids may cause cholestasis, hepatic peliosis, adenomas, and carcinomas. Hepatic peliosis is a rare syndrome characterised by vascular changes in the liver leading to the formation of bloodfilled enlarged sinusoids. The condition can lead to internal haemorrhage and death from hepatic failure. It may or may not revert by stopping anabolic androgenic steroids. Hepatic tumours including adenomas and carcinomas are the most serious hepatic complications of prolonged anabolic steroid use (over 2 years). Despite being benign neoplasms, hepatic adenomas carry the risk of sudden rupture and bleeding leading to haemoperitoneum. Spontaneous regression of adenomas may occur following discontinuation of the drugs. The diagnosis of intrahepatic cholestasis induced by the use of anabolic androgenic steroids is often overlooked, particularly if direct and specific inquiry about the use of these agents is not made. The diagnosis is usually based on temporal association between the use of anabolic androgenic steroids and the development of cholestatic jaundice. A liver biopsy is usually not essential but may prove useful for uncertain cases. Druginduced cholestasis can have several histological forms such as cholestatic hepatitis, bland cholestasis, and idiosyncratic liver injury, including vanishing bile duct syndrome. Cholestatic hepatitis is the most common form of drug induced cholestasis. The most common presenting symptoms in patients with pancreatic cancer are pain, jaundice, and weight loss. Abdominal pain is one of the most common manifestations of pancreatic cancer even with small pancreatic cancers. The pain is typically epigastric that is radiating to the back, usually insidious in onset. Pain in extrahepatic cholangiocarcinoma is a less prominent feature and present in 30–50% of patients. The pain is typically a dull ache in the right upper quadrant.

Further reading

Aithal GP, Watkins PB, Andrade RJ, et al. Case definition and phenotype standardization in druginduced liver injury. Clin Pharmacol Ther 2011; 89:80615.

Chazouilleres O, Housset C. Intrahepatic cholestasis. Textbook of Hepatology: From Basic Science to Clinical Practice, 3rd edition. Oxford: Wiley Blackwell Publishing; 2008. pp. 1479–1500.

Ibrahim WH, Choura M, Bshesh F, et al. Severe cholestasis with marked weight loss mimicking malignancy: An overlooked etiology. Libyan J Med Sci 2018; 2:73–76.

Kleiner DE. The pathology of druginduced liver injury. Semin Liver Dis 2009; 29:36472.

Nakeeb A, Pitt HA, Sohn TA, et al. Cholangiocarcinoma. A spectrum of intrahepatic, perihilar, and distal tumors. Ann Surg 1996; 224:463.

Porta M, Fabregat X, Malats N, et al. Exocrine pancreatic cancer: symptoms at presentation and their relation to tumour site and stage. Clin Transl Oncol 2005; 7:189–197.

Scenario no. 26

A patient with abnormal body movement

Candidate copy

Please read the GP referral letter for Mr Aslam
The time distribution for this station is as follows:
>   You have (---) minutes to take a history from the patient.
>   You have (---) minutes to collect your thoughts.
>   You have (---) minutes for discussion with the examiners.

Please do not examine the patient

> **Dear Doctor,**
> Thank you for seeing Mr Aslam, a 60-year-old man with hypertension and end-stage kidney disease for which he is on regular haemodialysis. His wife has witnessed abnormal jerky movements in his legs and is concerned that he is having fits.
> Yours faithfully,

Please interview the patient and based on history taking construct a differential diagnosis and plan of investigation. Provide explanation to the patient and answer any questions she may have.

Surrogate copy

Chief complaints and history of present illness

- You are Mrs Aslam, the wife of Mr Aslam.
- You are concerned about the abnormal jerky movements when your husband relaxes and especially when he lies down to go to sleep.
- They happen when your husband is relaxed even whilst sitting on a chair.
- They do not happen when he is active or walking.
- Your husband does not lose consciousness during the attacks.
- Your husband says he feels an itchy or buzzing sensation in his legs which gives him a strong urge to keep moving his legs.
- He feels that he needs to keep moving his legs for the sensations to go away.
- You are very worried as such abnormal movements may keep your husband awake all night.
- This has affected his job as shopkeeper as he keeps falling asleep during the day.

Review of systems

- Your husband does not lose control of urine or stool during the attacks.
- He does not lose consciousness.
- He does not have abnormal sensations or movement elsewhere in his body.
- He does not feel weakness in his legs or arms.

Past medical history

Your husband suffers from end-stage kidney disease due to severe hypertension and has been on haemodialysis 3 times per week for 1 year. He was diagnosed with high blood pressure 20 years ago, but this was not well controlled as he was not taking his blood pressure tablets regularly. Since he developed kidney disease, he started taking his medications regularly and now his blood pressure is controlled. He was diagnosed with depression 1 year ago and started on a tablet called mirtazapine 30 mg every night.

Drug history

- Amlodipine 10 mg daily
- Mirtazapine 30 mg every night
- Calcium carbonate daily
- Paracalcitol 1 microgram daily.

Family history

No similar illness in your husband's family.

Social history

- Your husband does not smoke.
- He does not drink alcohol.
- He is a shopkeeper.
- His job has been affected significantly by his illness because of lack of sleep.
- You have two daughters.

Your questions to the doctors and concerns

What has caused these movements and is there a treatment?

Steps in history taking in a patient with abnormal movements

Step 1: Introduction, greeting and confirmation of patient identity

- Good morning Mrs Aslam (shakehands with the patient), pleased to meet you.
- I am Dr X working in the medical outpatient clinic.
- Can I confirm that I am talking to Mrs Aslam, the wife of Mr Aslam?
- I have just read the referral letter from your GP who states that you are concerned about your husband's abnormal leg movements. I assume that your husband does not mind you talking to me about his illness.
- Can you tell me more about these abnormal movements?
- Allow the patient to speak.
- Avoid interruptions.
- Avoid medical jargon (e.g. dyskinesia, seizure, renal, etc.)
- *Use open-ended questions such as:* What else?

Step 2: Elaborating important points in the history of abnormal movements

History of presenting illness

- What is the onset of the movement like?
- Is it sudden or gradual?
- For how long does the abnormal movement last? (duration)
- Can you describe the abnormal movements?
  - *Movement disorders:*
    - *Tremor:* Rhythmic oscillations caused by intermittent muscle contractions.
    - *Tics:* Paroxysmal, stereotyped muscle contractions: Simple (single muscle group) or complex (multiple muscle groups). They can be temporarily suppressed.
    - *Myoclonus:* Shock-like, rhythmic twitches. Not suppressible.
    - *Chorea:* Dance-like, unpatterned movements, often approximate a purpose (e.g. adjusting clothes, checking a watch). Can be rapid and may involve proximal or distal muscle groups.
    - *Athetosis:* Writhing movements, mostly of arms and hands. Often slow.
    - *Dystonia:* Sustained or repetitive muscular contractions, often produces abnormal posture.
    - *Siballismus:* Wild, large-amplitude, flinging movements on one side of the body, commonly affecting proximal limb muscles but can also affect the trunk.
    - *Seizure:* Uncontrolled electrical activity in the brain, which may produce a physical convulsion, minor physical signs, thought disturbances, or a combination of symptoms.
    - *Epilepsy:* Recurrent, unprovoked seizures from known or unknown causes. Old definition of status epilepticus is 30 minutes of continuous seizure activity or a series of seizures without a return to full consciousness. Newer definition states 5 continuous minutes of generalised seizure activity or 2 or more separate seizure episodes without return to baseline.
    - *Restless leg syndrome (RLS):* A sleep disorder characterised by a strong urge to move the legs because of abnormal sensations in the legs. Moving the legs will

usually improve the sensations. They are voluntary and irresistible and tend to occur when the patient goes to bed.

- ■ *Periodic limb movement:* These are repetitive involuntary limb movement that occur during sleep.
- When does this abnormal movement happen?
  - *Before sleep or at rest:* RLS   - *Any time:* Seizure.
  - *During sleep:* Periodic leg movement syndrome
- Which parts of the body is involved in the abnormal movements?
  Arms, legs, face, one side of the body, generalised or starts in one place and then spreads.
- What are the precipitating factors?
  - *Strong light:* Seizure
  - *New stroke:* Seizure or hemiballismus.
- Was it associated with loss of consciousness?
- Was it associated with incontinence of urine or stool?
- Was it preceded by an aura?
- Was it associated with tongue biting or body injury?
- Is there any history of head trauma?
- What are the circumstances before, during and after the incident?

Review of systems

- *Cardiac symptoms:* Palpitations (arrhythmia)
- *Renal symptoms:* Frothy urine, reduced urine output, change in urine colour
- GIT symptoms
- *Thyroid symptoms:* Cold intolerance, fatigue, menorrhagia
- Symptoms of increased sleepiness and fatigue in case of RLS.

Past history

- Similar illness in the past.
- History of epilepsy.
- History of heart disease.
- History of hypertension.
- History of DM.
- History of stroke.
- History of Parkinsonism or movement disorders.
- History of head trauma.
- History of neoplasm, infections, metabolic disorders.

Menstrual history

Pregnancy.

Family history

Family history of similar illness, epilepsy or malignancy.

Drug history:

History of use of drugs that might precipitate or worsen abnormal movements such as levodopa, metoclopramide, antipsychotic medications.

Social history

- History of alcohol use.
- History of drug abuse (hepatitis).
- Recent travel.

Further information not covered (at end of history taking)

Ask the patient the following question: Is there anything else that you feel is important and would like to tell me about?

Step 3: Explaining the diagnosis and the plan of management

Mrs Aslam, from the history you gave, it seems your husband has developed abnormal movements in his legs which come on when he goes to sleep or relaxes but they do not happen when he is active. Your husband is awake during the attacks and he feels abnormal sensations in his legs which give him an urge to move his legs. Your husband has kidney failure and is on haemodialysis and depression for which he was prescribed mirtazapine. The most probable cause of your husband's abnormal movements is a condition called 'restless leg syndrome'. This can cause unpleasant sensations in the legs and an irresistible urge to move them. Symptoms commonly occur in the evening and are often most severe at night when a person is resting but can occur when someone is inactive and sitting for extended periods. RLS is one of several disorders which can affect sleep and lead to daytime sleepiness, which can strongly affect mood, concentration and performance at work. In most cases, the cause of RLS is unknown, although it may be related to a dysfunction in the part of the brain (basal ganglia) that controls movement. RLS occurs more commonly in patients with end-stage kidney disease on haemodialysis and those with iron deficiency or using antidepressant medication like mirtazapine. I will arrange tests of your husband's nerves in his legs as this end-stage kidney disease can lead to nerve damage and painful sensations. I would recommend that the psychiatrist changes the mirtazapine to another antidepressant that does not worsen RLS. I am going to check the iron level in the blood of your husband as low levels may also worsen RLS. I will also refer your husband to a colleague in neurology who specialises in treating RLS.

Check understanding and agreement on plan of management.

Does that make sense to you?

Step 4: Ask about and address patient's concerns

Do you have any questions or concerns?

Patient's concern: Doctor, is there any treatment for this problem?

Reply: Yes. One of the most important steps in treating RLS is to identify and treat the underlying cause. In the case of your husband, optimizing dialysis and avoiding precipitating drugs such as mirtazapine should improve this condition. Additionally, lifestyle changes such as quitting alcohol and tobacco (not relevant for your husband) and avoiding caffeine before sleep, changing or maintaining a regular sleep pattern, a program of moderate exercise, and massaging the legs, taking a warm bath, and leg-stretching exercises of moderate intensity may provide some relief from mild symptoms. There are also some devices that include a foot wrap that puts pressure underneath the foot and another that is a pad that delivers vibration to the back of the legs, which can provide relief. I have checked the iron level in the blood of your husband, and we will treat any iron deficiency, if necessary. If these measures do not work, then we can consider sleeping pills and certain antiseizure medications like gabapentin and pregabalin.

People with RLS may be sleep deprived and tend to feel sleepy and tired during the day. I strongly recommend that driving or activities that require you to be alert should be stopped for the time being until the RLS is treated.

After answering each concern confirm the agreement by saying, is that OK or does that sound good to you?

Step 5: Summarise the discussion, confirm patient's understandings and close the meeting.

Mrs Aslam, I would like to summarise our discussion to be sure you understand important information about your husband's illness. The most probable cause for the abnormal movements of your husband's leg is a condition called RLS. Firstly,

I would recommend that the psychiatrist changes the mirtazapine as it may worsen RLS. I will check the iron levels and treat them if they are low as this can worsen RLS. I will arrange for your husband to be seen in a specialist clinic in sleep medicine and RLS. I strongly recommend that your husband stops driving and other tasks which require him to be alert until the RLS is treated. I will see you in 2 weeks' time to give you further answers. Meanwhile, I am going to provide you with my contact number in case you have any further questions or concerns regarding your condition. Does that sound good to you? You can get information from the internet on RLS. Thank you and see you soon.

Discussion

Problem
Abnormal leg movements in a patient with end-stage renal disease on haemodialysis taking mirtazapine.

Diagnosis
Restless leg syndrome.

Other plausible diagnosis
- **Periodic limb movement disorder**
  These are involuntary movements when the patient is sleeping.
- **Peripheral neuropathy secondary to uraemia**
  Peripheral neuropathy should be excluded in patients with end-stage renal failure as it may cause abnormal sensations.
- **Nocturnal leg cramps**
  These are typically unilateral, painful and palpable involuntary muscle contractions that are of sudden onset.

Causes of abnormal body movements

Tremor
Involuntary rhythmic oscillation movement of a body part, usually the hands and arms.
Common types of tremor
- *Resting tremor:* Parkinson's disease and other parkinsonian syndromes are the most common cause.
- *Postural tremor:* It occurs when the affected part adopts a fixed position, for instance, asking the patient to keep arms stretched out fully in front of them.
- *Common causes:* Physiological tremor (anxiety disorders, thyrotoxicosis), alcohol withdrawal and benign essential tremor.
- *Intention tremor:* As target approaches, tremor increases. This is best elicited by performing the finger/nose test. Occurs with cerebellar diseases.

Dystonia
Sustained and repetitive movements produced by simultaneous contractions of opposing muscle groups, often produces abnormal posture (which may be painful).
Common types of dystonia
- *Cervical dystonia:* Also known as spasmodic torticollis. Muscles in the head and neck are involved, resulting in abnormal head positioning.
- *Blepharospasm:* Eyelids close involuntarily, leading to prolonged closure or excessive blinking.
- *Tardive dyskinesia:* Most commonly results as a side effect of dopamine antagonists. Repetitive movements such as involuntary grimacing, sticking out the tongue or smacking of the lips are seen.

- Athetosis is an older term (which is now thought to be part of the spectrum of dystonia) where the affected body part undergoes writhing movements, and the patient is unable to keep it in one position.

Chorea

Chorea is a sudden dance-like jerky involuntary movement that is random in distribution, not repetitive or nonrhythmic and nonsustained. It can affect any part of the body and is usually bilateral.

Causes of chorea:

- Benign hereditary chorea
- Huntington's disease
- Wilson's disease
- Hyperthyroidism
- Systemic lupus erythematosus
- Rheumatic fever (Sydenham's chorea)
- Pregnancy (Chorea gravidarum)
- Drugs—oral contraceptive, levodopa, anticholinergics
- Toxins—alcohol
- Stroke or tumour affecting contralateral basal ganglia.

Hemiballismus

Wide and large flinging movements, commonly affecting one side of the body (usually the proximal limb).

The most common cause of hemiballismus is a stroke.

Myoclonus

Shock-like arrhythmic twitches that are not suppressible.

Tics

Brief, intermittent, meaningless movements (motor tics) or sounds (phonic tics), preceded by premonitory urges (unpleasant sensations which are relieved by carrying out the tic). They can be wilfully suppressed and often disappear with distraction.

Seizure

Uncontrolled electrical activity in the brain, which may produce a physical convulsion, minor physical signs, thought disturbances, or a combination of symptoms.

Epilepsy

Recurrent, unprovoked seizures from known or unknown causes.

Restless legs syndrome

Restless legs syndrome is one of the commonest movement disorders affecting sleep and the prevalence may be 8–10% in the Caucasian population. The diagnosis is simple and depends on taking a proper medical history. The condition is largely underdiagnosed and can cause great distress to the sufferers. It is characterised by motor restlessness and a strong urge to move the lower limbs, usually associated with unpleasant feeling in the legs that improves somewhat with movement. These unpleasant feeling can be in the form of aching, tingling, or crawling sensations. Symptoms are worse or exclusively present at rest and are partially relieved with activity. Symptoms are worse in the evening or at night before going to sleep. In order to relieve these sensations, the patient keeps moving the limbs sometimes in sudden and jerky movements. The movements usually alleviate the abnormal sensations which recur upon stopping the movements. Due to the unpleasant sensations and the urge to repeatedly move the legs, patient's sleep is often disturbed, and this can result in burdensome interruption of sleep and impairment of daytime function as a result of sleep deprivation.

It can be either primary or secondary.

- Primary or idiopathic RLS usually begins slowly, before approximately 40–45 years of age and may disappear for months or even years. It is often progressive and gets worse with age
- Secondary RLS often has a sudden onset after the age of 40 years and is associated with specific medical conditions or the use of certain drugs including:
  - Chronic renal disease/uraemia
  - Iron deficiency anaemia
  - Pregnancy
  - Peripheral neuropathy
  - Antihistamines
  - Tricyclic antidepressant such as mirtazapine
  - Metoclopramide
  - Excessive caffeine ingestion at night.

Diagnostic criteria

Diagnostic criteria include:

- A strong urge to move the limbs, usually associated with unpleasant or uncomfortable sensations.
- It starts or worsens during inactivity or rest.
- It improves or disappears (at least temporarily) with activity.
- It worsens in the evening or night.
- These symptoms are not caused by any medical or behavioural condition.

Treatment

- *Identify the cause and treat it:* Renal failure, avoid precipitating drugs, treat peripheral neuropathy
- *Lifestyle changes:* Avoid or reduce the use of alcohol and tobacco, maintain a regular sleep pattern, a program of moderate exercise, and massaging the legs, taking a warm bath, or using a heating pad or ice pack. Aerobic and leg-stretching exercises of moderate intensity may provide some relief from mild symptoms.
- Food and Drug Administration approved medical devices include a foot wrap that puts pressure underneath the foot and another that is a pad that delivers vibration to the back of the legs.
- Iron therapy for iron deficiency anaemia.
- Gabapentin, pregabalin and other antiseizure medications.
- Benzodiazepines.
- Use of dopaminergic drugs such as levodopa and bromocriptine.

What is the difference between RLS and periodic limb movement syndrome (PLMS)?
Periodic limb movement syndrome differs from RLS in that RLS occurs while the patients are awake, the movements are a voluntary response to an uncomfortable feeling in the legs. PLMS, on the other hand, occurs when the patient is asleep and unaware, and the movements are involuntary. The diagnosis of PLMS requires a sleep study (Polysomnography) and the diagnostic criteria require the presence of more than 15 periodic limb movements per hour of sleep time in adults causing clinically significant sleep disturbance or impairment in mental, physical, social, occupational, educational, or behavioural well-being not explained by some other entity. PLMS may occur with RLS and the drugs used for treatment are similar.

Further reading

Byrne R, Sinha S, Chaudhuri KR. Restless legs syndrome: diagnosis and review of management options. Neuropsychiatr Dis Treat 2006; 2:155–164.

Khalil A, Malik S. Movement disorders and tremors. InnovAiT 2013; 6:416–424.

National Institute of Neurological Disorders and Stroke. (2017). Restless Legs Syndrome Fact Sheet. How is restless legs syndrome diagnosed? [online]. Available from https://www.ninds.nih.gov/Disorders/Patient-Caregiver-Education/Fact-Sheets/Restless-Legs-Syndrome-Fact-Sheet#4. [Last accessed October, 2019].

The American Academy of Sleep Medicine. The AASM Manual for the Scoring of Sleep and Associated Events: Rules, Terminology and Technical Specifications, Version 2.5. Darien, IL: American Academy of Sleep Medicine; 2018.

Scenario no. 27

A patient with uncontrolled asthma

Candidate copy

Please read the GP referral letter for Mr Nasser
The time distribution for this station is as follows:

    You have (---) minutes to take a history from the patient.
    You have (---) minutes to collect your thoughts.
    You have (---) minutes for discussion with the examiners.

Please do not examine the patient

> **Dear Doctor,**
>
> Thank you for seeing Mr Nasser, a 24-year-old man with bronchial asthma. His asthma diagnosis was confirmed by spirometry. He was taking fluticasone inhaler 250 mcg twice daily and when needed salbutamol. However, his asthma remains uncontrolled. Despite changing fluticasone to fluticasone salmeterol (250/50 mcg) twice daily, his asthma remains uncontrolled with daily wheezing and daily use of salbutamol inhaler.
>
> Yours faithfully,

> Please interview the patient and based on history taking construct a differential diagnosis and plan of investigation. Provide explanation to the patient and answer any questions she may have.

Surrogate copy

Chief complaints and history of present illness

- You are Mr Nasser, 24-years-old.
- You are concerned about your asthma as you have been getting frequent chest tightness and wheezing almost every day for the last 3 months.
- You wake up at night short of breath 4–5 times per week.
- You have frequent absences from work because of your asthma.
- You use your salbutamol inhaler every day more than 3 times per day.
- You visited the emergency department 3 weeks ago for asthma symptoms and were given some medications via nebuliser and sent home.
- You also have cough but without phlegm.
- You did not have a respiratory infection before this.
- You do not know what brings on your asthma symptoms.
- You have not observed any difference in asthma symptoms during different seasons.
- You have not observed any difference in your asthma symptoms indoor or outdoor.
- Your asthma is not related to exercise.

Only when asked:
- You have never been provided with an asthma action plan
- You do not have a peak flow meter at home.

Review of systems

Only when asked:
- You have recurrent sneezing and your nose is runny and itchy.
- You also feel the desire to clear your throat frequently.
- You do not have acidity or heartburn.
- Occasionally, your skin becomes itchy.
- Rest of the systemic review is normal.

Past medical history

- You have been diagnosed with asthma since the age of 13 years. Your asthma control was better until the age of 22 years. Since the age of 22 years, you started getting asthma symptoms again which worsened over the last 3 months. Your GP performed a spirometry test and confirmed it as asthma.
- Apart from your visit to the emergency room 3 weeks ago, you have never been admitted to the hospital or intensive care unit for asthma before.

Drug history

- At the beginning, your GP prescribed fluticasone inhaler and salbutamol inhaler.
- You were using both when needed.
- Your asthma did not get better on these medications.
- Your GP has changed fluticasone to fluticasone salmeterol in one inhaler and despite using the new drug, when needed, it did not help.
- *Only if doctor* requests to show how to use your inhaler: Just spray the inhaler in your mouth without taking a breath.

Family history

- Two of your uncles from your mother's side have asthma.
- Your cousin also has asthma.

Social history

- You do not smoke.
- You not drink alcohol.
- You work as a computer technician.
- You keep a cat at home.
- You have not observed moulds at home.

Your questions to the doctors and concerns

Why is my asthma not controlled?

Steps in history taking in a patient with uncontrolled asthma

Step 1: Introduction, greeting and confirmation of patient identity
- Good morning Mr Nasser (shakehands with the patient), pleased to meet you.
- I am Dr X working in the medical outpatient clinic.
- Can I confirm that I am talking to Mr Nasser?
- I have just read the referral letter from your GP who states that you are concerned about your asthma control.
- Can you tell me more about that?
- Allow the patient to speak.
- Avoid interruptions.
- Avoid medical jargon [e.g., gastroesophageal reflux disease (GERD), allergic rhinitis, pulmonary function test, etc.]
- *Use open-ended questions such as:* What else?

Step 2: Elaborating important points in the history of asthma

History of presenting illness
- What are the main symptoms of the patient?
  - Typical symptoms of asthma are chest tightness, wheezing, breathlessness and cough.
  - Sputum production is not typical for asthma and should raise the possibility of alternative diagnosis such as bronchiectasis).
- What are the exacerbating factors for your asthma symptoms?
  Such as food, pollens, trees, cat fur, dog fur, perfumes, smokes, etc.
- What are the relieving factors for your asthma symptoms?
- Have you observed any seasonal variation in your asthma symptoms?
  This may point to specific allergens (e.g. pollens).
- Is your asthma worse indoor or outdoor?
  Indoor: Suspect indoor allergens (house dust mites, cockroaches, etc.)
  Outdoor: Suspect outdoor allergens (grass, pollens, etc.)
- Do you wake up at night because of asthma symptoms?
  Nocturnal symptoms denote poorly controlled asthma.

- **Check asthma level of control over the previous 4 weeks**
  Use validated tools such as Global Initiative for Asthma (GINA) control tool or asthma control test.

Review of systems
- *Nose and throat:* Allergic rhinitis symptoms such as runny, itchy nose and postnasal drip.
- *Skin:* Urticaria, allergic skin rash
- *Cardiovascular:* Chest pain, PND, orthopnoea
- GIT symptoms: GERD
- *Locomotor:* Purpura (Churg–Strauss syndrome)
- *Symptoms of obstructive sleep apnoea:* Increased sleepiness, snoring, nocturnal apnoea and fatigue.

Past history
- When was the asthma diagnosed?
- Was asthma diagnosis confirmed by spirometry?
- This is a very important question as not all wheezes are caused by asthma and many patients who are thought to have uncontrolled asthma, have in fact alternative diagnoses causing the respiratory symptoms.
- Previous emergency room visits, hospital admissions and ICU admissions because of asthma.
- History of associated asthma comorbidities
  (Such as allergic rhinitis, postnasal drip, GERD, obstructive sleep apnoea). Such comorbidities, if left untreated, can cause worsening of asthma control [for uncontrolled asthma, search above the chest (nose/throat) and below the chest (stomach/GERD)].

Menstrual history
Effects of pregnancy and menstruation on asthma control.

Family history
Family history of asthma and allergic disease.
Drug history:
- Details of asthma medications

- Does the patient know the difference between reliever and controller medications?
- Does the patient use controller medication as a reliever (When there are symptoms only)?
  (Patient's wrong perception of the role of asthma medications, such as using controller as a reliever only, is an important cause of poor asthma control).
- Ask the patient to demonstrate the inhaler technique.
  History of use of drugs that worsen asthma control such as NSAID, beta-blockers and aspirin.

Social history
- History of smoking.
- Keeping pets or birds at home.
- *Housing condition:* Presence of moulds, cockroaches, grass and trees and high humidity may cause worsening of asthma control.

Further information not covered (at end of history taking)
Ask the patient the following question: Is there anything else that you feel is important and would like to tell me about?

Step 3: Explaining the diagnosis and the plan of management
Mr Nasser, your asthma seems to be out of control these days as you are having frequent day time symptoms, you wake up at night frequently with asthma symptoms and the asthma is preventing you from doing your daily work. There are good reasons why your asthma is not controlled. First is the way you are using your inhaler medication and the lack of knowledge about asthma medications. There are major mistakes in your inhaler technique.
This has to be corrected as it will not be possible for you to control asthma if the medication is not reaching your lungs in the proper way. I am going to demonstrate to you the proper technique and will also refer you to our asthma educator to further teach you on that. In addition, you mentioned that you are using the fluticasone inhaler for a few days and only when you have your asthma symptoms. Fluticasone is not a reliever medication for asthma. In fact, it is a controller medication that aims to prevent your asthma symptoms from coming on. That is why, it has to be taken for a longer period of time even when you are free of symptoms. The second reason is your uncontrolled nose allergy. You mentioned that you have a runny and itchy nose with a desire to clear your throat frequently. This suggests that you are suffering from a condition called 'allergic rhinitis' which may coexist with asthma. If left untreated, allergic rhinitis can cause worsening of your asthma control. I am going to prescribe a spray to be used in the nose and will explain how to use it. In order to improve your asthma care and help you to control your asthma, I am going to provide you with an asthma action plan. This is a written plan displayed in traffic light colours that tells you what to do and what medications you need to take at various stages of your asthma control. I am also going to provide you with a peak expiratory flow meter which is a small device you blow into every day to check the performance of your lungs. I understand that you are keeping a cat at home. I am going to perform some blood and allergy testing to look for different allergens that may bring on your asthma symptoms so that you can avoid them.
Check understanding and agreement on plan of management.
Does that make sense to you?

Step 4: Ask about and address patient's concerns
Do you have any questions or concerns?
Patient's concern: Why is my asthma not controlled?

Reply: Answered
After answering each concern, confirm agreement by saying, is that OK or does that sound good to you?

Step 5: Summarise the discussion, confirm patient's understandings and close the meeting

Mr Nasser, I would like to summarise our discussion to be sure that you understand important information about your asthma. The most probable causes for your uncontrolled asthma are the wrong inhaler technique, the lack of knowledge about types and roles of asthma medications, and the presence of untreated allergic rhinitis. I am going to demonstrate to you the proper technique of inhaler use and refer you to an asthma educator. We have to also treat your allergic rhinitis. I will provide you with a written asthma action plan that will show how to deal with your asthma. I will also provide you with a peak expiratory flow meter to use at home for measurement of lung performance. I will see you in 2 weeks to give you further answers. Meanwhile, I am going to provide you with my contact number in case you have any further questions or concerns regarding your condition. Does that sound good to you? You can get some videos from the internet on inhaler use and asthma control. Thank you and see you soon.

Discussion

Problem

Uncontrolled asthma.

Diagnosis

Poor inhaler technique and wrong perception of asthma medications.

Other plausible diagnosis

- Presence of uncontrolled allergic rhinitis
- Persistent allergen (e.g. cat fur).

Causes of uncontrolled asthma

- Wrong diagnosis (It is an asthma mimic and not asthma)
- *Persistent allergen:* Moulds, house dust mites, cockroaches, animal fur, etc.
- Poor inhaler technique
- Wrong perception and knowledge about asthma and asthma medications.
- *Presence of untreated comorbidities:* Allergic rhinitis, post-nasal drip, GERD or obstructive apnoea
- Severe form of asthma.

Six important actions to be taken in any asthma case clinic visit

- *Assess asthma control:* Using validated tool such as GINA control tool or asthma control test.
- *Allergen search:* Look for allergens that precipitate symptoms.
- *Ability to use inhaler:* Check inhaler technique.
- *Adherence to medication:* Check adherence and knowledge about asthma medications.
- *Asthma comorbidities:* Treat asthma comorbidities that make asthma worse such as allergic rhinitis treatment, post-nasal drip, GERD, obstructive apnoea and obesity.
- *Asthma action plan:* Written plan should be provided to every patient with asthma.

Correct steps for use of metered-dose inhaler

- Remove the cap.
- Shake the inhaler.
- Breath out.
- Put the mouth piece inside the mouth and apply good seal.
- Press the canister at the start of inspiration and breathe in slowly.
- Hold breath for 10 seconds.

Note: Dry powder inhalers (DPI) require forceful and deep inhalation for the powder to reach the lungs.

Table 3 Stepwise approach for managing asthma	
Step 1	As needed SABA
	Consider low dose ICS
Step 2	As needed SABA
	Low dose ICS
Step 3	As needed SABA
	Low dose ICS + LABA
Step 4	As needed SABA
	Medium or high dose ICS + LABA
Step 5	As needed SABA
	Add on such as: • Tiotropium • Anti-IgE • Anti-IL5

(ICS: inhaled corticosteroid; LABA: long-acting beta agonist; SABA: short-acting beta agonist; IgE: immunoglobulin E; IL: interleukin)

Stepwise approach to asthma management

The stepwise approach for managing asthma is given in **Table 3**.

Further reading

Global Initiative for Asthma. (2018). Global strategy for asthma management and prevention, 2018. [online]. Available from https://ginasthma.org/wp-content/uploads/2018/04/wms-GINA-2018-report-tracked_v1.3.pdf. [Last accessed October, 2019].

Ibrahim WH, Suleiman NN, El-Allus F, et al. The burden of adult asthma in a high GDP per capita country: the QASMA study. Ann Allergy Asthma Immunol 2015; 114:12–17.

Scenario no. 28

A patient with hand pain

Candidate copy

Please read the GP referral letter for Ms Salma.
The time distribution for this station is as follows:

> You have (---) minutes to take a history from the patient.
> You have (---) minutes to collect your thoughts.
> You have (---) minutes for discussion with the examiners.

Please do not examine the patient

Dear Doctor,

Thank you for seeing Ms Salma, a 24-year-old woman. She has been complaining of bilateral hand pain and paresthesia on exposure to cold over the past 3 months. These symptoms are distressing as they interfere with her job as a secretary.

Yours faithfully,

Please interview the patient and based on history taking construct a differential diagnosis and plan of investigation. Provide an explanation to the patient and answer any questions she may have.

Surrogate copy

Chief complaints and history of present illness

- You are Ms Salma, 24-year-old.
- You are concerned about hand pain over the last 3 months.
- The pain involves both of your hands.
- The pain occurs in episodes.
- It is worse at the tip of your fingers.
- It sometimes involve your toes as well but less frequently than your fingers.
- The pain is aching and associated with sensations of pins and needles.
- The pain episodes are usually precipitated by exposure them to cold and gets better when you warm your hands.

Only when asked:
You experience a change in the colour of your fingers when you expose them to cold. Initially, the colour of your fingers turn white (pale), then it becomes blue. It takes 15–20 minutes after warming to become red.

Review of systems

Only when asked:
- You have recurrent joint pains involving knees and fingers.
- On occasions, you suffer difficulty in swallowing (involves both solid and liquid food).
- Your hair has been falling out.
- You suffer recurrent mouth ulcers.
- You do not have a skin rash.
- You do not have sensitivity to light.

Rest of systemic review is normal.

Past medical history

You have had migraine for 5 years. The migraine attacks are usually severe and have been increasing in frequency for the last 6 months.

Drug history

Only if the doctor asks about medications, you mention that you are taking migraine tablets called Migril (Ergotamine and caffeine) to relieve your migraine attacks. You have been using these tablets frequently for the past 3 months.

Family history

Your aunt has a disease called systemic lupus erythematosus (SLE).

Social history

- You smoke 20 cigarettes every day for the past 4 years.
- You do not drink alcohol.
- You do not take recreational drugs (cocaine).
- You work as a secretary in an office.
- Your hand pains have made your job difficult and you are thinking of resigning.

Your questions to the doctors and concerns

> What causes this condition?
> Is there any treatment for this condition?

Steps in history taking in a patient with Raynaud's phenomenon

Step 1: Introduction, greeting and confirmation of patient identity

- Good morning Ms Salma (shakehands with the patient), pleased to meet you.
- I am Dr X working in the medical outpatient clinic.
- Can I confirm that I am talking to Ms Salma?
- I have just read the referral letter from your GP who states that you are concerned about your hand pains.
- Can you tell me more about this pain?
- Allow the patient to speak.
- Avoid interruptions.
- Avoid medical jargon (e.g. Raynaud's, SLE, scleroderma, etc.)
- *Use open-ended questions such as:* What else?

Step 2: Elaborating important points in the history of abnormal movements

History of presenting illness

- Analyse pain using LIQOR AAA?
  Location of the pain, Intensity, Quality, Onset, Radiation, Aggravating factors, Alleviating factors and Associated symptoms.
- Ask about the sequence of changes in the colour of fingers when exposed to cold? Raynaud's phenomenon typically starts with sudden pain in the fingers on exposure to cold. Typical colour changes of the fingers begin as pallor/white (due to vasoconstriction) and then turn bluish (due to tissue hypoxia). After rewarming, the skin becomes erythematous (from reperfusion).
- Pain may be associated with paraesthesia in the form of pins and needles.
- Toes may also be involved.

Review of systems

Ask about symptoms of rheumatologic diseases such as SLE, scleroderma, mixed connective tissue disease:

- Mouth ulcers
- Hair fall
- Photosensitive skin rash
- Dysphagia
- Joint pain.

Past history

Past history of connective tissue disorders.

Family history

Family history of connective tissue diseases.

Drug history

Drugs that can cause or exacerbate Raynaud's phenomenon:

- Ergotamine
- Cocaine
- Beta-blockers
- Clonidine
- Certain chemotherapeutic agents.

Social history

- History of smoking.
- History of cocaine abuse.
- *Occupation:* Using vibrating tools.

Further information not covered (at end of history taking):

Ask the patient the following question: Is there anything else that you feel is important and would like to tell me about?

Step 3: Explaining the diagnosis and the plan of management

Ms Salma, you complain of pain in your fingers that gets worse after cold exposure. Your finger colour also changes during exposure to cold. The cause of your pain is a condition called 'Raynaud's phenomenon'. Have you heard of this condition before? Raynaud's phenomenon is a condition named after Dr Maurice Raynaud, the man who first described it in 1862. In this condition, the small blood vessels of the fingers (and toes) become narrow (constrict), most commonly when they are in a cool environment. These changes result in a decrease in blood flow to the fingers and toes and subsequently the changes in the skin colour you experience during the attack. There are some conditions that need to be excluded as possible causes of Raynaud's phenomenon. Among these conditions are a group of diseases called 'autoimmune diseases'. I am going to request some blood tests to make sure that you do not have any of these diseases.

Does that make sense to you?

Step 4: Ask about and address patient's concerns

Do you have any questions or concerns?

Patient's concern: What causes Raynaud's phenomenon?

Reply: This is a very good question. It is important to know there are two types of Raynaud's phenomenon—these are referred to as 'primary' and 'secondary'. Primary Raynaud's occurs in patients who do not have another rheumatic disease. Secondary Raynaud's is 'secondary' to another condition. These conditions are numerous and can include several autoimmune conditions. The most common rheumatic diseases associated with Raynaud's include scleroderma and lupus, but can include other forms of rheumatic diseases.

Patient's concern: Is there any treatment for this condition?

Reply: Besides treating the disease that has caused it, there are different measures used to treat Raynaud's phenomenon:

- When possible, please avoid cold exposure and sudden temperature changes such as holding ice cream, suddenly entering a cold place or putting hands in a freezer.
- Please dress warmly (including warm gloves and socks).
- Smoking is a very important risk factor for Raynaud's phenomenon. I strongly encourage you to stop smoking.
- Your migraine tablet 'Migril' contains substances that constrict your blood vessels. These substances are ergotamine and caffeine. I strongly recommend that you discuss with your migraine doctor to change this medication.
- I also recommend that you reduce drinks and food that is rich in caffeine.
- Most patients respond very well to these measures. However, for those who do not respond, we may start certain medications that prevent the blood vessels from getting narrow.

After answering each concern, confirm agreement by saying, is that OK or does that sound good to you?

Step 5: Summarise the discussion, confirm patient's understandings and close the meeting

Ms Salma, I would like to summarise our discussion to be sure that you understand important information about your illness. The most probable cause for the pain in your fingers is Raynaud's phenomenon. I am going to order some blood tests for you to make sure that there is no autoimmune disease causing this. Please avoid exposure to cold, wear warm gloves and socks, stop smoking, and avoid medications and drinks that trigger Raynaud's. I will arrange another appointment in 2 weeks' time to review with you the results of blood tests. Meanwhile, I am going to provide you with my contact number in case you have any further questions or concerns regarding your condition. Does that sound good to you? You can get some information from the internet on Raynaud's phenomenon. Thank you and see you soon.

Discussion

Problem

Pain and paraesthesia in fingers.

Diagnosis

Raynaud's phenomenon.

Other plausible diagnosis

- Systemic lupus erythematosus
- Systemic sclerosis
- Drug-induced Raynaud's phenomenon.

Discussion

Aetiology of Raynaud's phenomenon

- *Primary (idiopathic)*
  - Accounts for the majority of cases of Raynaud's phenomenon (90%).
  - Affects younger age groups (15–30 years).
  - More common in women (disease of young women).
  - About 1 in every 10 women in some western countries has primary Raynaud's.
  - Typically does not cause digital ulcer or gangrene.
- *Secondary causes*
  - *Connective tissue diseases:* Systemic sclerosis, mixed connective tissue disease, SLE, Sjogren's syndrome
  - Hand–arm vibration syndrome ('vibration white finger')
  - Extrinsic vascular compression (e.g. cervical rib)
  - Buerger's disease, atherosclerosis
  - Paraproteinaemia, malignancy
  - *Certain drugs and chemicals:* Beta-blockers, ergotamine, cisplatin, clonidine, vinyl chloride.

Differentiating primary from secondary Raynaud's phenomenon

- Comprehensive history and physical examination looking for symptoms and signs of other autoimmune diseases, medications, smoking, etc.
- Performing nailfold capillaroscopy and testing for autoantibodies (in particular, those associated with systemic sclerosis. Patients with Raynaud's phenomenon and either abnormal nailfold capillaroscopy or a systemic sclerosis-specific antibody (and especially with both) have a high risk of transitioning to an autoimmune connective tissue disease.

Treatment of Raynaud's phenomenon

Nonpharmacologic measures (General/lifestyle measures)
- Avoidance of cold exposure
- Avoidance of vasoconstricting drugs
- Avoidance of smoking
- Avoidance of trauma.

Pharmacologic therapies
- *Calcium channel blockers:* Nifedipine 10–40 mg twice daily, amlodipine 5–10 mg once daily
- *Phosphodiesterase 5 inhibitor:* Sildenafil 20 mg or 25 mg three times daily to 50 mg three times daily
- *Angiotensin II receptor blockers:* Losartan 25–100 mg once daily
- *Selective serotonin reuptake inhibitor:* Fluoxetine 20 mg once daily
- Intravenous prostanoid therapy.

Procedural therapies, including surgery
- Botulinum toxin injections
- Digital sympathectomy and amputation.

Further reading

American College of Rheumatologists. (2019). Raynaud's phenomenon. [online]. Available from https://www.rheumatology.org/I-Am-A/Patient-Caregiver/Diseases-Conditions/Raynauds-Phenomenon. [Last accessed October, 2019].

Herrick AL. Evidence-based management of Raynaud's phenomenon. Ther Adv Musculoskelet Dis 2017; 9:317–329.

Hughes M, Herrick AL. Raynaud's phenomenon. Best Pract Res Clin Rheumatol 2016; 30:112–132.

Part 3

Communication skills

The seven-step approach to the communication skill scenario

Always read the scenario carefully and make sure you understand the instructions before you start. All the information provided is relevant. Make notes and a framework for your discussion. Sometimes a hidden agenda is incorporated, pay attention to that.

Introduction and identification

- **Prepare the environment**
  Sit at the same level as the patient with comfort and avoid barriers like tables.

- **Introduce yourself to the patient**
  Shake hands (be aware of social and religious reasons preventing some patients from shaking your hand).
  Hello Mr Z, I am doctor X, working in the medical outpatient clinic.

- **Enquire from the patient if he would like someone else to be present during the discussion**
  Can I confirm that I am talking to Mr Z?
  Would you like to invite anybody else to this discussion?

- **Confirm the objective of the interview**
  We are here today to discuss the results of your investigations and diagnosis. Is that alright?

Check patient's understanding and expectations

- Tell me Mr Z, how much do you know about your health?
- Do you know why the test was ordered for you?
- What do you suspect might be wrong with your lungs?

Discussion with the patient (information giving)

- Give the patient the information (avoid medical jargon and explain what you mean)
- Pay attention to the hidden agenda in the scenario.

Hidden agenda is important information you should discuss with the patient and is usually not mentioned directly in the scenario. It is usually related to one of the following topics:
- Effect of the disease on pregnancy and effects of pregnancy on the disease
- Use of contraceptive pills (interaction with drugs/need for birth control)
- Driving and the illness (disease interferes with ability to drive vehicles)
- Effect of the disease on occupation
- Effect of the disease on other people in the community (infectious disease)
- Alcohol and smoking
- Travel and flights (stroke, pulmonary embolism, acute coronary syndrome)
- Sexual relations
- The need for vaccination

- The need for cancer screening/family screening
- Organ donation/do not attempt resuscitation (DNAR).

Explore and respond to the patient's concerns

Is there any question or concern you want to discuss?

Show empathy

I can understand Mr Z how difficult it is to hear that you have this condition, we are here to help you.

Summarise and confirm understanding

So Mr Z, I would like to briefly summarise our discussion as it is important for me to be sure that you have understood all the information. You were admitted to the hospital with a cough, fever, and mild breathing difficulty. Because of your long-standing history of smoking, we did some breathing function tests and these show that you have a condition called chronic obstructive pulmonary disease (COPD). Your disease is at a mild stage right now and should respond to inhalers. We will show you how to use these inhalers. It is really important that you stop smoking, have a regular flu vaccine, and enter an exercise program to help your breathing.

    Is everything clear so far?

    Please tell me if you want to discuss anything more at this moment.

Offer help and follow-up and close the discussion

Examples of such help and follow-up plans are:
- Should you have any further questions later, please do not hesitate to contact me on my office phone number.
- I will also arrange another appointment in 2 weeks, in case you have further questions or concerns.
- I will arrange an appointment with a colleague specialised in lung diseases to further discuss with you the treatment options.
- I will refer you to the smoking cessation clinic.
- I will also provide you with some website addresses and printed material which will give you more idea about your condition.

Do's and don'ts in communication skill (and history taking) stations

- Do read carefully the scenario in the time allocated and mark each point
- Do remember that all information given in the scenario is important
- Do introduce yourself to the patient
- Do use open-ended question at the beginning
- Do use simple language
- Do mention the purpose of the interview
- Do explain the problem and management
- Do address the patient's concerns
- Do show empathy
- Do know your limitations (refer to colleagues/seek help for ethical/legal dilemmas)
- Do summarise at the end and ask the patient if they have any further concerns
- Do not develop speech diarrhoea in the station
- Do not use medical jargon

- Do not interrupt the patient/surrogate
- Do not confront the patient/surrogate
- Do not panic when you face an angry patient/surrogate
- Do not forget to address patient's concerns/questions
- Do not talk about your colleagues or criticise them.

Facing a difficult patient

Difficult patient encounters occur in about 15% of patients.

There are many reasons why some patients may seem difficult and include:
- Presence of underlying mood, anxiety disorder or psychosocial disorders
- Fear and anxiety regarding their current illness
- Alcoholism
- Physician's experience (less-experienced physicians report encountering more difficult patients)
- Unmet requests after healthcare visits
- Long waiting time in healthcare facilities can also create difficult patient encounters.

Difficult patient encounters may take different forms such as:
- Dealing with anxious patients
- Dealing with angry patients
- Dealing with quiet patients
- Dealing with overconfident patients or even violent patients
- Dealing with ethical dilemmas.
  Whatever the type of difficult patient encounter faced, physicians should always bear in mind that they are obliged ethically and morally to help patients and solve their medical problems, whenever possible.

How to respond to a difficult patient's encounter?
- Listen to your patient's concern or complaint, express your understanding of their feelings and emotional response to the condition and always show empathy.
- Always stay calm and professional when encountering a difficult patient.
- Use simple sentences to show your empathy. An angry patient, for example, may be reassured by a simple sentence from his/her physician such as 'I understand your frustration and I am here to help you' or 'I am sorry to hear you are frustrated, I am here to help you.'
- Avoid arguing, blaming or confronting patients. Such unprofessional behaviour may worsen a difficult situation.

Types of communication skills scenarios in postgraduate clinical examinations

Information giving/explaining

Explaining diagnosis

Common scenarios:

- Asthma
- Chronic obstructive pulmonary disease
- Idiopathic pulmonary fibrosis
- Multiple sclerosis
- Diabetes
- Hypertension
- Epilepsy
- Systemic lupus erythematosus

- Congestive heart failure
- End-stage renal disease
- Obstructive sleep apnoea
- Myocardial infarction and prevention of recurrence
- Stroke and prevention of recurrence
- Lymphoma
- Colon cancer
- Inflammatory bowel disease
- Motor neuron disease
- Huntington's chorea
- Leukaemia.

Explaining management and treatment of a disease

- Warfarin
- New oral anticoagulants
- Low-molecular weight heparin during pregnancy
- Initiating insulin therapy.

Explaining the results of investigations

(Abnormal laboratory tests or imaging)
- Incidental finding of a solitary pulmonary nodule on CT scan
- Abnormal liver function or kidney function
- Discuss a CT/MRI scan result that shows a possibility of malignancy or a chronic illness.

Planning discharge from the hospital

- Discharge plan of a patient after acute coronary syndrome
- Discharge plan of a patient after ischaemic stroke
- Discharge plan of a patient after a massive pulmonary embolism.

Breaking bad news

- Chronic illness
- Cancer
- Discussing an acutely ill patient's condition with the family.

Dealing with angry patient and their family and managing complaints

- A son/daughter who feels his/her parent was mismanaged
- A patient who is angry because of a delay in management.

Discussing 'do not resuscitate order' and 'end-of-life issues'

- Do not resuscitate order
- Brain death
- Persistent vegetative state
- Organ donation.

Obtaining patient's consent for a procedure

- Kidney biopsy
- Enteral tube feeding (PEG)
- Liver biopsy
- Haemodialysis/peritoneal dialysis

Special legal and ethical issues

- HIV testing
- Fitness to drive
- A colleague (nurse) with a needle stick injury
- Unprofessional attitude/behaviour of a colleague
- Patient refusing treatment
- Discharge against medical advice
- Interfering relatives

Further reading

Gough M, Hoffenberg R, Ledingham J. The value of history taking. BMJ 2003; 327:1117.

Haas L, Leiser J, Magill M, et al. Management of the Difficult Patient. Am Fam Physician 2005; 72:2063–2068.

Maguire P. Key communication skills and how to acquire them. BMJ 2002; 325:697–700.

Paley L, Zornitzki T, Cohen J, et al. Utility of clinical examination in the diagnosis of emergency department patients admitted to the department of medicine of an academic hospital. Arch Intern Med 2011; 171:1395–1356.

Peterson MC, Holbrook JH, von Hales D, et al. Contributions of the history, physical examination, and laboratory investigation in making medical diagnoses. West J Med 1992; 156:163–165.

Part 4

Communication skills and ethics scenarios

Scenario no. 1

Type of scenario: Information giving/breaking bad news of chronic disease

Candidate information

Your role: You are the doctor in the medical outpatient clinic.
Problem: Explanation of newly diagnosed chronic disease.
Patient: Mr Muhammad, a 50-year-old gentleman.

Please read the scenario printed below. When the bell sounds, enter the room. You have (---) minutes for your consultation with the patient/relative, (---) minutes to collect your thoughts, and (---) minutes for discussion.

Please do not examine the patient
Please do not take a history

> Mr Muhammad is a 50-year-old gentleman who was admitted recently to the acute medical unit with a productive cough, sputum, and fever for which he was treated with a course of antibiotics. He has had a cough for the last 2 years along with mild exertional dyspnoea and weight loss of 5 kg in the last year. He is a smoker of 20 pack-years. His chest X-rays was normal. His pulmonary function tests showed he has mild chronic obstructive pulmonary disease (COPD). Now he is worried that he may have a cancer as he has been smoking for a long time.
>
> **Your task:** Is to answer the patient's questions and help him to understand the new diagnosis and further plan of management if needed.

Approach

Always read the scenario carefully and make sure you understand the instructions before you start. Any information provided is important. Make notes and a framework for your discussion. Sometimes, a hidden agenda is incorporated; pay attention to that.

Introduction and identification

- **Prepare the environment**
  Sit at the same level as the patient with comfort and avoid barriers like tables.

- **Introduce yourself to the patient**
  Shake hands.
  Hello Mr Muhammad, I am Dr X, working in the medical outpatient clinic.

- **Enquire from the patient if he would like someone else to be present during the discussion**
  Can I confirm that I am talking to Mr Muhammad?
  Would you like to invite anybody else to this discussion?

- **Confirm the objective of the interview**
  We are here today to discuss the results of your investigations and diagnosis. Is that alright?

Check patient's understanding and expectation

Tell me Mr Muhammad how much do you know about your health status?
Do you know why the breathing test was ordered for you?
What do you think might be wrong with your breathing and chest?

Discussion with the patient (information giving)

- **Give the patient the information (avoid medical jargon)**
  As you know Mr Muhammad, you were admitted to the hospital with a cough, fever, and some mild breathing difficulty. Since you have had the cough and breathing difficulties for about 2 years and you have been smoking for almost 20 years, we did the chest X-ray which was normal. However, the breathing tests show that you have a problem with your lungs called 'chronic obstructive pulmonary disease (COPD)'.

- **Explore the patient's ideas about COPD**
  Have you heard of COPD before? Pause....

- **Explain to the patient in simple terms about chronic obstructive pulmonary disease or COPD (avoid medical jargon)**
  Chronic obstructive pulmonary disease is a long-standing narrowing of the windpipes in the chest caused by smoking. Smoking causes inflammation of the windpipe and smaller air passages in the lungs leading to narrowing and damage of these passages with time. These changes cause the cough and reduce the amount of oxygen in the air passing to your body and increase the chance of getting chest infections. The special breathing tests (lung function tests) confirmed that the type of airway narrowing is due to COPD.

- **Pause and ask the patient if they understand everything so far.**

- **Explain how the assessment of severity of COPD is done**
  Based on your symptoms, the chest X-ray findings, and the lung function tests, I can say that you have a mild form of COPD.

- **Explain the treatment options**
  The treatment of COPD involves four lines of therapy: Avoiding the cause, which means you have to stop smoking; medication to widen the narrowed airways and improve oxygen delivery to the blood, some exercise and vaccination programs, and if necessary, surgery. Since your COPD is mild at the moment, surgery is not indicated. Regarding medications, inhalers will help to keep your windpipes open and relieve your symptoms. Have you seen someone using inhalers before? It is important that you use the inhalers properly and we will teach you how to do this.

- **Explain the importance of smoking cessation**
  Mr Muhammad, smoking has played a major role in your illness; therefore, quitting smoking is a crucial step in managing your illness. Continuing to smoke will make the COPD worse, leading to worsening of your symptoms and the need for oxygen therapy at home. It can also increase your risk of developing lung cancer and heart disease.
  Are you willing to discuss the ways to stop smoking?
  If he agrees, discuss with him the type of help offered by the smoking cessation clinic and refer him.
  If he is not willing to discuss this, then give him informative material regarding the clinic and suggest you will discuss this further in the next appointment.

- **Advise about vaccination**
  Another important point to mention is that your symptoms can worsen with infections. There are vaccines which can help in reducing the chances of getting such infections. The main vaccinations are against bacteria called pneumococci and the flu shot. They are safe with no major side effects. If you are willing to take them, I can arrange that for you.

- **Pulmonary rehabilitation**
  As you have some on-going breathing difficulty and you were admitted recently to hospital, I will refer you to an exercise programme which will help to improve your breathing difficulty. Does that make sense to you?

- **Lung cancer screening**
  (See patient's concerns).

- **Check the patient understanding.**
  Is everything clear so far?

Explore and respond to patient's concerns

Do you have any questions or concerns to discuss?

- **Do I have cancer? Why am I losing weight?**
  This is an important question. Smoking can cause lung cancer. What is reassuring in this regard is that your chest X-ray did not show any evidence of cancer. COPD itself can cause weight loss. I would emphasize that the chances of getting lung cancer become higher if you continue to smoke.
  - **Inform about screening for lung cancer**
  - **Eligibility:** Age 55–74 years with ≥30 pack-year smoking history and either continuing to smoke or have quit within the past 15 years (American College of Chest Physicians, 2013).

- **He may ask you regarding the duration of treatment**
  Mr Muhammad, your illness is long-standing and it cannot be cured, so it needs long-term use of inhalers, which can be changed or used more or less frequently based on your breathing function tests.

- **He may ask regarding long-term effect of inhalers**
  You do not require a steroid inhaler just now which can have some mild side effects; otherwise all other inhalers have no major side effect.

- **He may ask about ways to help him quit smoking and electronic cigarettes**
  There are a number of ways to help you quit smoking. We have a specialised clinic with colleagues who are expert in this. I am going to write a referral letter to one

of them to see you soon. One of the methods is the nicotine replacement method where some of the nicotine that gives you the craving to smoke is given in the form of nicotine gum, patch or lozenges. There are serious concerns from experts regarding the effectiveness and safety of electronic cigarettes.

Show empathy

I understand Mr Muhammad how difficult it must be to hear that you have COPD. We are here to help you.

Summarise and confirm understanding

So, Mr Muhammad, I would like to briefly summarise our discussion as it is important for me to be sure that you understand important points about your illness. Following your admission to the hospital with cough, fever, and mild breathing difficulty, the breathing function tests showed that you have mild COPD. This can be treated with inhalers and we will teach you how to use them.

We have also discussed the importance of smoking cessation, vaccination, and the exercise programme.

Is everything clear so far?

Do you have any further questions at this moment?

Offer help and follow-up and close the discussion

Should you have any further questions, please do not hesitate to contact me on my office telephone number.

I will arrange another appointment in 2 weeks to review how you are getting on.

I am going to arrange an appointment with our lung specialist and refer you to the smoking cessation clinic.

I will provide you with some website addresses and printed material to read more about your diagnosis.

Discussion

Ethical principles

- **What are the main ethical principles in this scenario?**

  Patient autonomy: A doctor should provide the patient with the necessary information to help him make his future decisions. Doctor should be honest and truthful when discussing the risks and complications regarding treatment. The patient has the right to know about the diagnosis and prognosis of his COPD. He has the right to agree or refuse smoking cessation or further treatment.

  Beneficence and non-maleficence:
  - Smoking cessation will stop further damage to the lungs.
  - Vaccination will limit infections and hospitalisation.
  - Compliance with medication will improve lung function.

  Justice: Should include justice to the patient and community. The patient should be treated in a fair manner without discrimination.

Hidden agenda

- Explaining the diagnosis and management plan.
- To adequately relieve the anxiety of malignancy.
- To emphasize the importance of smoking cessation.

What are the risk factors for COPD?

- Smoking
- Alpha-1 antitrypsin deficiency
- Pollution.
- Burning biofuel mass/cooking with wood burning, etc.

How to diagnose COPD?
- Presence of chronic symptoms
- Exposure to risk factor(s)
- Spirometry is essential to confirm the diagnosis.

What are the spirometric criteria for the diagnosis of COPD?
- Forced expiratory volume in one second (FEV1)/forced vital capacity (FVC) <70%
- *Lack of reversibility*: FEV1 does not increase by 12% and 200 mL after bronchodilator.

Stages of COPD
The assessment of COPD severity depends on three factors:
1. Patient's symptoms (using the modified British Medical Research Council Questionnaire or the CAT questionnaire)
2. FEV1 value on spirometry (GOLD stage)
3. Risk of exacerbation.

Gold stage based on FEV1%:
- *Stage 1 Mild*: FEV1 ≥80%
- *Stage 2 Moderate:* 50% to <80%
- *Stage 3 Severe*: 30% to <50%
- *Stage 4 Very severe*: <30%

Complications of COPD/COPD comorbidities
Pulmonary complications:
- Risk of disease exacerbation.
- Hypercapnic respiratory failure
- Cor-pulmonale and pulmonary hypertension
- Lung cancer.

Systemic complications:
- Muscle wasting
- Coronary artery disease and metabolic syndrome
- Depression
- Osteoporosis.

Management of COPD
- **Pharmacologic treatment:**
  Recommendation is based on the stage of the disease.
  - *Stage A:* Short-acting beta-agonists (SABA) or long-acting muscarinic antagonists (LAMA)
  - *Stage B:* LAMA + long-acting beta-agonists (LABA)
  - *Stage C:* LAMA + LABA +/– inhaled corticosteroids (ICS)
  - *Stage D:* LAMA + LABA + ICS + Roflimulast/Macrolide.

- **Non-pharmacologic treatment:**
  - Smoking cessation
  - Vaccination
  - Pulmonary rehabilitation
  - Non-invasive ventilation (BIPAP/CPAP)
  - Long-term oxygen therapy (LTOT)
  - Lung cancer screening.

- **Surgical treatment:**
  - Lung volume reduction surgery
  - Lung transplantation.

- **What are the indications of LTOT in COPD?**
  - Pao_2 ≤55 mmHg or $SpaO_2$ ≤88% (should be confirmed twice over a 3-week period).

- Pao_2 between 50 mmHg and 60 mmHg or $SpaO_2$ of 88% in the presence of pulmonary hypertension, oedema due to CCF or polycythaemia (Hct >55%).
- Once placed on LTOT, ABG should be repeated at 60 to 90 days to determine if the patient still requires LTOT.
- LTOT should be used >15 h/day.
- Patient should avoid smoking when using O_2 to prevent fire.

- **What are the indications of non-invasive ventilation in COPD?**
  - During exacerbations to correct hypoxemia, hypercapnia or respiratory acidosis.
  - Stable COPD if there is a persistent daytime $Paco_2$ ≥52 mmHg.

- **Other possible scenarios on this subject in clinical examinations**
  Other scenarios may involve a case of advanced COPD that requires LTOT, non-invasive ventilation or DNAR.

Further reading

Booker R. Effective communication with the patient. Eur Respir Rev 2005; 14:93–96.

Global Initiatives for Chronic Obstructive Lung Disease (GOLD). Global strategy for the diagnosis, management and prevention of chronic obstructive pulmonary disease, 2018.

Scenario no. 2

Type of scenario: Information giving/breaking bad news of chronic disease

Candidate information

Your role: You are a doctor in the medical outpatient clinic.
Problem: Explanation of newly diagnosed chronic disease.
Patient: Mrs Smith, a 28-year-old lady.

Please read the scenario printed below. When the bell sounds, enter the room. You have (---) minutes for your consultation with the patient/relative, (---) minutes to collect your thoughts, and (---) minutes for discussion.

Please do not examine the patient
Please do not take a history

> Mrs Smith is a 28-year-old woman, who has had joint pains and rash on her face for the last 12 months. She was seen by her GP and her investigations suggest that she has systemic lupus erythematosus (SLE) which is limited to her joints and skin without multisystem involvement. She is here today to discuss the results of her investigations. She is working as an office secretary and is very concerned about her illness.
>
> **Your task:** Is to answer the patient's questions and help her to understand what SLE is and discuss how it will be managed.

Approach

Always read the scenario carefully and make sure you understand the instructions before you start. Any information provided is important. Make notes and a framework for your discussion. Sometimes, a hidden agenda is incorporated, pay attention to that.

Introduction and identification

- **Prepare the environment**
  Sit at the same level as the patient with comfort and avoid barriers like tables.

- **Introduce yourself to the patient**
  Shake hands
  Hello Mrs Smith, I am Dr X, working in the medical outpatient clinic.
  Can I confirm that I am talking to Mrs Smith?
  Would you like to invite anybody else to this discussion?

- **Confirm the objective of the interview**
  We are here today to discuss the results of your investigations and diagnosis. Is that alright?

Check patient's understanding and expectation

Tell me Mrs Smith, how much do you know about your health status?
Do you know anything about the results of your investigations?
What do you think could be wrong with your skin and joints?

Discussion with the patient (information giving)

- **Give the patient the information (avoid medical jargon)**
  Mrs Smith, you have had joint pains and a rash on your face for 12 months. Your GP requested some investigations, which confirm that you have a problem called 'systemic lupus erythematosus (SLE)' or lupus. Pause....

- **Explore with the patient her understanding of SLE**
  Have you ever heard of SLE before? Pause....

- **Explain to the patient in simple terms about SLE (avoid medical jargon)**
  Systemic lupus erythematosus or lupus is a disease in which your immune system produces proteins that attack your own body tissues. These proteins are called 'antibodies'. These antibodies cause damage to different tissues and organs including the joints, skin, lungs, heart, brain, and kidneys. So far, we do not know why this happens and many scientists are currently investigating the reason behind this. In your case, the disease is in its milder form as it has affected only the skin and joints. Although there is no cure for SLE, there are different medications that can reduce the activity of the disease and relieve the symptoms it causes.

- **Pause and ask the patient if she understands what you have said so far.**

- **Explain how the severity of lupus is assessed and how it can progress?**
  People with lupus tend to have disease flares during which their symptoms might worsen. This may be followed by a period of remission, when their symptoms improve. Lupus can be mild in some people and more severe and complicated in others when several organs are affected. There are a wide variety of treatments to reduce the symptoms and pain as well as minimise organ damage. Many people can go into a stable state (remission) which requires no treatment, sometimes for years.

- **Explain the treatment options**
  The medications used in the treatment of lupus vary depending on the degree of activity and severity of disease. Some patients may just need painkillers and anti-inflammatory drugs, whilst others may require medications to reduce the immune response of the body. Because your disease is mild, I am going to prescribe some painkillers to relieve your joint pains and will refer you to my colleague (called a rheumatologist) who specialises in diseases like SLE. It is important to understand that SLE needs regular follow-up in a specialised rheumatology clinic to monitor disease activity and treatment with drugs to prevent damage to your organs.

  You need to remain active and do regular exercise to strengthen your bone and muscles and we will also give you some bone strengthening medication (to avoid osteoporosis).

- **Advice about vaccination**
  It is important to note that SLE and the medications used to treat it may make you more susceptible to infections. To lower the risk of infections, you need vaccination against bacteria called pneumococci and a yearly flu shot. If you agree, we can arrange to give you these in this clinic.

- **Pregnancy and birth control**
  See response to patient's concerns.

- **Check patient understanding.**
  Is everything is clear so far?

Explore and respond to patient's concerns

Are there any questions or concerns you would like to discuss at this moment?

- **I am concerned about my job. I am having pain in my hands and I cannot continue my work as a secretary because it involves typing, what should I do?**
  I understand your concern. As your disease is mild and is limited to your skin and joints, I am expecting that you will see significant improvement in the next couple of weeks with the medications we prescribe. I would advise that you continue your job and we can see how you get on. You may consider taking a short sick leave until your pain is better.

- **How long will I be on this treatment?**
  Systemic lupus erythematosus is a long-standing illness. Some patients can have mild disease while others have a more severe form that involves multiple body organs and requires multiple medications. Your rheumatologist will decide for how long you will need the medications based on the disease activity and your response to these medications.

- **I am planning a pregnancy. Is it safe to do so?**
  This is an important question as lupus can affect pregnancy in different ways and pregnancy itself can cause the activity of the disease to flare up. Most women with SLE can get pregnant and carry to term and have a normal delivery. However, some with active disease may develop complications such as miscarriages, high blood pressure and heart disease in their infants. Some medications used to treat lupus may also harm the fetus. I would strongly recommend that you have close follow-up with the rheumatologist and obstetrician at least 6 months before deciding to become pregnant. Certain antibodies need to be checked in your blood and the doses of lupus medications need to be adjusted to ensure that they do not harm the baby.

- **What kind of birth control methods should I use?**
  Some birth control pills can increase the chances of getting a clot in your limbs while others are relatively safer (progesterone-only pills). There are also certain devices

that can be placed in the womb. I will refer you to an obstetrician, who is an expert, to advise you on different kinds of birth control methods.

- **Are these medications safe during pregnancy?**
  Once your disease is controlled for about 6 months on treatment then a careful evaluation and risk assessment regarding medications and disease activity can be undertaken to plan your pregnancy. Some medications are safe during pregnancy with no major side effect, while others are harmful and should not be given during pregnancy and you need to discuss this with your rheumatologist.

Show empathy

I understand Mrs Smith how difficult it is to hear about a new illness like SLE. We are here to help you.

Summarise and confirm understanding

Mrs Smith, I would like to summarise our discussion to be sure that you understand important information about your illness. Your joint pains, skin rash, and investigations suggest that you have a condition called lupus or systemic lupus erythematosus. This is an abnormality of the immune system and we do not fully understand what causes this. Your disease is currently mild, and you need to remain active and do regular exercise to maintain the strength of your bone and muscles. I will prescribe you some pain medication and the rheumatologist will decide regarding further medications to suppress your overactive immune system and stop further damage. You will also need to have vaccinations and take some birth control methods until your disease is under control for at least 6 months.

    Is this clear so far?

    Would you like to discuss anything else at this moment?

Offer help and follow-up

Should you have any further questions, please do not hesitate to contact me on my office telephone number. I will arrange an appointment in 2 weeks to see how you are getting on.

    I will refer you to a gynaecologist for selective birth control methods and the rheumatologist for an expert opinion on further managing of your SLE.

    I will also provide you with some website addresses and printed material to read more about your condition.

Discussion

Ethical principles

- **What are the main ethical principles in this scenario?**
  Patient's autonomy: The doctor should provide the patient with the necessary information to help her make an informed decision on her condition. The doctor should be honest and truthful when discussing the risks and complications of the disease and treatment. The patient has the right to know about the diagnosis and prognosis of her SLE. She has the right to agree or refuse medications.

  Justice: The patient should be treated fairly and equally. Expensive immunosuppressive medications and biologic therapies can be used to treat lupus and the patient has the right to get these medications if necessary.

  Beneficence and non-maleficence: Use medications with the least side effects if possible. Advice regarding pregnancy is important to avoid lupus complications during pregnancy. Refer to the rheumatologist and gynaecologist for expert management, especially during pregnancy.

Hidden agenda

- Explaining the diagnosis and management plan.
- Her main concern regarding joint pain and her job as a secretary.
- Her wish to become pregnant.

Systemic Lupus International Collaborating Clinics (SLICC) 2012 Diagnostic Criteria (4 of 11)

- Malar rash
- Discoid rash
- Photosensitivity
- Recurrent painless oral ulcer
- Arthritis
- Serositis (pleuritis/pericarditis)
- Renal disorder
- Neurologic disorder (seizures/psychosis)
- Hematologic disorders (haemolytic anaemia/leucopenia/lymphopenia/thrombocytopenia)
- ANA
- Immunologic disorder (anti-dsDNA/anti-Sm/antiphospholipid/low complement).

Management of lupus

- *Non-pharmacological therapy:*
  - Sun protection
  - Diet
  - Exercise
  - Appropriate immunization
  - Contraception counselling
  - Pregnancy planning
- *Pharmacological therapy:*
  - Non-steroidal anti-inflammatory drugs (NSAIDs)
  - Hydroxychloroquine
  - Low-dose steroid <7.5 mg
  - *Immunosuppressive*: Azathioprine, methotrexate (MTX), mycophenolate mofetil, cyclophosphamide, rituximab, and other biologics.

Further reading

Lateef A, Petri M. Managing lupus patients during pregnancy. Best Pract Res Clin Rheumatol 2013; 27:435–447.
Petri M, Orbai AM, Alarcón GS, et al. Derivation and validation of the Systemic Lupus International Collaborating Clinics classification criteria for systemic lupus erythematosus. Arthritis Rheum 2012; 64:2677–2686 .

Scenario no. 3

Type of scenario: Taking consent for a procedure

Candidate information

Your role: You are the doctor on the medical ward.
Problem: Taking consent for a procedure.
Patient: Miss Ayesha, a 20-year-old lady.

Please read the scenario printed below. When the bell sounds, enter the room. You have (---) minutes for your consultation with the patient/relative, (---) minutes to collect your thoughts, and (---) minutes for discussion.

Please do not examine the patient
Please do not take a history

> Miss Ayesha is a 21-year-old lady who was diagnosed with SLE a month ago. She was commenced on ibuprofen tablets by her GP to control her joint pain while waiting for a rheumatology appointment. She was admitted after an emergency referral by her GP because of fatigue, nausea, and vomiting with bilateral lower limb oedema and a serum creatinine of 400 µmol/L. An ultrasound of her kidneys revealed normal-sized kidneys and it has been decided that she needs a kidney biopsy.
>
> **Your task:** Is to take consent for the renal biopsy, answer the patient's questions and concerns, and help her to understand what is happening.

Approach

Always read the scenario carefully and make sure you understand the instructions before you start. Any information provided is important. Make notes and a framework for your discussion. Sometimes, a hidden agenda is incorporated, pay attention to that.

Introduction and identification

- **Prepare the environment**
  Sit at the same level as the patient with comfort and avoid barriers like tables.

- **Introduce yourself to the patient**
  Shake hands
  Hello Miss Ayesha, I am Dr X and I am the doctor on the medical ward.
  Can I confirm that I am talking to Miss Ayesha?
  Would you like to invite anybody else to this discussion?

- **Confirm the objective of the interview**
  I am here to discuss and obtain your consent for a kidney biopsy. Is that alright?

Check patient's understanding and expectation

Tell me Miss Ayesha how much do you know about your health status?
Do you know anything about the results of your investigations?
What do you suspect might be wrong with your health?

Discussion with the patient

- **Explain the indication (avoid medical jargon)**
  Miss Ayesha, as you are aware, you have lupus for which your GP prescribed some painkillers. You now complain from fatigue and swelling of your legs. Your GP requested some tests which show that your kidneys are not functioning normally. The scan of your kidneys looks fine, but there are two possible reasons for your abnormal kidney function. It could be a result of taking too many painkillers which can affect kidney function, or it could be because of the effects of lupus on the kidneys, a condition called lupus nephritis. Lupus nephritis needs immediate treatment and

if left untreated, it can cause permanent damage to the kidneys. The only way we can work out the underlying cause of the abnormal kidney function is by taking tiny pieces of your kidneys and examine them under a microscope. This procedure is called a kidney biopsy.

- **Explore the patient ideas about a kidney biopsy**
  Have you ever heard of a kidney biopsy before? Pause....

- **Explain to the patient in simple terms about the procedure (avoid medical jargon)**
  A kidney biopsy involves taking one or more tiny pieces (samples) of your kidney to look at them under a microscope.

Before the procedure we will do some blood tests to make sure you do not have any bleeding tendency in order to avoid any bleeding during and after the biopsy. We will also do a urine test to look for a urine infection. It is very important that you stop your painkillers and you should not be on any blood thinning medications.

During the procedure you will be asked to lie on your stomach. If you need, your doctor can give you a sedative through a vein in your hand or arm to help you relax. These medications will make you feel a little drowsy but will decrease any pain or discomfort during the procedure. The doctor will clean the area with antiseptic and will give you an injection to numb the pain at the site of kidney biopsy. A small needle will be inserted through the skin into the kidney and a small piece of tissue will be removed from the kidney. To keep the kidney in one position during the biopsy you will be asked to take in a deep breath and hold it as the doctor puts in the needle.

After the procedure you will need to rest in bed for 12–24 hours and you will stay overnight in the hospital for observations to make sure there is no bleeding and your pain is controlled. You should not take NSAIDs, aspirin or any other blood thinning medication after the procedure for 1 week. You should not do any exercise or lift heavy things for 2 weeks. Please inform the doctor immediately if you feel dizzy or feverish or if you develop severe pain at the site of the biopsy or see frank blood in your urine or you are unable to urinate.

Based on your age, the chances of a complication are very low. There are no alternatives to the kidney biopsy as this is the only definitive way of identifying underlying lupus nephritis, which without treatment can progress to end-stage kidney failure. We cannot start you on a very high dose of immunosuppressive medication without knowing the exact cause of the kidney problem because immunosuppressive medications have their own risks, complications, and side effects.

- Pause and ask the patient if she understands what you have told her.
- Explain possible complications of the procedure.
- Potential complications include:
  - Pain that can be easily controlled.
  - You may observe some blood in the urine. This is common and usually stops within a few days. Severe bleeding can rarely occur, within 24 hours of the procedure, which is why we will keep you in hospital overnight and if needed, can give you a blood transfusion.
  - Very rarely, injury to the blood vessels of the kidneys can create a track between the artery and vein called an 'arteriovenous fistula'.
- Check patient understanding
  Is everything clear so far?

Explore and respond to patient's concerns

Do you have any questions or concerns to discuss at this moment?
- **Will my kidney function recover?**
  At the moment and before obtaining the kidney biopsy, it is difficult to predict, but recovery of the kidney function will depend on establishing the underlying cause and appropriate treatment.

- **Will I need dialysis in the future?**
  This is an important question, but it is difficult to answer at this moment as we are not sure of the underlying cause of your abnormal kidney function. Your kidney biopsy will allow us to assess the chances of recovery compared to disease progression. I will explain to you in more detail after we have the results of the kidney biopsy.

Show empathy

Miss Ayesha, I can understand how difficult it is to hear that the lupus might have affected your kidneys. We are here to help you.

Summarise and confirm understanding and consent

Miss Ayesha, I would like to summarise our discussion to be sure that you understand important information about your illness. You were diagnosed with SLE for which, you have been taking painkillers. You currently feel very tired and your legs became swollen. Your GP found that your kidney function is abnormal. Although the initial scan of your kidneys looks fine, you need to have a kidney biopsy to determine what has caused the abnormal kidney function. I have also explained the procedure and its complications.

  Is everything clear so far?
  Please let me know if you need to discuss anything else at this moment.
  Now Miss Ayesha, if you agree to have a kidney biopsy done, may I request you kindly sign the consent form.

Offer help and follow-up

  If you have any further concerns, please contact me on this number.
  A colleague of mine who is specialised in kidney disease will discuss further with you about kidney biopsy.
  I will provide you with printed material on kidney biopsy so that you can read more about the procedure.

Discussion

Ethical principles

- **What are the main ethical principles in this scenario?**
  Patient's autonomy: The patient has the right to agree or refuse the procedure. The doctor should provide the patient with the necessary information about the risks and benefits of the procedure to help her make her decision. Doctors should be honest and truthful when discussing the risks of the procedure.

  Justice: The patient should undergo further investigations to enable timely diagnosis and treatment without discrimination.

  Beneficence and non-maleficence: Advice to undergo a kidney biopsy will be in the best interest of the patient as this will allow the correct diagnosis and early treatment. Failure to diagnose and stage lupus nephritis will impose a major risk of developing end-stage renal failure. Alternatively, starting immunosuppressant drugs without knowing the diagnosis could cause harm if the diagnosis is not lupus nephritis.

Hidden agenda

- Explain the kidney biopsy procedure including the indications, contraindications as well as complications.
- Explain to the patient how serious lupus nephritis is.

Lupus nephritis

Lupus nephritis is very serious complication of SLE. It is a major risk factor for morbidity and mortality. About 10% of patients with lupus nephritis will develop end-stage renal disease (ESRD). The risk of ESRD is higher in certain subsets of patients with lupus nephritis. In class 4 lupus nephritis, the risk may be as high as 44% over 15 years. Lupus nephritis is defined as abnormal urinalysis (proteinuria) with or without an elevated plasma creatinine concentration in a patient with SLE. If kidney involvement is suspected, a kidney biopsy should be considered.

- Classification of lupus nephritis
  Lupus nephritis is classified based on histopathology:
  - *Class I*: Minimal mesangial lupus nephritis
  - *Class II*: Mesangial proliferative lupus nephritis
  - *Class III*: Focal lupus nephritis
  - *Class IV*: Diffuse lupus nephritis
  - *Class V*: Lupus membranous nephropathy
  - *Class VI*: Advanced sclerosing lupus nephritis.
- Management of lupus nephritis
  - Pulsed steroid for 3–5 days
  - Cyclophosphamide
  - Mycophenolate mofetil
  - Cyclosporine
  - Rituximab.

Further reading

National Kidney Foundation. Renal biopsy. [online] Available from https://www.kidney.org/atoz/content/kidney-biopsy [Last accessed October, 2019].

Weening JJ, D'Agati VD, Schwartz MM, et al. The classification of glomerulonephritis in systemic lupus erythematosus revisited. J Am Soc Nephrol 2004; 15:241–250.

Almaani S, Meara A, Rovin BH. Update on lupus nephritis. Clin J Am Soc Nephrol 2017; 12:825–835.

Alarco´n GS. Multiethnic lupus cohorts: what have they taught us? Rheumatol Clin 2011; 7:3–6.

Tektonidou M, Dasgupta A, Ward M. Risk of end-stage renal disease in patients with lupus nephritis, 1970-2015: A systematic review and Bayesian meta-analysis. Arthritis Rheumatol 2016; 68:1432–1441.

Scenario no. 4

Type of scenario: Information giving/breaking bad news of chronic disease

Candidate information

Your role: You are a doctor in the medical outpatient clinic.
Problem: Explanation of a newly diagnosed neurologic disease.
Patient: Mrs Al-Murri, a 28-year-old lady.

Please read the scenario printed below. When the bell sounds, enter the room. You have (---) minutes for your consultation with the patient/relative, (---) minutes to collect your thoughts, and (---) minutes for discussion.

Please do not examine the patient
Please do not take a history

Mrs Al-Murri is a 28-year-old lady who recently came to the emergency department because of blurring of vision in her left eye. Previously, she had been seen in the emergency department with mild tingling and numbness in her arms and discharged home. This time she underwent a lumbar puncture in the emergency department and an MRI brain that showed multiple demyelinating plaques in the periventricular area consistent with multiple sclerosis. She came today to discuss the results of her investigations.

Your task: Is to answer the patient's questions and help her to understand the new diagnosis and further plan of management.

Approach

Always read the scenario carefully and make sure you understand the instructions before you start. Any information provided is important. Make notes and a framework for your discussion. Sometimes, a hidden agenda is incorporated, pay attention to that.

Introduction and identification

- **Prepare the environment**
  Sit at the same level as the patient with comfort and avoid barriers like tables.

- **Introduce yourself to the patient**
  Be aware of social and religious reasons preventing her from shaking your hand.
  Hello Mrs Al-Murri, I am Dr Z, working in the medical outpatient clinic.
  Can I confirm that I am talking to Mrs Al-Murri?

- **Ask the patient if she would like someone else to be present during the discussion**
  Would you like to invite anybody else to this discussion?

- **Confirm the objective of the interview**
  We are here today to discuss the results of your investigations and diagnosis. Is that alright?

Check patient's understanding and expectation

Tell me how much do you know about your health status?
Do you know anything about the results of your investigations?
What do you suspect might be wrong with your vision?

Discussion with the patient

- **Give the patient the information (avoid medical jargon)**
  Mrs Al-Murri, when you came to the emergency room the first time, you were complaining from some tingling and numbness in your arms and the second time you had a problem with sight in the left eye. My colleagues in the emergency department performed a lumbar puncture to remove some of the fluid around your spinal cord and a MRI scan of your brain. The results of these tests confirm that you have a disease called multiple sclerosis (MS). Pause....

- **Explore the patient's ideas about multiple sclerosis**
  Have you ever heard of multiple sclerosis before? Pause....

- **Explain to the patient in simple terms about multiple sclerosis (avoid medical jargon)**
  Multiple sclerosis is a disease of the nerves in the body. In multiple sclerosis, the immune system attacks the covering of the nerves (myelin sheath) and causes

inflammation and damage of this sheath. Nerves in the brain, spinal cord, eyes, and other parts of the body can be affected. This nerve damage slows down the passage of signals to the brain and leads to a number of symptoms such as numbness and tingling in the legs and hands, blurring of vision, and sometimes weakness and imbalance when walking. So far, the cause of multiple sclerosis is unknown but extensive research is going on to identify the cause. Unfortunately, MS is not a curable disease. The disease activity tends to be episodic and may cause only minimal symptoms or it can present with severe progressive disability. In some patients, the disease remains stable without symptoms for a long time.

- **Pause and ask the patient if everything is clear so far.**

- **Explain the treatment options**
  Pharmacological treatment: Mrs Al-Murri, there are several types of MS and your disease appears to be the relapsing remitting type which means that you will have flare ups of the disease followed by episodes of stable disease. Different treatments are available for different stages of the disease. For acute attacks, you may need high doses of steroid injection over 3–5 days and for more stable patients, there are injectable and oral options. I will refer you to a neurologist who will assess you and start the necessary medication to control your disease.

  Non-pharmacological treatment: I will also refer you to a physiotherapist as regular exercise will decrease your body aches, fatigue, and muscle stiffness as well as improve your mood and quality of life. I will also refer you to an occupational therapist to help you adjust your home and work environment and deal with your daily activities.

- **Check the patient understanding.**
  Does that make sense to you?

Explore and respond to patient's concerns

Do you have any questions or concerns at this moment?

- **Why was MS not diagnosed during my first visit?**
  MS is sometimes difficult to diagnose, especially as numbness and tingling are common symptoms and can be caused by many diseases. However, on the second time, the sudden loss of eye sight made MS a likely diagnosis that was confirmed by the lumbar puncture and MRI scan.

- **How long will I be on MS treatment?**
  This is a good question. MS is a long-standing disease. Some patients have episodic disease, whilst others have more progressive disease. Acute flares of the disease need admission and high-dose steroid for 3–5 days. Stable patients have different options for oral and injectable medication depending on your disease status. The disease requires lifelong follow-up and management.

- **Will I be disabled soon doctor?**
  It is very difficult to predict what will happen as there are different types of MS. The type of MS you have is most likely the episodic (relapsing and remitting) one. This has a good quality of life and survival as compared to the progressive form in which the patient becomes disabled very quickly. With the advent of new more powerful medications, we can reduce the number of disease attacks and delay disability.

- **I am planning to become pregnant. Is it safe to do so?**
  This is a very important question. The chances of acute attacks of MS during pregnancy decrease but increase just after delivery (postpartum). Some of the

medications used to control MS are also harmful to the baby and such drugs should be discontinued for at least 3 months before pregnancy planning. It is very important that you discuss with your neurologist and obstetrician any plans for pregnancy.

- **Other possible questions:**
  - **Are MS medications safe during breast feeding?**
    Some of the medications are safe as they are secreted at very minimal level in breast milk while others are harmful as they are secreted in significant amounts in breast milk. Just after delivery, your neurologist and obstetrician will decide which medications will be suitable for you while breastfeeding.
  - **What is the chance that my children will get MS?**
    First-degree relatives are affected more (7%) than other family members (2.5%) in their lifetime compared to the general population and monozygotic twins are affected even more (20–25%).

Show empathy

I understand Mrs Al-Murri how difficult it is to hear about a diagnosis of MS. We are here to help you.

Summarise and confirm understanding

So Mrs Al-Murri, I would like to summarise our discussion to be sure that you understand important information about your illness. You came initially to the emergency department with numbness and tingling in your arm and later with temporary loss of vision in your left eye. Further tests showed that you have MS. Your disease seems to be the episodic one (relapsing and remitting) and does not appear to be progressive. I have also explained the need for regular follow-up and timely treatment especially when you have an acute attack.

Is everything clear so far?
Would you like to discuss anything else at this moment?

Offer help and follow-up

If you have any further questions, please do not hesitate to contact me on my office telephone number. I will arrange another appointment in 2 weeks to review your progress.

I will refer you to a neurologist for an expert opinion and to plan further management and follow-up.

I will refer you to a physiotherapist to help you undertake regular exercise.

I will also provide you with some website addresses and printed material on MS.

Discussion

Ethical principles

- **What are the main ethical principles in this scenario?**
  Patient's autonomy: The patient has the right to know about the diagnosis and prognosis of her disease. The doctor should provide the patient with the necessary information to help her make an informed decision about her disease and its management. The doctor should be honest and truthful about the diagnosis, treatment, and outlook of the disease.

  Justice: There are multiple medications that are effective for different stages of the disease. It is better to start with medication that is least expensive and with fewer side effects. Patient should be diagnosed and treated without discrimination.

  Beneficence: Patients should be offered all available options and the treatment chosen should be in the best interest of the patient. Haematopoietic stem cell transplantation

(HSCT) is being used with excellent outcomes in patients with active inflammation and mild disability. It carries major risks in relation to the procedure itself which need to be explained to the patient.

Non-maleficence: Medications that are harmful during pregnancy or breastfeeding should be avoided.

Hidden agenda

- Discussing different types of MS.
- Discussing MS and pregnancy.
- Discussing MS and breastfeeding.

What is multiple sclerosis?

Multiple sclerosis is a chronic inflammatory autoimmune disease which can cause demyelination and axonal loss in the nervous system. People with MS typically develop symptoms in their late 20s, experiencing visual and sensory disturbances, limb weakness, gait problems and bladder and bowel dysfunction.

Types of MS

- **Relapsing remitting MS (RRMS)**
  The most common pattern of disease is where periods of stability (remission) are followed by an exacerbation of symptoms (relapses). About 85% of people with MS have RRMS at onset.

- **Secondary progressive MS**
  Around two-thirds of people who start with RRMS may develop secondary progressive MS. This occurs when relapses are associated with progressively less complete recovery, and subsequently individuals gradually develop worsening symptoms without remissions.

- **Primary progressive**
  About 10–15% of people with MS have primary progressive MS where symptoms develop and worsen over time from the start, without ever experiencing relapses and remissions.

- **Progressive-relapsing MS**

Diagnostic criteria of MS

Multiple sclerosis should not be diagnosed on the basis of MRI findings alone as there are other diseases that can cause demyelinating lesions in the brain that mimic MS. Assessing that episodes are consistent with an inflammatory process, excluding alternative diagnoses and establishing that lesions have developed at different times, and are in different anatomical locations is important for a diagnosis of relapsing-remitting MS. Establishing progressive neurological deterioration over 1 year or more is important for a diagnosis of primary progressive MS.

- **2010 Revised McDonald criteria for diagnosis of MS**
  These criteria require the following combination of evidence for diagnosis: evidence of damage (clinical attacks and/or lesions) in two or more separate areas of the CNS (including the brain, spinal cord, and optic nerves), plus evidence that the damage happened one or more months apart, plus evidence that the damage did not happen because of another disease (exclusion of other diseases).

- **Possible investigation to do based on presentation**
  - *MRI brain and spine:* Demonstration of typical lesion suggestive of MS as per McDonald criteria.

- *CSF analysis:* To look for oligoclonal bands (usually lymphocytic otherwise unremarkable). It is not a must for diagnosis of MS.
- *Visual evoked potential:* It is the detection of an electrical event in the CNS which is generated by peripheral visual stimulation.

Management of MS

- **Establish multidisciplinary plan of care**
- **Pharmacologic management**
  - *Treat acute exacerbations* with methylprednisolone (plasma exchange only if severe neurological symptoms and having a poor response with glucocorticoid)
  - *Disease-modifying therapies* for controlling the disease: Interferon beta, glatiramer acetate, natalizumab, alemtuzumab, fingolimod, etc. Disease modifying treatments have beneficial effect especially in relapsing and remitting MS. The main aim of these medications is to decrease relapse rate and to slow the progression of the disease.
  - *Symptom management* for muscle stiffness (baclofen, botulinum toxin), bladder dysfunction (oxybutynin, tamsulosin), and neuropathic pain (carbamazepine).
- **Non-pharmacological therapy**
  - Physiotherapy
  - Exercise
  - Occupational therapy
  - Support groups, local services, social services, and national charities are organised and how to get in touch with them.
  - Legal requirements such as notifying the Driver and Vehicle Licensing Agency (DVLA) and legal rights including social care, employment rights, and benefits.
  - Offer Flu vaccine
  - Advise people with MS not to smoke and explain that it may increase the progression of disability.

Further reading

Finkelsztejn A, Brooks JB, Paschoal FM Jr, et al. What can we really tell women with multiple sclerosis regarding pregnancy? A systematic review and meta-analysis of the literature. BJOG 2011; 118:790–797.

National Institute for Health and Care Excellence (NICE). (2014). Clinical guideline 186: Management of multiple sclerosis in primary and secondary care. [online] Available from https://www.nice.org.uk/guidance/cg186 [Last accessed October, 2019].

Nielsen NM, Westergaard T, Rostgaard K, et al. Familial risk of multiple sclerosis: a nationwide cohort study. Am J Epidemiol 2005; 162:774–778.

Polman CH, Reingold SC, Banwell B, et al. Diagnostic criteria for multiple sclerosis: 2010 Revisions to the McDonald criteria Ann Neurol 2011; 69:292–302.

Scenario no. 5

Type of scenario: Information giving/breaking bad news of chronic disease

Candidate information

Your role: You are a doctor in the medical outpatient clinic.
Problem: Explanation of newly diagnosed chronic disease.
Patient: Mrs Jamal, a 28-year-old lady

Please read the scenario printed below. When the bell sounds, enter the room. You have (---) minutes for your consultation with the patient/relative, (---) minutes to collect your thoughts, and (---) minutes for discussion.

Please do not examine the patient
Please do not take a history

> Mrs Jamal is a 28-year-old construction engineer who was recently appointed on her new job. She has had a second grand mal seizure in the last 2 months without any identifiable cause on her initial investigations. Her brain scan, lumbar puncture, metabolic profile and EEG result are all normal. She is married and has no other prior illnesses.
>
> **Your task:** Is to explain the results of her investigations, possible diagnosis, and further plan of management.

Approach

Always read the scenario carefully and make sure you understand the instructions before you start. Any information provided is important. Make notes and a framework for your discussion. Sometimes, a hidden agenda is incorporated, pay attention to that.

Introduction and identification

- **Prepare the environment**
  Sit at the same level as the patient with comfort and avoid barriers like tables.

- **Introduce yourself to the patient**
  Offer to shake her hand, but be aware of social and religious reasons preventing her from shaking your hand
  Hello Mrs Jamal, I am Dr X, working in the medical outpatient clinic.
  Can I confirm that I am talking to Mrs Jamal?

- **Ask the patient if she would like someone else to be present during the discussion**
  Would you like to invite anybody else to this discussion?

- **Confirm the objective of the interview**
  We are here today to discuss the results of your investigations and diagnosis. Is that alright?

Check patient's understanding and expectation

Tell me Mrs Jamal, how much do you know about your health status?
Do you know why we requested all these investigations?
What do you suspect might be wrong with your health?

Discussion with the patient (information giving)

- **Give the patient the information (avoid medical jargon and explain what they mean)**
  As you know Mrs Jamal, you came with a second episode of abnormal movements with loss of consciousness which we call a seizure. These two seizures have occurred in the last 2 months. Although your brain scan, blood tests and EEG to detect abnormal brain activity were normal we suspect that you have epilepsy.

- **Explore the patient's ideas about epilepsy**
  Have you ever heard of epilepsy before? Pause....

- **Explain to the patient in simple terms about epilepsy (avoid medical jargon)**
  Epilepsy is a disease that can cause excess electrical activity in the brain. Because of this excess activity, patients can have attacks of sudden loss of consciousness, abnormal involuntary movement in different parts of the body or abnormal body sensations. These attacks are called seizure episodes. The occurrence of a single seizure does not necessarily indicate that a person has epilepsy. However, if a person experiences regular seizures, then this is called epilepsy. Epilepsy may happen without an obvious cause which is called idiopathic epilepsy, or it can be related to abnormalities in the brain structure or blood tests.

- **Pause and ask the patient if everything clear so far.**

- **Explain management and preventive measures of seizure**
  Since you have already had two seizure episodes, it is recommended that you start taking anti-epileptic medication to minimise the risk of recurrence of a seizure. There are multiple anti-epileptic medications that can be used. I am going to seek the help of a colleague who specialises in epilepsy regarding the best option for you. Besides the regular use of antiepileptic medication, the major problem for patients with seizures is the inability to predict when another seizure is going to happen. It is therefore important to observe the following precautions:
  - As your job is a construction engineer, there is a risk, when going to high places that you may develop a seizure and fall from such high places. Therefore, I strongly recommend that you avoid going to high places. We can write a letter to your employer explaining such risks. You may shift to office work (If she does not agree, discuss further the risks and offer discussion with her GP and her employer).
  - It is very important that you minimise alcohol consumption and avoid excess alcohol as it can provoke a seizure.
  - Get adequate sleep and avoid abnormal sleeping habit/sleep deprivation/avoid shift working as sleep deprivation may provoke a seizure.
  - Avoid swimming alone in swimming pools to avoid the risk of drowning in case a seizure happens.
  - When taking a bath, avoid locking the door of the bathroom and using a bathtub to avoid drowning in case a seizure happens.
  - Avoid operating heavy machinery, power tools, and other dangerous equipment.
  - Avoid noise, loud sound, and exposing yourself to disco/flashing lights as these can provoke seizure activity.

- Be careful when using over-the-counter medication/herbal and dietary supplements as some may interact with epilepsy medications.
- For any new medication, inform the prescribing doctor that you have epilepsy and you are taking antiepileptic medication.
- Consult your doctor if you have any infection (can precipitate a seizure).
- If time allows, discuss about vaccination, mainly pneumococcal vaccination and annual influenza vaccination.
- *Driving and epilepsy: (DVLA guideline—UK)*
  - Group-1 (car/motor cycle): No seizures for 5 years
  - Group-2 (Bus/Lorry): No seizures for 10 years
- *First unprovoked seizure:*
  - Group-1 (Car/motor cycle): No seizures for 6 months
  - Group-2 (Bus/lorry): No seizures for 5 years.

- **Pregnancy and birth control pills**
  See later.

- **Check the patient's understanding.**
  Is that clear so far?

Explore and respond to patients' concerns

Do you have any question or concern you would like to discuss at this moment?

- **If all the investigations are normal, then why should I have epilepsy?**
  This is a good question. More than 50% of patients with epilepsy have no identifiable cause and investigations will be normal. Normal investigations, therefore, do not exclude epilepsy. If any patient has two or more episodes of seizure, then treatment is recommended to reduce risk of recurrence and complications related to seizure.

- **Why were these medications not started at the time of the first seizure?**
  After the first seizure, the doctor will assess the risk of recurrent seizures. If the risk is low and the investigations are normal, careful observation without anti-epileptic medications may be considered. A second seizure tells us there is a risk of recurrent seizures and therefore, it is recommended to start treatment.

- **How long will I continue anti-epileptic medication?**
  Many patients require these medications for at least 3–5 years. Generally speaking, if the patient is seizure-free for 2 years and the doctor estimate a low risk of recurrence then anti-epileptic medications can be withdrawn gradually, followed by careful observation. A low risk of recurrence is usually indicated by normal brain imaging, normal EEG, and easy control of seizures on a single medication.

- **I want to become pregnant. Is there any problem with that?**
  This is a very important question and needs to be addressed. Your disease does not prevent you from becoming pregnant. More than 90% of patients with epilepsy do well during their pregnancy. However, you need to inform your neurologist and gynaecologist before pregnancy planning as some of the epilepsy medications are unsafe during pregnancy and can be harmful to the baby. Breastfeeding for most women taking anti-epileptic drugs is generally safe.

- **What about birth control methods?**
  It is very important to understand that most of the medications used to control epilepsy cause failure of the effectiveness of birth control pills. You may use birth control pills along with some barrier methods (condoms male/female, sponge etc.) for double protection. Your gynaecologist will give you further advice on that.

Show empathy

I understand Mrs Jamal how difficult it is to hear about this new diagnosis. We are here to help you.

Summarise and confirm understanding

Mrs Jamal, I would like to summarise our discussion to be sure that you understand important information about your illness. You had two episodes of abnormal body movements called seizure activity or epilepsy and we will prescribe for you a medication to reduce the chances of having further attacks.

We have discussed regarding medications, certain precautions, vaccination, and pregnancy planning along with birth control methods.

Is everything clear so far?

Please let me know if you want to discuss anything else at this moment.

Offer help and follow-up

Should you have any further questions, please do not hesitate to contact me on my office telephone number. I will also arrange an appointment in 2 weeks to review your progress.

I will arrange an appointment with a neurology colleague who will further discuss with you the management plan.

I will also provide you with some website addresses and printed material about epilepsy.

Discussion

Ethical principles

- **What are the main ethical principles in this scenario?**
  Patient's autonomy: The patient has the right to know about the diagnosis, treatment, and prognosis of her disease. The doctor should provide the patient with the necessary information to help her in making her decision. The doctor should be honest and truthful in discussing the risks and advising regarding the diagnosis and treatment.

  Beneficence and non-maleficence: Start with a single anti-epileptic medication with the least side effects. Explain the important precautions to avoid injuries or drowning during seizure attack. Provide advice regarding the risks associated with her job.

  Provide advice on triggering factors of seizure. Offer vaccinations to prevent some infections that can trigger seizure. Explain about pregnancy planning and birth control methods.

  Justice: Discussing the risks of driving in an epileptic patient is a form of justice to the patient and community, as it is risky for the epileptic patient and the community. The patient should receive the necessary care and treatment without discrimination.

Hidden agenda

- Discussing certain precautions to minimise injuries in epileptic patients.
- Discussing effects of the job on epilepsy.
- Discussing epilepsy and driving.
- Discussing epilepsy/anti-epileptic medications and pregnancy.
- Discussing contraceptive methods in epileptic women.

What is epilepsy?

An epileptic seizure is defined as 'a transient occurrence of signs and/or symptoms due to abnormal excessive or synchronous neuronal activity in the brain'. Epilepsy is diagnosed when an individual has—(1) at least two unprovoked or reflex seizures >24 hours apart, (2) one unprovoked or reflex seizure and a probability of having another seizure similar to the general recurrence risk after two unprovoked seizures ($\geq$60%) over the next 10 years, or (3) an epilepsy syndrome.

Classification of seizure disorders is discussed in **Table 1**.

Table 1 Classification of seizure disorders			
Generalised epilepsy	**Focal epilepsy (patient is aware or has impaired awareness)**	**Combined generalised and focal epilepsy**	**Unknown if generalised or focal epilepsy**
Motor:	**Motor:**		
Tonic-clonic	Automatism		
Tonic	Atonic		
Clonic	Clonic		
Myotonic	Myoclonic		
Atonic	Spasms		
Non-motor:	**Non-motor:**		
Typical	Autonomic		
Atypical	Sensory		
Myoclonic	Emotional		
Eyelid myoclonia	Behavioural arrest		
	Cognitive		

General causes of seizure:

- Genetic
- Structural
- Metabolic
- Immune related
- Infectious
- Unknown.

Diagnostic investigation: To look for an identifiable cause:

- Metabolic profile
- Lumbar puncture
- MRI brain
- EEG.

Management

Choice of anti-epileptic medication depends on the individual case and to treat any identifiable underlying cause.

Further reading

Driving and Vehicle Licensing Authority (DVLA)–UK. Epilepsy and driving. [online] Available from https://www.gov.uk/epilepsy-and-driving [Last accessed October, 2019].

Falco-Walter JJ, Scheffer IE, Fisher RS. The new definition and classification of seizures and epilepsy. Epilepsy Res 2018; 139:73–79.

Fisher RS, Acevedo C, Arzimanoglou A, et al. ILAE official report: a practical clinical definition of epilepsy. Epilepsia 2014; 55:475–482.

National Institute for Health and Care Excellence (NICE). (2012). Epilepsies: diagnosis and management Clinical guideline 2012. [online] Available from https://www.nice.org.uk/guidance/cg137/resources/epilepsies-diagnosis-and-management-pdf-35109515407813 [Last accessed October, 2019].

Scenario no. 6

Type of scenario: Information giving/breaking bad news

Candidate information

Your role: You are a doctor in the medical outpatient clinic.
Problem: Breaking bad news.
Patient: Mrs Walter, a 70-year-old lady.

Please read the scenario printed below. When the bell sounds, enter the room. You have (---) minutes for your consultation with the patient/relative, (---) minutes to collect your thoughts, and (---) minutes for discussion.

Please do not examine the patient
Please do not take a history

> Mrs Walter is a 70-year-old lady who is being followed in the clinic for the investigation of iron deficiency anaemia. She was investigated with a gastroscopy as a part of the workup for anaemia. Colonoscopy was not done due to her frail health condition. Gastroscopy showed an ulcer in the stomach and a biopsy was taken which proved to be a malignant growth. A CT scan revealed an ovarian cystic lesion and multiple nodules in the lungs, likely metastatic. She is very weak and rarely goes out of her house. Mrs Walter has come to the clinic for a follow-up appointment along with her daughter.
>
> **Your task:** Is to answer the patient's questions and help her to understand the new diagnosis and further plan of management.

Approach

Always read the scenario carefully and make sure you understand the instructions before you start. Any information provided is important. Make notes and a framework for your discussion. Sometimes, a hidden agenda is incorporated; pay attention to that.

Introduction and identification

- **Prepare the environment**
  Sit at the same level as the patient with comfort and avoid barriers like tables.

- **Introduce yourself to the patient**
  Shake hands
  Hello Mrs Walter, I am Dr X, working in the medical outpatient clinic.
  Can I confirm that I am talking to Mrs Walter?

- **Enquire from the patient if she would like someone else to be present during the discussion**
  Would you like to invite anybody else to this discussion? I heard that your daughter is here and you want to include her in our discussion?

- **Confirm the objective of the interview**
  We are here today to discuss the results of your investigations and diagnosis. Is that alright?

Check patient's understanding and expectation

Tell me Mrs Walter, how much do you know about your health status?
What do you suspect might be wrong with your health?

Discussion with the patient

- Give the patient the information (avoid medical jargon and explain what they mean)
  As you know Mrs Walter, we have been investigating the reasons for your low blood count over the last few weeks. As an important step of the workup we looked inside your stomach using with a gastroscopy (which is a camera attached to a long pipe). The gastroscopy showed an abnormal growth inside your stomach. We took tiny pieces from the growth and examined them under the microscope. I am afraid that the result is not good. Pause... I mean it is confirmed now to be a cancer of the stomach. Pause.....Check, and be prepared for patient's reaction. Would you like to continue the discussion? Or, would you like to further discuss your diagnosis at this moment?
  (If the answer is yes, proceed to the next stage of the discussion).

- **Explore the patient ideas about cancer**
  Have you ever heard of stomach cancer before? Pause....
  Do you know what cancer is? Pause.... Ask the patient.

- **Explain to the patient in simple terms about her cancer (avoid medical jargon)**
  I know this is bad news for you; but we will be working together to help you.
      Cancer starts when cells in the body begin to grow out of control. Cancer can arise anywhere in the body. When it originates from the stomach, we call it stomach or 'gastric' cancer. Cancer cells can spread to other parts of the body. For this reason, we performed a CT scan of your whole body and found that you have some cysts in your ovary; and multiple abnormal spots in your lungs which means that your cancer has already spread to other parts of your body.

- **Pause and ask the patient if everything is clear so far.**

- **Explain the treatment options**
  There are different treatment options for stomach cancer. As your stomach cancer has already spread to other parts of your body, surgical removal of the stomach cancer is not a treatment option in your case. Another treatment option is called chemotherapy where anticancer drugs are injected into a vein or given by mouth as pills. These drugs enter the bloodstream and reach all areas of the body, making this treatment useful for cancer that has spread to organs beyond where it started. This treatment can be given alone or with radiation therapy. However, such medications are very toxic and people with poor overall health may not tolerate their side effects. Another treatment option is called palliative care where a team of specialists work together with you and your family to provide an extra layer of support and treat your symptoms such as pain. We have a team of specialists including doctors specialising in treating stomach cancer (Multidisciplinary team). I will refer you to this team to arrange a meeting with you and decide on the best treatment for you.

- **Check the patient understanding**
  Does that make sense to you?

Explore and respond to patient's concerns

Is there any question or concern you would like to discuss at this moment?

- **What should I do for the low blood count?**
  We think that you have had blood loss from the cancer area. We will prescribe some iron tablets and vitamins to improve your blood count and overall health as well as a drug that reduces the acid production in your stomach (PPI) to help reduce the blood loss.

- **Doctor, do you think I will die soon?**
  As you know Mrs Walter, cancer is an aggressive disease particularly if it has spread to other organs in the body. Without treatment it progresses very fast. Nobody can predict the exact time of death, but I think a more accurate answer can be provided by our cancer specialists who are experts in this field.

Show empathy

I understand Mrs Walter how difficult it is to hear that you have cancer. We are here to help you.

Summarise and confirm understanding

Mrs Walter, I would like to briefly summarise our discussion to be sure that you understand important information about your illness. You had a low blood count for which a gastroscopy was done. The gastroscopy showed an abnormal growth in your stomach. Examination of tiny pieces of this growth confirmed that it is stomach cancer. Your cancer has spread to other parts of your body and complete removal of cancer is not possible. A specialised team that manages people with stomach cancer will see you soon and will discuss with you the different treatment options and the one that suits you most.
    Is that clear so far?
    Please let me know if you want to discuss anything else at this moment.

Offer help and follow-up

This is my office number. Please do not hesitate to contact me should you have any further question or concern.
    My nurse will call you shortly for an appointment with our multidisciplinary team.
    I will arrange another meeting in 1 week, in case you have any more questions or concerns.
    I will provide you with some website addresses and printed material containing information on stomach cancer.

Discussion

Ethical principles

- **What are the main ethical principles in this scenario?**
  Patient's autonomy: The patient has the right to know about the diagnosis and prognosis of her disease. The doctor should provide the patient with the necessary information to help her make her decision. The doctor should be honest and truthful in discussing the diagnosis and treatment.

  Beneficence and non-maleficence: Patient has the right to know what is in her best interest. In this case, as the patient has metastatic disease, she may be eligible for palliative treatment based on specialist assessment. Any intervention resulting in harm to the patient should not be undertaken. In this case, as the patient has metastatic disease, surgery is not in the best interest of the patient and could be harmful (non-maleficence). Similarly, she is not a candidate for radical treatment as such aggressive treatment may carry more harm (poor performance score).

Justice: All the available resources should be provided to her without any discrimination and that should include specialised palliative care. The patient should know about the risks associated with more aggressive therapies.

Hidden agenda

- Discussing different management options including palliative care.
- Considering the poor overall health of the patient.
- Recognising that final management decision should be by a specialised multidisciplinary team.
  Gastric cancer displays significant global variation in incidence. The highest rates are seen in Eastern Asia, Eastern Europe, and South America, with lower rates in North America and Western Europe.

- **Risk factors for gastric cancer include:**
  - Male gender (incidence is twice as high)
  - *Helicobacter pylori* infection
  - Tobacco use
  - Alcohol use, high-salt diet
  - Atrophic gastritis
  - Partial gastrectomy
  - Ménétrier's disease.

Familial aggregation is seen in 10% of cases, and an inherited genetic predisposition is found in a small proportion of cases (1–3%); relevant syndromes include hereditary non-polyposis colorectal cancer, familial adenomatous polyposis, colorectal cancer, hereditary diffuse gastric cancer, gastric adenocarcinoma, proximal polyposis of the stomach, and Peutz–Jeghers syndrome.

Types of gastric cancer

- Adenocarcinomas (90% of gastric cancers)
  Diffuse (undifferentiated) and intestinal (well-differentiated) types
- Gastrointestinal stromal tumours (GISTs)
- Gastric lymphoma
- Neuroendocrine tumours.

Surgical resection of gastric cancer, particularly at the early stages, is potentially curative. However, the majority of patients still relapse following resection, and therefore, combined modality therapies are standard for ≥ Stage IB disease.

Double or triple platinum/fluoropyrimidine combinations are recommended for fit patients with advanced gastric cancer.

Trastuzumab is recommended in conjunction with platinum and fluoropyrimidine-based chemotherapy for patients with human epidermal growth factor receptor 2 (HER2)-positive advanced gastric cancer.

When making a decision regarding chemotherapy, the functional age of the patient must also be considered, as comorbidities and performance status may have an equal effect on tolerance of chemotherapy as age. Geriatric assessment may be helpful before initiating treatment in older patients.

Further reading

Smyth EC, Verheij M, Allum W, et al. Gastric cancer: ESMO clinical practice guidelines. Ann Oncol 2016; 27:v38–v49.
Get palliative care. [online] Available from https://getpalliativecare.org/whatis/ [Last accessed October, 2019].

Scenario no. 7

Type of scenario: Refusal of therapy

Candidate information

Your role:	You are a doctor in the medical ward.
Problem:	Explain management of a disease/refusal of therapy.
Patient:	Mrs Ali, a 36-year-old lady.

Please read the scenario printed below. When the bell sounds, enter the room. You have (---) minutes for your consultation with the patient/relative, (---) minutes to collect your thoughts, and (---) minutes for discussion.

Please do not examine the patient
Please do not take a history

> Mrs Ali is a 36-year-old lady who was admitted last night to the acute medical unit with vomiting, abdominal pain, and dehydration. She was found to have hyperglycaemic hyperosmolar non-ketotic coma (HONK) and was managed accordingly. The plan now is to prepare her for discharge. Her diabetes mellitus (DM) is uncontrolled with an average glycated haemoglobin (HbA1c) of 12%. She uses gliclazide 120 mg daily, metformin 1,000 mg BID, and sitagliptin 100 mg daily. She was offered insulin therapy by her GP on multiple occasions in the past but she refused it. She is now concerned about the control of her diabetes. Her body mass index (BMI) is 28.
>
> **Your task:** Is to answer the patient's questions and help her to understand regarding treatment of her uncontrolled disease and a further plan of management if needed.

Approach

Always read the scenario carefully and make sure you understand the instructions before you start. Any information provided is important. Make notes and framework of your discussion. Sometimes, a hidden agenda is incorporated, pay attention to that.

Introduction and identification

- **Prepare the environment**
  Sit at the same level as the patient with comfort and avoid barriers like tables.

- **Introduce yourself to the patient**
  Shake hands
  Hello Mrs Ali, I am Dr X, working on the medical ward.
  Can I confirm that I am talking to Mrs Ali?

- **Enquire from the patient if she would like someone else to be present during discussion**
  Would you like to invite anybody else to this discussion?

- **Confirm the objective of the interview**
  We are here today to discuss your diabetes and further plan of management. Is that alright?

Check patient's understanding and expectation

Tell me Mrs Ali how much do you know about your health status?
What do you suspect might be wrong with your diabetes? And why are your blood sugars not controlled?

Discussion with the patient (information giving)

- **Give the patient the information (avoid medical jargon)**
  Are you feeling better today Mrs Ali? You were quiet unwell yesterday with recurrent vomiting and tummy pain. The blood and urine tests confirmed that your blood sugar was very high and you had developed a serious diabetes complication called hyperglycaemic hyperosmolar non-ketotic coma (abbreviated as HONK).

- **Explore the patient's ideas about hyperglycaemic hyperosmolar non-ketotic coma**
- Have you ever heard of this before? Pause....

- **Explain to the patient in simple terms about HONK (avoid medical jargon)**
  Hyperosmolar hyperglycaemic non-ketotic coma or HONK is one of the life-threatening emergency complications of diabetes. In this condition, because blood sugar becomes very high, the body tries to remove excess sugar in the urine. The water in your body is lost along with the sugar in the urine and results in severe and serious fluid and salt loss. This can lead to loss of consciousness, seizure, clots in the body, and sometimes death. Your doctors have worked hard to replace the fluid lost and lower your sugar which makes you feel better today. However, if your sugar is not kept under control, there is a significant chance that you develop HONK again or other long-term complications of diabetes in the future such as kidney, heart or eye diseases.

- **Pause and ask the patient if everything clear so far.**

- **Explore the reasons for insulin refusal**
- As mentioned Mrs Ali, the main reason for your current illness is the high sugar in your blood. Your last HbA1c was 12% which is very high. I understand that you were taking multiple pills for your sugar and your GP has offered insulin therapy to you, but you were not willing to use it. Could you tell me the reasons that made you decide not to take insulin?

- **Patient's concern**
  Yes doctor, that is correct. I did not start insulin because my GP informed me it may increase my weight. As you can see doctor, I am already overweight.

- **Express understanding of concerns, emphasise importance of therapy, and provide alternatives**
  I understand your concern. It is true that insulin can increase your body weight. At the same time, high sugar can lead to serious complications. Besides complications like HONK, high sugars can cause damage to the nerves, kidneys, eyes, heart, and other vital organs in your body. Of course being overweight can affect body image, joints, and blood pressure. Since your HbA1c is very high, insulin therapy is very important for you as other medications are unlikely to bring your sugar down to the required level. However, there are alternative ways by which we can control blood sugar and at the same time help you reduce or maintain your weight. One of those options is by changing your current diabetic pills to medication that will

help you reduce weight alongside a single dose of insulin. One such medication is called liraglutide, given as a single daily injection or there are now also once weekly injections like dulaglutide and semaglutide. These drugs are very effective in losing weight and controlling blood sugar. It is very important to note that the weight reduction will be greater with good diet control and physical activity. I am going to request a dietician to see you and advise you on, diet, exercise and physical activity. There are also other drugs such as SGLT-2 inhibitors that can be given along with insulin to help you reduce weight.

- **Explain about insulin therapy**
  Furthermore, insulin can be given using sophisticated pens with a very thin needle that causes very minimal pain. There are different insulin types based on the duration of action. Long-acting insulin enters the bloodstream 1–2 hours after injection and may be effective for as long as 24 hours. Rapid-acting insulin begins to affect blood glucose about 15 minutes after injection and works for a few hours so it is injected before a meal. The timing of insulin injection, storage, and use will be explained to you by our diabetes educator shortly. As with any drug or treatment, side effects and complications are possible. The most important side effect is low blood sugar. However, with careful follow-up and advice this complication can be avoided especially if we use continuous glucose sensors.

- **Check the patient understanding**

Explore and respond to patient's concerns

Do you have any questions or concerns you would like to discuss at this moment?
- **What about bariatric surgery in my case?**
  Treatment with bariatric surgery has been shown to be very effective in controlling blood sugar and reducing weight. However, bariatric surgery is costly and has associated risks. Currently, bariatric surgery may be considered for adults with a BMI ≥ 35 kg/m^2 and T2DM. Your current BMI is 28. There is insufficient evidence to recommend surgery for you.

Show empathy

I understand Mrs Ali how difficult this all is but we are here to help you.

Summarise and confirm understanding

Mrs Ali, I would like to summarise our discussion to be sure that you understand important information about your diabetes. You were admitted to the hospital with a serious complication of DM called HONK that resulted from uncontrolled blood sugar. If your diabetes remains uncontrolled, it can result in serious complication. It is important, therefore, to bring your blood sugar down to the desirable level for which you need insulin therapy. However, because of your concern regarding weight gain, we can prescribe other diabetic medications that can lower your weight in addition to insulin.

If you agree to start insulin therapy, our diabetes specialist will discuss the options for the different types of insulin therapy and the other medications.

Please let me know if you want to discuss anything more at this moment.

Offer help and follow-up

This is my telephone number. Please do not hesitate to contact me should you have any further questions.

You will be seen shortly by our diabetes specialist educator, and dietician.

I will arrange another meeting in the diabetes clinic in a week to review your progress.

I will provide you with some website addresses and printed material on DM and insulin therapy.

Discussion

Ethical principles

- **What are the main ethical principles in this scenario?**

  Patient's autonomy: The patient has the right to know about the diagnosis and complications of her disease. Doctor should provide the patient with the necessary information to help her make her decision. Doctor should be honest and truthful in discussing the risks and advise regarding the diagnosis and treatment. The patient has the right to refuse or accept insulin therapy.

  Beneficence: In this case, insulin therapy is beneficial to avoid further complications of diabetes.

  Non-maleficence: Alternative therapy that could reduce the risk of insulin-induced weight gain should be offered to the patient. Continuing her current oral agents alone is not in the best interest of the patient.

  Justice: All treatment options that can be of benefit should be provided to the patient without discrimination. Glucagon-like peptide-1 (GLP-1) agonists such as liraglutide should be offered. Bariatric surgery is expensive and not indicated in her case. Therefore, it should be reserved for those who need it.

Hidden agenda

- Exploring the reasons behind refusal of therapy.
- Explaining the importance of insulin in her case.
- Discussing new alternative therapies that help to reduce weight such as GLP-1 agonists and SGLT-2 inhibitors.

Dealing with patients who resist starting recommended therapy or refuse medical advice

- Doctor should explore the reason for resisting starting therapy. Most of the time, the information about the therapy has not been communicated well to the patient.
- Express empathy and understanding of the patient's concerns.
- Explain to the patient and ensure that they understand why the medication is important to them.
- Explain the possible consequences of not taking the medication.
- Consider various alternatives to address the situation such as: changing to alternative medication regimen, helping to avoid possible side effects, further patient education, referral to a specialist, providing nursing services, relieving phobia, etc.

Reasons for diabetic patients to refuse insulin therapy

- Injection phobia
- Pain
- Weight gain
- Job working environment
- Social stigma.

Job working environment and injection phobia can be reduced by using new sophisticated insulin injection devices that can be carried in pockets like pens. They have tiny needles that cause minimal pain. Injecting insulin in the tummy is less painful compared to other sites. Regarding the job working environment, it can be adjusted by changing insulin timing or arranging with the employer to make the job environment suitable for patients who are taking insulin.

Effects of diabetic medication on weight

Diabetic medications associated with weight loss:
- Metformin
- Alpha-glucosidase inhibitors

- Glucagon-like peptide-1 agonists
- Amylin mimetic
- Sodium–glucose cotransporter-2 inhibitors.

Diabetic medications that are weight neutral:
- Dipeptidyl peptidase-4 inhibitors.

Diabetic medications that increase weight:
- Insulin secretagogues
- Thiazolidinediones
- Insulin.

Classification of diabetes mellitus

- Type 1 diabetes mellitus (due to autoimmune β-cell destruction, usually leading to absolute insulin deficiency).
- Type 2 diabetes mellitus (due to a progressive loss of β-cell insulin secretion frequently on the background of insulin resistance).
- Gestational diabetes mellitus (GDM) (diabetes diagnosed in the second or third trimester of pregnancy).
- Specific types of diabetes due to other causes, e.g. monogenic diabetes syndromes [such as neonatal diabetes and maturity-onset diabetes of the young (MODY)], diseases of the exocrine pancreas (such as cystic fibrosis and pancreatitis), and drug- or chemical-induced diabetes (such as with glucocorticoid use, in the treatment of HIV/AIDS, or after organ transplantation).

How is diabetes diagnosed?

One of the following criteria:
- Fasting plasma glucose (FPG) ≥126 mg/dL (7.0 mmol/L) (Fasting is defined as no caloric intake for at least 8 hours).
- Two-hour PPG ≥200 mg/dL (11.1 mmol/L) during an oral glucose tolerance test (OGTT).
- A1c ≥6.5%
- In a patient with classic symptoms of hyperglycaemia or hyperglycaemic crisis, a random plasma glucose ≥200 mg/dL (11.1 mmol/L).

Patients with prediabetes are defined by the presence of IFG and/or IGT and/or A1c 5.7–6.4%.

HbA1c goals when treating diabetes mellitus

- A reasonable A1c goal for many non-pregnant adults is <7%.
- More stringent A1c goals (<6.5% if this can be achieved without significant hypoglycaemia or other adverse effects of treatment) for selected individual patients with short duration of diabetes, T2DM treated with lifestyle or metformin only, long life expectancy, or no significant cardiovascular disease.
- Less stringent A1c goals (such as <8%) may be appropriate for patients with a history of severe hypoglycaemia, limited life expectancy, advanced microvascular or macrovascular complications, extensive comorbid conditions, or long-standing diabetes in whom the goal is difficult to achieve despite diabetes self-management education, appropriate glucose monitoring, and effective doses of multiple glucose-lowering agents including insulin.

Complications of diabetes mellitus

Microvascular complications

- **Retinopathy**
  Annual dilated eye examination by ophthalmologist or retinal screening.

- **Nephropathy**
  Annual urine testing
  Blood pressure should be less than 130/80 mmHg in adults.

- **Neuropathy**
  Assess for painful neuropathy symptoms and monofilament examination.

Macrovascular complications

- Cardiovascular disease
- Stroke
- Other possible problems are:
  - Dental issues, gum disease
  - Glaucoma, cataract
  - High cholesterol.

Management of diabetes mellitus

- **Pharmacological therapy**
- **Risk factor management**
  - Quit smoking
  - Control blood pressure
  - Control lipid level
  - Regular exercise
  - Diet control (not to take high sugar diets)
  - Weight loss
- **Monitoring for and preventing complications**
  - HbA1c every 3 months
  - Check lipids; consider statins or fibrates.
  - Check blood pressure; consider starting an angiotensin converting enzyme (ACE) inhibitor or angiotensin-receptor blocker (ARB).
  - *Retinopathy:* Annual retinal screening
  - *Nephropathy:* Urine protein/creatinine ratio and eGFR
  - *Neuropathy:* Annual monofilament examination.
- **Patient education**
  - Diabetes self-management education and support
  - Symptoms of hyper-and hypoglycaemia
  - Blood sugar targets
  - Diabetes complications
  - Regular self-foot care and examination
  - Proper nail cutting
  - Proper body hygiene.
- **Vaccination**
  - Annual vaccination against influenza
  - Vaccination against pneumococcal disease
  - Hepatitis B vaccine.

Driving and diabetes mellitus

- Patients on temporary insulin therapy, less than 3 months, do not need to inform DVLA.
- Patients on insulin therapy, more than 3 months, need to inform DVLA.
- If patient develops any complication (retinopathy/nephropathy/neuropathy etc.), he/she must inform the DVLA and stop driving until reassessed and a further decision is taken.
- Patients must have adequate awareness of hypoglycaemia to be able to drive.

Diabetes and pregnancy

- Preconception counselling should address the importance of glycaemic control as close to normal as is safely possible. Ideally A1c should be <6.5% (48 mmol/mol) to reduce the risk of congenital anomalies.

- Women with pre-existing diabetic retinopathy need close monitoring during pregnancy because of the risk of progression of diabetic retinopathy associated with rapid improvement in glycaemic control during pregnancy.
- Blood sugar monitoring in pregnancy is through self-monitoring of fasting and postprandial blood glucose and there is an increasing use of continuous glucose monitoring systems (CGMS). HbA1C is slightly lower in pregnancy due to increased red blood cell turnover.
- The A1c target in pregnancy is 6–6.5%.
- HbA1c <6% may be optimal if this can be achieved without significant hypoglycaemia, but the target may be relaxed to <7% (53 mmol/mol), if necessary, to prevent hypoglycaemia.
- Insulin is the first-line agent recommended for the treatment of DM in pregnancy. Some studies support the efficacy and safety of metformin and glyburide for the treatment of GDM. However, both agents cross the placenta and there is no agreement regarding the comparative advantages and disadvantages of the two oral agents.
- Self-monitoring blood sugar targets in pregnancy:
  - Fasting <95 mg/dL (5.3 mmol/L) and either
  - One-hour postprandial <140 mg/dL (7.8 mmol/L) or
  - Two-hour postprandial <120 mg/dL (6.7 mmol/L).

Further reading

American Diabetic Association. Standards of Medical Care in Diabetes 2018. Diabetes Care 2018; 41:S1–S159.

Driving and Vehicle Licensing Agency (DVLA)–UK. Diabetes and driving. [online] Available from https://www.gov.uk/diabetes-driving [Last accessed October, 2019].

Smith-Marsh DE. What you need to know about insulin. Endocrineweb. [online] Available from https://www.endocrineweb.com/guides/insulin/what-you-need-know-about-insulin [Last accessed October, 2019].

Abu Hassan H, Tohid H, Mohd Amin R, et al. Factors influencing insulin acceptance among type 2 diabetes mellitus patients in a primary care clinic: a qualitative exploration. BMC Fam Pract 2013; 14:164.

Scenario no. 8

Type of scenario: Information giving/ethical dilemma

Candidate information

Your role: You are the doctor in the medical outpatient clinic.
Problem: Explanation of newly diagnosed chronic disease.
Patient: Mr Taylor, a 45-year-old gentleman.

Please read the scenario printed below. When the bell sounds, enter the room. You have (---) minutes for your consultation with the patient/relative, (---) minutes to collect your thoughts, and (---) minutes for discussion.

Please do not examine the patient
Please do not take a history

Mr Taylor is a 45-year-old gentleman, working as a driver. He was admitted with high blood pressure and headache 3 months ago. His examination at that time revealed:

BP: 180/110 mmHg

HR: 89 beats/min

BMI: 42

He was commenced on medication and is currently taking amlodipine 10 mg, perindopril 10 mg, and indapamide 1.5 mg daily. His hypertension is uncontrolled. Recently, he had a road traffic accident because he slept on the wheel while driving. A sleep study was requested and the results showed an apnoea–hypopnoea index of 48 per hour and a desaturation index of 55 per hour. Now he is worried about his job.

Your task: Is to answer the patient's concerns and help him to understand the new diagnosis and further plan of management, if needed.

Approach

Always read the scenario carefully and make sure you understand the instructions before you start. Any information provided is important. Make notes and a framework for your discussion. Sometimes, a hidden agenda is incorporated, pay attention to that.

Introduction and identification

- **Prepare the environment**
  Sit at the same level as the patient with comfort and avoid barriers like tables.

- **Introduce yourself to the patient**
  Shake hands
  Hello Mr Taylor, I am Dr X, working in the medical outpatient clinic.
  Can I confirm that I am talking to Mr Taylor?

- **Enquire from the patient if he would like someone else to be present during the discussion**
  Would you like to invite anybody else to this discussion?

- **Confirm the objective of the interview**
  We are here today to discuss the results of your investigations and diagnosis. Is that alright?

Check patient's understanding and expectation

Tell me Mr Taylor, how much do you know about your health status?
Do you know why we requested the sleep studies for you?
What do you suspect might be wrong with your health and your blood pressure?

Discussion with the patient

- **Give the patient the information (avoid medical jargon)**
  Mr Taylor, your blood pressure is uncontrolled despite using 3 medications and you frequently complain of headache. Recently, you had a road traffic accident because you slept while driving. Based on your history and clinical examination, we requested a sleep study, which confirms that you have a condition called 'obstructive sleep apnoea (OSA)'.

- **Explore the patient's ideas about OSA**
  Have you ever heard of OSA before? Pause....

- **Explain to the patient in simple terms about OSA (avoid medical jargon)**
  Obstructive sleep apnoea means a temporary pause of breathing during sleep.
  Normally, the muscles around the tongue and throat function to keep the throat and
  windpipe open during sleep and allow air in and out easily. In OSA, these muscles
  lose control and block the throat. As they block the throat, breathing stops during
  sleep and the oxygen level in your blood drops. This happens repeatedly while the
  person is sleeping with repeated cessation of breathing and frequent awakenings
  during sleep (gasping for air). As you keep waking up frequently to breath, you
  become sleep-deprived and feel very tired and fatigued during the day. In addition, it
  leads to elevation in the blood pressure which is difficult to control.

- **Pause and ask the patient if everything is clear so far.**

- **Explain how the assessment of OSA is done**
  Based on your symptoms, physical examination, and uncontrolled blood pressure, a
  sleep study was done for you and this confirmed that you have severe OSA.

- **Explain the importance of treating OSA and the risks associated with untreated
  OSA**
  It is very important to treat OSA and ensure that your oxygen concentration during
  sleep normalises. Untreated OSA can cause significant harm to your body and serious
  long-term consequences for your health which include:
  - High blood pressure
  - Heart disease, e.g. heart attack and
    heart failure
  - Stroke
  - Diabetes
  - Depression
  - Risk for accidents and injuries
  - Memory problems
  - Erectile dysfunction

  Therefore, we need to plan treatment for you as soon as possible.

- **Explain the treatment options**
  First of all, I would advise you to lose weight as obesity is a major risk factor for OSA.
  I will refer you to our obesity clinic where my colleagues will explain to you the
  different options for treating obesity.

  Secondly, I would advise lifestyle modifications like positional sleep (it is better to
  sleep on your side rather than on your back) and sleep hygiene (the environment
  of the room you sleep in should have no noise and optimal temperature without
  disturbance).

  Thirdly, you need a continuous positive airway pressure (CPAP) machine with a mask
  to put over your face while you sleep. This machine will push air inside your airways
  whilst you sleep by keeping your throat open. Our respiratory therapist will explain to
  you how to use this machine properly.

- **Advice regarding driving**
  Mr Taylor, I understand that your job is as a company driver. Is that correct?

  What are you driving (group 1—car/motorcycle, group 2—HGV/lorry etc.)?

  Are you the only support for your family or is your wife working?

  I am sorry to inform you that as per regulation, you cannot drive until your
  obstructive sleep apnoea is controlled and properly treated. This is because of the
  risk of falling asleep whilst driving which may result in a serious accident harming
  yourself and others. I note that you previously had a minor accident. You have to
  inform the DVLA regarding your OSA. Once your disease is controlled, DVLA may
  allow you to resume driving.

If the patient refuses to stop driving or refuses to inform DVLA.

Empathise and listen to him.

Explore the reasons that prevent him from stopping driving or informing DVLA.
Explain to the patient the consequences of continuing to drive while OSA is untreated and provide alternative options:

- He will be fined by the DVLA if he does not inform them.
- He will lose his insurance.
- Most importantly, he can cause serious accidents and put his and other people's lives at risk.
- Discuss alternative options such as using public transport.
- Consider referring to a social worker if he has socioeconomic concerns.
- Ask his GP to issue a letter that will help with his current job.

- **OSA and alcohol/OSA and general anaesthesia**
  Mr Taylor, do you drink alcohol? How much do you drink?
  Alcohol can make OSA worse as it affects the sleep pattern and the time it takes for you to fall asleep. The best advice is to abstain from alcohol, but if it is not possible, then at least minimise alcohol consumption and avoid drinking several hours prior to bedtime.
  I would also advise you to inform your doctor about your OSA before any surgery especially if you need general anaesthesia as it will be difficult to manage your airway during anaesthesia.

- **Check patient understanding**
  Does that make sense to you?

Explore and respond to concerns

Do you have any question or concerns you would like to discuss at this moment?

- **How long shall I use CPAP?**
  Some patients improve by losing weight while others need CPAP for quite a long time and even lifelong. Your sleep specialist may consider repeating the sleep test after losing weight to see how much your sleep apnoea has improved. Besides improving your sleep, CPAP has many other beneficial effects such as helping to control your BP, preventing memory problems, improving your heart function, and sexual performance.

- **Is there any other alternative? What if I do not want to use the machine?**
  There are alternative therapies but they are used only for mild disease and would not be effective in your case as you have severe OSA. A mandibular advancement device can be put in the mouth while you are sleeping. Basically, it advances your lower jaw while keeping the throat open. There is no evidence of its effectiveness in severe OSA.
  Another alternative is a type of surgery called uvulopalatopharyngoplasty (UPPP) which involves cutting part of the soft palate to increase the size of the throat, but again there is no evidence that it is more effective than CPAP.

Show empathy

I understand Mr Taylor it must be difficult to hear that you have OSA. We are here to help.

Summarise and confirm understanding

Mr Taylor, I would like to briefly summarise our discussion to be sure that you understand important information about OSA. You have high and uncontrolled blood pressure and you have had a road traffic accident because you fell asleep while driving. The sleep study showed that you suffer from severe OSA. I have explained to you the entire treatment plan including losing weight, having comfortable sleep, avoiding alcohol, and the need to use the CPAP machine during sleep. Furthermore, you have to stop driving until your OSA is controlled and you need to inform the DVLA regarding your OSA.

Is everything clear so far?

Would you like to discuss anything else at this moment?

Offer help and follow-up

This is my telephone number. Please do not hesitate to contact me should you have any further questions.

I will arrange an appointment with a sleep specialist and a sleep therapist to discuss OSA and its management in detail.

I will also request an appointment for you in the obesity clinic.

I will arrange to review you in 2 weeks.

I will provide you with some website addresses and printed material about OSA.

Discussion

Ethical principles

- **What are the main ethical principles in this scenario?**

  Patient's autonomy: The patient has the right to know about the diagnosis and complications of his disease. The doctor should provide the patient with the necessary information to help him make his decision. The doctor should be honest and truthful in discussing the risks and advice regarding the diagnosis and treatment. The patient has the right to refuse or accept CPAP or other forms of therapy.

  Beneficence: In this scenario, lifestyle modification (losing weight, diet control, and positional sleep), sleep hygiene, and CPAP therapy are beneficial for the patient.

  Non-maleficence: Significant risks and harms can arise from untreated OSA with harm to the patient and community.

  A mandibular advancement device and surgery are not effective in severe OSA.

  Justice: A CPAP machine is expensive but essential for this patient. Hence, the patient has the right to use it. Justice to the community is also applicable as driving by patients with untreated OSA can be dangerous to the community.

Hidden agenda in this scenario

- Driving and OSA
- Job and social issues in patients with OSA.

- **What is OSA?**

  Collapse of the airway causing cessation of breathing during sleep

- **What is obesity hypoventilation syndrome? (Pickwickian syndrome)**

  As the name indicates 'alveolar hypoventilation during the daytime secondary to obesity'

  Classic features of obesity hypoventilation syndrome:
  - BMI $\geq$30 kg/m^2
  - Daytime $P\text{aco}_2$ >45 mmHg
  - Associated sleep-related breathing disorder
  - Absence of other known causes of hypoventilation.

- **What are the risk factors for OSA?**
  - *Structural abnormality:*
    - Crowded airway (enlarged tonsils, adenoids, nasal polyps, etc.)
    - Retrognathia

- - ■ Micrognathia
    - ■ Macroglossia
    - ■ Short thick neck.
  - – *Increased neck circumference:*
    - ■ Family history of OSA
    - ■ Obesity
    - ■ Male gender.

- **What are the symptoms of OSA?**
  - – Loud snoring during sleep
  - – Episodes of apnoea and hypopnoea during sleep
  - – Choking during sleep
  - – Un-refreshing sleep
  - – Early morning headache
  - – Daytime hypersomnolence
  - – Daytime fatigue/tiredness
  - – Nocturia
  - – Loss of concentration
  - – Memory loss
  - – Irritability
  - – Decreased sexual drive.

Probability and screening for sleep apnoea

S-T-O-P B-A-N-G Questionnaire
- **S**noring
- **T**ired
- **O**bserved apnoea
- **P**ressure
- **B**ody mass index > 35 kg/m^2
- **A**ge >50 years
- **N**eck size is large (neck circumference 17 inches/43 cm in male or 16 inches/41 cm in female)
- **G**ender: Male

Low-risk OSA: 0–2
Intermediate risk OSA: 3–4
High-risk OSA: 5–8

How to assess daytime sleepiness?

Epworth Sleepiness Scale
- Sitting and reading.
- Watching television.
- Sitting inactively in a public place, e.g. in a meeting.
- Lying down to rest in the afternoon.
- Sitting talking to someone.
- Sitting quietly after a lunch without alcohol.
- In a car, stopped in traffic or at lights.
- In a car, as a passenger for an hour.

For each section above, use the relevant number
  0 = would never doze
  1 = slight chance of dozing
  2 = moderate chance of dozing
  3 = high chance of dozing

What are the investigations needed in OSA?

- *Complete blood count*: To look for erythrocytosis/secondary polycythaemia
- *Urea electrolyte and HCO$_3$*: To assess compensation of chronic hypercapnia

- *Liver function tests*: Look for non-alcoholic fatty liver disease (NAFLD) as evidence of metabolic syndrome.
- *Thyroid function tests*: Hypothyroidism can be associated with OSA.
- *Arterial blood gas*: To look for chronic hypercapnia due to OHS.
- *Sleep study*: To confirm OSA.
- *Chest X-ray*: In OHS, it may give information about some of the causes of hypoventilation that need to be ruled out, like diaphragmatic paralysis, thoracic cage abnormality, low lung volume, cardiomegaly, and heart failure.
- *ECG*: To look for CAD and arrhythmias (AF).

Management of sleep apnoea

Lifestyle modification

- Weight loss
- Diet
- Positional sleep
- Sleep hygiene
- Avoid alcohol.

CPAP therapy and NIV

These are the treatment of choice in severe OSA.
Oral appliance therapy like mandibular advancement device:
- Oral appliances are considered for patients with mild-to-moderate OSA.
- May also be considered for patients with severe OSA, who are unable to tolerate or cannot wear CPAP devices.

Surgery

- UPPP in selected cases only
- Upper airway stimulation (UAS) therapy.

Driving and OSA

DVLA Rule: (Gov./UK)
Group 1—Car/Motorcycle:
- No driving until symptoms are controlled
- Review every 3 years.
Group 2—HGV/Bus/Lorry:
- No driving until symptoms are controlled
- Review annually.

Further reading

Chung F, Abdullah HR, Liao P. STOP-Bang Questionnaire: A practical approach to screen for obstructive sleep apnoea. Chest 2016; 149:631–638.

Chung F, Yegneswaran B, Liao P, et al. STOP questionnaire: a tool to screen patients for obstructive sleep apnoea. Anaesthesiology 2008; 108:812–221.

Driver and Vehicle Licensing Agency (UK). Obstructive sleep apnoea and driving. [online] Available from https://www.gov.uk/obstructive-sleep-apnoea-and-driving [Last accessed October, 2019].

Kapur VK, Auckley DH, Chowdhuri S, et al. Clinical Practice Guideline for Diagnostic Testing for Adult Obstructive Sleep Apnoea: An American Academy of Sleep Medicine clinical practice guideline. J Clin Sleep Med 2017; 13:479–504.

Qaseem A, Holty JE, Owens DK, et al. Management of obstructive sleep apnoea in adults: A clinical practice guideline from the American College of Physicians. Ann Intern Med 2013; 159:471–483.

Scenario no. 9

Type of scenario: Information giving/discharge management plan

Candidate information

Your role: You are the doctor in the cardiology unit.
Problem: Explanation of a new diagnosis.
Patient: Mr Lee, a 52-year-old businessman.

Please read the scenario printed below. When the bell sounds, enter the room. You have (---) minutes for your consultation with the patient/relative, (---) minutes to collect your thoughts, and (---) minutes for discussion.

Please do not examine the patient
Please do not take a history

Mr Lee is a 52-year-old businessman. He has smoked 20 cigarettes per day for the last 30 years. He was admitted 2 days ago with severe chest pain and breathing difficulty and found to have an anterior myocardial infarction. He underwent coronary angioplasty with two stents placed in his coronary vessels. His echocardiography showed some segmental wall motion abnormality and ejection fraction of 48%. He is pain-free now and stable. He wants to be discharged soon as he wants to travel for a business meeting. He is waiting for you in his room.

Your task: Is to answer the patient's questions and concerns and help him to understand the further plan of management if needed.

Approach

Always read the scenario carefully and make sure you understand the instructions before you start. All information provided is important. Make notes and a framework for your discussion. Sometimes, a hidden agenda is incorporated; pay attention to that.

Introduction and identification

- **Prepare the environment**
  Sit at the same level as the patient with comfort and avoid barriers like tables.

- **Introduce yourself to the patient**
  Shake hands.
  Hello Mr Lee, I am Dr X, working in the cardiology unit.
  Can I confirm that I am talking to Mr Lee?

- **Enquire from the patient if he would like someone else to be present during discussion**
  Would you like to invite anyone else to this discussion?

- **Confirm the objective of the interview**
  We are here to discuss your disease and further management. Is that alright?

Check patient's understanding and expectation

Tell me Mr Lee, how much do you know about your health status?

Do you know what was wrong with your heart when you were admitted?

Discussion with the patient

- **Give the patient the information (avoid medical jargon)**

  As you know Mr Lee, you came initially with chest pain and breathing difficulty and our tests showed that you have had a heart attack. I assume that other colleagues explained to you what a heart attack is. If not, I can further explain it. Is that alright?

  A heart attack is a sudden blockage of one of the three main blood vessels supplying blood to the heart. Because of the blockage, blood flow to the heart muscle supplied by that vessel will stop or diminish resulting in intense pain in the chest. In addition, the heart muscles that suffer lack of blood supply will not be able to perform their normal pumping action resulting in the feeling of breathing difficulty.

- **Giving information about what happened in the hospital**

  Mr Lee, I assume someone has also discussed with you the management plan when you were admitted. If not, I will further discuss with you. Is that alright?

  As you know Mr Lee, your heart doctor has unblocked the blocked heart vessels by performing angioplasty in which, a small wire with a balloon at the tip was inserted via the vessels in your groin and pushed to the heart vessels. The balloon was inflated to open the blocked heart vessels and small mesh-like stents were placed in each blocked vessel to keep the lumen open.

- **Discussion about further management plan/discharge planning**

  Mr Lee, now let us discuss your further treatment plan.

  - *Medications*: There are important medications that you need to take after discharge. These medications are very important to help keep your blood vessels open and avoid the formation of clots inside the stents and vessels. Other medications are important to help keep your heart muscle strong. It is very important that these medications are taken as directed. Some of these medications need to be taken for life, while others can be stopped after a year.

    - *Medications that need to be taken lifelong post-ST-elevation myocardial infarction (STEMI)*:
      - Aspirin
      - High dose statin
      - Beta-blockers.

    - *Medications that need to be taken for 12 months*: Dual antiplatelet therapy (DAPT) with aspirin and clopidogrel is recommended in patients with STEMI who undergo primary percutaneous coronary intervention (PCI) for up to 12 months.

  Clopidogrel is recommended for 1 month in patients treated with fibrinolysis without subsequent PCI (expanding the duration of DAPT up to 12 months should be considered in these patients).

  For patients undergoing fibrinolysis and subsequent PCI, DAPT is recommended for 12 months.

    - *Medications that are prescribed based on the situation*: Angiotensin-converting enzyme (ACE) inhibitors are recommended, starting within the first 24 hours of STEMI in patients with evidence of heart failure, left ventricular (LV) systolic dysfunction, diabetes, or an anterior infarct.

- **Explain the importance of smoking cessation**

  Mr Lee, smoking, no doubt, has contributed to your illness, and therefore, quitting smoking is a crucial step in reducing the chances of a second heart attack. Are you willing to discuss how we can help you to stop smoking? If he agrees, discuss with him the benefits of smoking cessation and referral to the smoking cessation clinic. If he is not willing to discuss it now, offer some informative material on smoking cessation and postpone the discussion to another meeting.

- **Lifestyle modification**
  - *Diet*: You need to eat a healthy diet. You will be referred to a dietician for further advice on a healthy diet. Generally speaking, you need to avoid greasy, fried and fatty foods, and eat more vegetables and fruits.
  - *Alcohol:* You need to limit your alcohol intake [maximum of 2 glasses (20 g of alcohol) daily for men and 1 for women].
  - *Heart rehabilitation program and exercise:* The heart rehabilitation programme is a special programme for patients with a heart attack after discharge (usually for 8–24 weeks). It helps you to perform exercise and physical activity that suits you, avoid the risk factors that caused the heart attack, manage your stress and provides psychological support.
  - *Blood pressure control:* Your blood pressure should be well controlled. Your systolic blood pressure (SBP) target should be <140 mmHg.
  - *Lipid control:* Your low-density lipoprotein cholesterol (LDL-C) should be <1.8 mmol/L (70 mg/dL).
  - *Weight loss:* Discuss if the patient is obese.
  - *Rest and avoiding stress:* Avoiding stress is important in preventing a further heart attack.
  - *Air travel:* I understand Mr Lee you are a busy person and travelling to a meeting may be important for you. However, the advice for air travel after a heart attack varies depending on the severity of the heart attack, the length of travel, and the degree of anxiety associated with travel. As your heart muscles are weak after the heart attack and we plan to start you on a heart rehabilitation programme soon, I recommend that you postpone your travel for at least 4 weeks. You may consider other ways of being involved in the business meeting without the need to travel, e.g. by video call or chat, etc.
  - *Sexual activity:* Mr Lee, I need to discuss an important personal issue, regarding your sexual activity, is that alright? Sexual activity can be resumed once you feel you can do your usual daily activities without chest pain. However, if you develop chest pain on exercise, please do not resume sexual activity until a doctor can assess and advise you further.
  - *Driving:* Do you drive a car? If yes, which type?
  I am sorry Mr Lee to inform you it may not be possible for you to drive for 4 weeks after your heart attack. (If he refuses to do so, explain the risks and document in patient's file after informing him).
      DVLA (Gov./UK) rules: If the patient is a group-2 driver, he should stop driving and inform the DVLA.
      Group-1 (car/motorcycle): He does not need to notify DVLA, but should stop driving for:
    - 1-week post angioplasty
    - 4 weeks if you have had angioplasty and it was not successful
    - 4 weeks if you had a heart attack and did not have angioplasty.
      Group-2 (bus/lorry): Patient needs to inform the DVLA and stop driving for 6 weeks after the myocardial infarction or angioplasty and then they need to be reassessed after 6 weeks.
- **Check patient understanding**
  Does that make sense to you?

Explore and respond to patient's concerns

Do you have any questions or concerns?
- **When can I resume sexual activity?**
  Already discussed
- **How long do I need to take these medications?**
  Already discussed
- **Can I drive my car?**
  Already discussed

Show empathy

I understand Mr Lee it must be difficult to hear about your heart problems. We are here to help you.

Summarise and confirm understanding

Mr Lee, I would like to briefly summarise our discussion to be sure that you understand important information about your illness. You were admitted to hospital with chest pain and breathing difficulty. You were diagnosed with an acute heart attack and it was treated successfully with angioplasty and stenting of the blocked vessels. I have explained to you the need to take your medication regularly and to undertake lifestyle modification.

We have discussed the importance of a balanced diet, weight loss, heart rehabilitation programme, smoking cessation, air travel, sexual activity and driving.

Is everything clear so far?

Would you like to discuss anything else at this moment?

Offer help and follow-up

This is my telephone number. Please do not hesitate to contact me should you have any other questions or concerns.

You will be contacted very soon to start your heart rehabilitation programme.

You will also be seen shortly in the heart clinic.

I will arrange another meeting within 2 weeks in case you have any more questions or concerns.

If at any time you feel your heart is racing, or you develop chest pain at rest, please call our emergency telephone number.

I will also provide you with some website addresses and printed material to read more about your diagnosis.

Discussion

Ethical principles

- **What are the main ethical principles in this scenario?**
  Patient's autonomy: The patient has the right to know about the diagnosis and prognosis of his disease. The doctor should provide the patient with the necessary information to help him make his decisions. The doctor should be honest and truthful in discussing the risks and advice regarding the diagnosis and treatment. The patient has the right to refuse or accept the advice or therapy.

  Beneficence and non-maleficence: Avoiding harm and doing good to the patient are important ethical principles. In this scenario, air travel may carry some risk to the patient because of his impaired ejection fraction due to STEMI. Controlling risk factors and taking the recommended medications are in the best interest of the patient and should be encouraged. The patient should be informed about the possible side effects of the medications. Advice regarding sexual activity and driving is also in the best interest of the patient.

Justice: The patient has the right to receive the medications and treatment without discrimination. The heart rehabilitation programme is expensive but is important.

Hidden agenda in this scenario

- Explaining the management plan.
- Acute MI and air travel.
- Acute MI and driving.

Definition of myocardial infarction

Myocardial infarction (heart attack) is the irreversible death (necrosis) of heart muscle secondary to a prolonged lack of oxygen (ischaemia).

Causes/associations of acute coronary syndrome

- Genetic susceptibility
- Age
- Male sex
- Hypertension
- Diabetes mellitus
- Dyslipidaemia and familial hypercholesterolemia
- Smoking
- Stress.

Clinical classification of MI

- Type 1 MI: Coronary artery pathology, intraluminal thrombus
- Type 2 MI: Ischaemia secondary to imbalance between oxygen supply and demand.
- Type 3 MI: Sudden cardiac death when biomarker values are unavailable.
- Type 4a MI: Related to PCI.
- Type 4b MI: Related to stent thrombosis.
- Type 5 MI: Related to coronary artery bypass grafting (CABG).

Long-term management and discharge plan post-ACS

Dual antiplatelet therapy post-STEMI:
- DAPT, combined aspirin, and clopidogrel are recommended in patients with STEMI who have undergone primary PCI, for up to 12 months.
- Clopidogrel is recommended for 1 month in patients treated with fibrinolysis without PCI (expanding the duration of DAPT up to 12 months should be considered in these patients). DAPT is recommended for 12 months for patients undergoing fibrinolysis and PCI.
- Aspirin is recommended indefinitely in all patients with STEMI.

Resumption of activity post-STEMI

- *Decisions should be individualised, based on:*
  - LV function
  - Completeness of revascularisation and rhythm control
  - The job characteristics.
- Extended sick leave is usually not beneficial.
- Light-to-moderate physical activity after discharge should be encouraged.
- Sexual activity can be resumed early according to physical ability.

Air travel

- There is limited evidence on air travel post-STEMI.
- The following factors should be considered:
    - Clinical circumstances
    - The length of travel
    - Degree of anxiety associated with travel.
    - For uncomplicated completely revascularised MI with left ventricular ejection fraction (LVEF) >40%, the risk is low, and travelling is regarded as safe after hospital discharge (from day 3 onwards).
    - In complicated STEMI, including patients with heart failure, LVEF <40%, residual ischaemia, and arrhythmia, travelling should be deferred until the condition is stable.

Blood pressure control

Blood pressure should be well-controlled. In addition to lifestyle changes, including reduced salt intake, increased physical activity, and weight loss, pharmacotherapy with a SBP target of <140 mmHg should be initiated.

Diet, alcohol and weight control

Current guidelines on prevention post-STEMI recommend:

- A diet similar to the Mediterranean diet, which includes a maximum of 10% of total energy intake from saturated fat, by replacing it with polyunsaturated fatty acids and as little as possible of trans fatty acids.
- Salt intake of <5 g/day
- 30–45 g fibre per day
- 200 g fruits and 200 g vegetables per day
- Fish 1–2 times per week (especially oily varieties)
- 30 g unsalted nuts daily
- Limited alcohol intake [maximum of 2 glasses (20 g of alcohol) daily for men and 1 for women]. Moderate alcohol consumption in abstainers is not recommended.
- Discourage sugar-sweetened drinks.
- Overweight and obesity should be managed.

Blood sugar management

Blood sugar should be controlled post-STEMI. Hypoglycaemia must be avoided particularly in the first few months post-STEMI.

Further reading

Ibanez B, James S, Agewall S, et al. The Task Force for the management of acute myocardial infarction in patients presenting with ST-segment elevation of the European Society of Cardiology (ESC). 2017 ESC Guidelines for the management of acute myocardial infarction in patients presenting with ST-segment elevation: Eur Heart J 2018; 39:119–1 77.

Scenario no. 10

Type of scenario: Ethical dilemma

Candidate information

Your role:	You are the infectious disease registrar on call.
Problem:	Counselling after needle stick injury.
Patient:	Dr Johnson, a 27-year-old junior doctor.

Please read the scenario printed below. When the bell sounds, enter the room. You have (---) minutes for your consultation with the patient/relative, (---) minutes to collect your thoughts, and (---) minutes for discussion.

Please do not examine the patient
Please do not take a history

> Dr Johnson is a 27-year-old doctor working as an emergency room resident. She saw a patient in the emergency department who was admitted with gastroenteritis and dehydration and had recently been diagnosed with HIV infection. While taking blood for laboratory testing, Dr Johnson got a needle stick injury. She is concerned about her risk of infection with HIV.
>
> **Your task:** Is to answer Dr Johnson's concerns, and explain to her the next steps to manage the situation.

Approach

Always read the scenario carefully and make sure you understand the instructions before you start. All the information provided is important and relevant. Make notes and a framework for your discussion. Sometimes, a hidden agenda is incorporated; pay attention to that.

Introduction and identification

- **Prepare the environment**
  Sit at the same level as the patient with comfort and avoid barriers like tables.

- **Introduce yourself to the patient**
  Shake hands.
  Hello Dr Johnson, I am Dr X, the infectious disease registrar on call.
  Can I confirm that I am talking to Dr Johnson?

- **Enquire from the patient if she would like someone else to be present during the discussion**
  Would you like to invite anybody else to this discussion?

- **Confirm the objectives of the interview**
  Dr Johnson, we are here to discuss the incident in the emergency department, is that alright?

Check patient's understanding and expectation

Could you kindly tell me about the incident?

Discussion with the patient

- **Important questions to ask in case of needle stick injury**
    - Where was the site of injury?
    - Which needle were you using?
    - Was it used for intramuscular or intravenous injection?
    - Was the injury superficial or deep?
    - Did you notice blood coming from the site of the injury?
    - What did you do when you got the needle stick injury?
    - Did you wash the injured site with free-flowing water? Did you allow the blood to come out freely? (If yes, tell her that she did the right thing and the chances of getting infection become very low. The average transmission after needle stick injury is 0.3% and if you did the right steps after needle stick injury, the chances become even lower).

- **Explore the idea about the source patient status**
    - Does the patient have established HIV, hepatitis B or hepatitis C?

- **Explore the idea about the injured status?**
    - Do you (Dr Johnson) have any diseases like HIV, hepatitis B or C?
    - Did you have vaccination for hepatitis B?
    - If yes, when did you have it? Do you know what your anti-HBsAg titre level is?
    - Have you had a booster dose?
    - Have you had a screening test before? If yes, when was it done? What was the result?

- **Discuss further management**
    - *Perform initial screening tests for the injured*
      If you have not had any screening, then we should do an initial screen now to establish that you do not already have any infections.
          If she refuses to do so, inform her that if immediate screening tests are not done and she is later found to be positive for HIV, hepatitis B or C, she may not opt for compensation. We will repeat the test after 3 months and 6 months. If after 6 months, the tests are negative, then the chances of acquiring HIV are negligible.
    - *Counsel the source patient for undertaking blood tests*
      Counsel the source patient (HIV patient) regarding testing for blood-borne infections such as hepatitis B and C, and their HIV status.
    - *Discuss prophylaxis*
      Dr Johnson, we will give you some prophylactic medications against HIV for 4 weeks to decrease the chances of transmission of HIV. But before doing so, may I ask if you are pregnant? This is because some of the medications are contraindicated during pregnancy and we can give you alternative medication.
    - *Advice regarding sexual activity and blood transfusion*
      Dr Johnson, you should avoid sex until your test results come negative. (If that is not possible, then offer advice regarding safe sex practices such as using barrier methods/male condoms, to avoid transmission to sexual partner).
      Another important issue is to avoid giving blood for the time being.
- **Check patient understanding**
  Does that sound clear to you?

Explore and respond to patient's concerns

Do you have any questions or concerns?

- **Am I allowed to carry on working?**
  You do not need to stop working unless you are found to have HIV. You will be followed up by the occupational health department and hospital staff clinic and they will provide you with further advice once the test result is ready.

- **I missed my menstrual period. What if I am pregnant?**
  Regarding the HIV prophylactic medications, see below in the discussion.

- **Will I get AIDS if my HIV test comes back positive?**
  Not all HIV-positive patients get acquired immunodeficiency syndrome (AIDS). This means that only those HIV-positive patients whose immune systems become weak will develop AIDS.
  Furthermore, the treatment of HIV infection allows people to live normal active lives with HIV.

Show empathy

Dr Johnson, I understand your worries and concerns. We are here to help.

Summarise and confirm understanding

Dr Johnson, I would like to briefly summarise our discussion, as it is important for me to be sure that you understand important information about you needle stick injury. You got a needle stick injury from an HIV-positive patient. I will request some initial screening tests to confirm that you do not already have HIV and I will give you some medications for 4 weeks that will help prevent the transmission of HIV.

I suggest that you inform your husband/sexual partner and practice safe sex until we establish that you are HIV-negative. Please avoid any blood donation during this period.

You will be followed up by occupation health and the hospital staff clinic regularly.

Your tests will be repeated at 3 months and 6 months.

Is everything clear so far?

Please let me know if you want to discuss anything else at this moment.

Offer help and follow-up

I will call the occupational health department on their emergency number to see if they have any further advice and will arrange an appointment with them in 24 hours.

This is my telephone number. Please do not hesitate to contact me should you have any further questions.

I will arrange another appointment in 2 weeks.

I will also provide you with some website addresses and printed material to read more about needle injuries.

Discussion

Ethical principles

- **What are the main ethical principles in this scenario?**
  Patient's autonomy: The patient has the right to know about the management of her current health issue. The doctor should provide the patient with the necessary information to help her make her decision. The doctor should be honest and truthful in discussing the risks and advice regarding treatment. The patient has the right to refuse or accept the advice or other therapy.

Beneficence: In this scenario, performing a screening test for HIV, hepatitis B and C is in the best interest of the patient for future consideration of compensation. Giving 4 weeks of prophylactic HIV medications will reduce the chances of transmission of HIV.

Non-maleficence: Harmful interventions should be avoided. In this scenario, there are some prophylactic medications that could be harmful during pregnancy.

Justice: The scenario involves justice to the patient by providing all necessary management without discrimination and justice to the community by preventing her husband/sexual partner from acquiring the infection in case she tests positive for HIV.

Hidden agenda in this scenario

- Plan of management and relieving anxiety
- Confidentiality
- Job issue
- Practicing safe sex
- HIV prophylaxis in pregnancy.

HIV transmission

- *Blood transfusion:* 90%
- *Needle stick (percutaneous; through the skin):* 0.3%
- *Sexual activity:* 0.3%
- *Vertical transmission:* 15–45%.

Risk of hepatitis B transmission

- *Transfusion:* 52–69% transmission if transfused with HBsAg (+) blood.
- Needle stick
- *HBeAg (+):* 37–62%
- *HBeAg (–):* 23–37%
- *Heterosexual exposures:* 18–44.2%
- Vertical transmission up to 30%.

Hepatitis C transmission

- Needle stick 0–10%
- *Heterosexual exposure:* 2–6%
- *Vertical transmission:* 5%.

Management of postoccupational exposure

- Irrigate the area with a large amount of saline or clean water.
- Determine the HIV, HBV, and HCV status of the source patient.
- Enquire about Hepatitis B, C, and HIV status of the healthcare worker.
- Assess the need for providing prophylaxis based on medical history. The goal is to initiate post-exposure prophylaxis within 1 to 2 hours of exposure; data from animal studies suggest decreased efficacy with delayed initiation. Postexposure prophylaxis is typically not recommended after a delay of more than 72 hours.
    - *For HBV prophylaxis:*
        - Previously vaccinated with known response to vaccine: No therapy required.
        - Previously vaccinated without known response to vaccine: Send anti-HepBs titre; administer prophylaxis (one dose of HBIG); booster is required.
        - Unvaccinated: Provide one dose of HBIG and initiate vaccination series.
    - *For HIV prophylaxis:*
        - Tenofovir plus emtricitabine plus either raltegravir or dolutegravir (all for 28 days). (Zidovudine is no longer recommended)
        - For pregnant women:
            - Dolutegravir should be avoided in pregnancy
            - Use tenofovir plus emtricitabine plus raltegravir.
    - Postexposure prophylaxis for hepatitis C is not established yet.

- Follow-up with occupational health or infectious disease in 24–72 hours
- Discuss need for safe sex practices until follow-up laboratory testing is negative for HIV
- Repeat blood tests at 3 and 6 months
- Always report such exposures
- Educate the healthcare worker.

Further reading

Guidelines for the Emergency Management of Injuries and Post-exposure Prophylaxis (PEP). Hepatitis B virus: epidemiology and transmission risks. [online] Available from http://www.hpsc.ie/a-z/EMIToolkit/appendices/app21.pdf. [Last accessed October, 2019].

Kuhar DT, Henderson DK, Struble KA, et al. Updated US Public Health Service guidelines for the management of occupational exposures to human immunodeficiency virus and recommendations for post exposure prophylaxis. Infect Control Hosp Epidemiol 2013; 34:875–892.

Stobart-Gallagher MA. Needle-stick guideline treatment & management. (2017). [online] Available from https://emedicine.medscape.com/article/784812-treatment [Last accessed October, 2019].

Zehnder NG. What should I do if I get a needle stick? The Hospitalist 2010; 2010.

Scenario no. 11

Type of scenario: Ethical dilemma/consent for investigation

Candidate information

Your role: You are the doctor in the medical outpatient clinic.
Problem: Taking consent for investigation.
Patient: Mr Akash, a 40-year-old gentleman.

Please read the scenario printed below. When the bell sounds, enter the room. You have (---) minutes for your consultation with the patient/relative, (---) minutes to collect your thoughts, and (---) minutes for discussion.

Please do not examine the patient
Please do not take a history

> Mr Akash is a 40-year-old gentleman with a past history of intravenous drug abuse. Recently, he was complaining of difficulty in swallowing and was found to have oesophageal candidiasis. Your consultant is considering doing HIV testing on him.
>
> **Your task:** Is to help him understand about HIV testing and answer any question or concern he may have about his management.

Approach

Always read the scenario carefully and make sure you understand the instructions before you start. All information provided is important. Make notes and a framework of your discussion. Sometimes, a hidden agenda is incorporated; pay attention to that.

Introduction and identification

- **Prepare the environment**
  Sit at the same level as the patient with comfort and avoid barriers like tables.

- **Introduce yourself to the patient**
  Shake hands.
  Hello Mr Akash, I am Dr X, working in the medical outpatient clinic.

- **Enquire from the patient if he would like someone else to be present during the discussion**
  Can I confirm that I am talking to Mr Akash?
  Would you like to invite anybody else to this discussion?

- **Confirm the objective of the interview**
  We are here today to discuss the need to perform some important investigations for you. Is that alright?

Check patient's understanding and expectation

Tell me Mr Akash, how much do you know about your health status?
What do you suspect might be wrong with your swallowing?
Has anyone discussed with you regarding the need for further investigations?

Discussion with the patient (information giving)

- **Give the patient the information (avoid medical jargon)**
  As you know Mr Akash, you came initially with swallowing difficulty and we found that you had a fungal infection of your food pipe. You told us that you were self-injecting drugs in your veins which you stopped 2 months ago.
  If you allow me, I want to ask some private questions. Is that alright?
  - Did you share needles with your friends when you were injecting drugs?
  - Do you know if any of these friends have HIV, hepatitis B or C?
  - Are you married or do you have a sexual partner?
  - How many sexual partners do you have (if yes, does any of them have HIV?).
  - Have you received a blood transfusion or had an accident before?

Mr Akash, fungal infection of the food pipe is rare. When it happens in a young person like you, we should make sure that the person does not have low immunity. HIV can cause low immunity and given your history of drug abuse, we need to make sure you do not have HIV.

- **Explore the patient's ideas about HIV infection**
  Have you heard of HIV infection before? Pause....

- **Explain to the patient in simple terms about HIV (avoid medical jargon)**
  The human immunodeficiency virus is a virus that attacks the infection-fighting system of the body. This virus destroys the immune system which becomes so weak that it cannot fight infection and certain illnesses appear like certain pneumonias and fungal infection of the food pipe, etc. Once these illnesses appear it is called "acquired immunodeficiency syndrome" (AIDS).
  Early diagnosis of HIV is important as it allows earlier treatment and better long-term health and infection-free life. Therefore, performing HIV testing now is very important for your future health. If the test is negative, then we will just treat your food pipe infection. If it is positive, then along with treatment of your food pipe infection, we also need to start HIV treatment which will help you live a normal life. Does that make sense to you?
  Your HIV test result will be kept confidential and will be discussed only with you.

- **Pause and ask the patient if everything is clear so far**

- **Explain how a HIV test is done**
  For HIV testing, we just need a small amount of your blood and the test will take a maximum of 2 days. Once the result is ready, I will call you to come to the hospital to discuss the result and any further management plan. Is that alright?

- **Further advice until the HIV result**
  Mr Akash, there are important points that I need to mention here while waiting for HIV test. HIV is found in semen, blood, vaginal and anal fluids, and breast milk. Therefore, please avoid sex until we have the result of HIV (If not possible, then at least practice safe sex for the time being by using barrier methods especially male condoms, to avoid transmission of the infection to your sexual partner). Please avoid donating blood for the time being. Is that alright?

- **Check patient understanding**

Explore and respond to patient's concerns

Do you have any questions or concerns?

- **Can HIV be treated?**
  Yes, treatment is available. However, the treatment has to be taken lifelong to keep the virus inactive and stop it from destroying the immune system.

- **I do not want to tell my wife/sexual partner if the test comes back positive**
  - Enquire about the reasons
  - Discuss the risk to others in case the test is positive
  - Suggest to the patient to invite his sexual partner/wife to a meeting with you to discuss the issue
  - Encourage use of protective measures (safe sex practice).

- **What about my health insurance if I decide to go for HIV testing?**
  Your previous health insurance policies will be considered. You can discuss future insurance policies with the insurance company.

Show empathy

I understand Mr Akash your worries and concerns. We are here to help you.

Summarise and confirm understanding

Mr Akash, I would like to briefly summarise our discussion, as it is important for me to be sure that you understand important information about your current health status. You had difficulty with your swallowing and you were found to have a fungal infection of your food pipe. Based on your previous history of self-injecting drugs and your presentation, we decided to test you for HIV as early identification and treatment helps to stop or reduce the activity of the virus and prevents destruction of the immune system. You have to avoid sex and blood donation until the results are out.
    Is this clear so far?
    Please let me know if you want to discuss anything more at this moment.

Offer help and follow-up and close the discussion

This is my telephone number. Please do not hesitate to call me should you have any further questions.
    I will arrange another meeting in 3 days in case you have any questions or concern and to give you your HIV result.
    I will also provide you with some website addresses and printed material to read more about your condition.

Discussion

Ethical principles

* **What are the main ethical principles in this scenario?**

  Patient's autonomy: The patient has the right to know about the management of his current health issue (swallowing problem and the potential reasons underlying it). The doctor should provide the patient with the necessary information to help him make his decision regarding HIV testing. The doctor should be honest and truthful in discussing the risks and advice regarding further management. The patient has the right to refuse or accept HIV testing.

  Beneficence and non-maleficence: In this scenario, performing a screening test for HIV is in the best interest of the patient, as early diagnosis and early treatment of HIV will help him live a normal life. Not offering HIV testing will result in treatment delay and put him at risk of serious infections.

  Justice: The scenario involves justice to the patient by providing all the necessary management without discrimination and providing further investigation urgently. It also involves justice to the community by preventing his wife and other sexual contacts from acquiring the infection.

  The patient should be advised to inform his sexual partners and his GP if the test comes back positive. If the patient refuses to disclose his HIV status and is practicing unsafe sex or sharing needles, then the doctor can justify breaching confidentiality and disclosure in the public interest (if failure to disclose may expose others to risk of death or serious harm). The doctor should inform the patient that such action will be taken if it is safe to do so.

Hidden agenda

* Plan of management and relieving anxiety
* Taking consent for HIV testing
* Confidentiality
* Practicing safe sex
* Considering the risks to others if the test is positive.

HIV transmission

* *Blood transfusion:* 90%
* *Needle stick (percutaneous; through the skin):* 0.3%
* *Sexual activity:* 0.3%
* *Vertical transmission:* 15–45%.

HIV/AIDS defining illnesses

Certain diseases and conditions occur in HIV-positive patient and are called AIDS defining illnesses and the person is labelled as having AIDS.

Certain AIDS defining illnesses based on CDC are:

* Candidiasis of bronchi, trachea, or lungs
* Candidiasis, oesophageal (thrush)
* *Mycobacterium avium* complex or *M. kansasii*, disseminated or extrapulmonary
* *Mycobacterium tuberculosis*, any site (pulmonary or extrapulmonary)
* *Mycobacterium*, other species or unidentified species, disseminated or extrapulmonary
* *Pneumocystis* pneumonia
* Recurrent pneumonia
* *Herpes simplex:* Chronic ulcer(s) (greater than 1 month's duration); or bronchitis, pneumonitis, or oesophagitis
* Histoplasmosis, disseminated or extrapulmonary
* Coccidioidomycosis, disseminated or extrapulmonary

- Cryptococcosis, extrapulmonary
- Invasive cervical cancer
- Chronic intestinal cryptosporidiosis (greater than 1 month's duration)
- Cytomegalovirus disease (other than liver, spleen, or nodes)
- Cytomegalovirus retinitis (with loss of vision)
- HIV-related encephalopathy
- Kaposi's sarcoma
- Burkitt's lymphoma
- Primary CNS lymphoma
- Progressive multifocal leucoencephalopathy
- Recurrent *Salmonella* septicaemia
- Toxoplasmosis of brain
- Wasting syndrome due to HIV.

Management of oesophageal candidiasis

- Fluconazole 200–400 mg/day for 14–21 days
- If refractory to a 1-week course of fluconazole, then voriconazole/posaconazole
- *If IV therapy is needed:* Use echinocandins such as caspofungin.

Classes of HAART therapy

- Nucleoside reverse transcriptase inhibitors
- Non-nucleoside reverse transcriptase inhibitors
- Protease inhibitors
- Integrase inhibitors
- Fusion inhibitors
- Chemokine receptor antagonists
- Entry inhibitors (CD4-directed post-attachment inhibitors).

Further reading

Centres for Diseases Control and Prevention (CDC). HIV/AIDS. [online] Available from https://www.cdc.gov/hiv/ [Last accessed October, 2019].

Centres for Diseases Control and Prevention (CDC). HIV Basics. [online] Available from https://www.hiv.gov/authors/cdc-s-hiv-basics [Last accessed October, 2019].

National Institute for Health and Clinical Excellence (NICE)-UK. HIV and AIDS. [online] Available from https://www.nice.org.uk/guidance/conditions-and-diseases/infections/hiv-and-aids#panel-pathways [Last accessed October, 2019].

Pappas PG, Kauffman CA, Andes DR, et al. Clinical practice guideline for the management of candidiasis: 2016 update by the Infectious Diseases Society of America. Clin Infect Dis. 2016; 62:e1–e50.

Scenario no. 12

Type of scenario: Breaking bad news

Candidate information

Your role:	You are the medical registrar in oncology.
Problem:	Breaking bad news about the death of your patient to his sister.
Patient:	Mr Yasir, a 49-year-old man.
Relative:	Miss Ayesha (The sister of Mr Yasir)

Please read the scenario printed below. When the bell sounds, enter the room. You have
(---) minutes for your consultation with the patient/relative, (---) minutes to collect your
thoughts, and (---) minutes for discussion.

Please do not examine the patient
Please do not take a history

> Mr Yasir is a 49-year-old man who was admitted to the oncology ward for severe
> breathlessness. He is known to have advanced lymphoma which has been deemed
> non-responsive to chemotherapy and radiotherapy. Over the last 6 months, he has had
> frequent admissions to the hospital because of multiple infections. The chest radiograph
> showed multiple lung nodules consistent with metastasis. His general condition on
> admission was very poor with marked weight loss and breathlessness. Despite O_2
> and other supportive therapies, his condition deteriorated rapidly, and he died in the
> oncology ward. His sister is waiting outside and is very upset and anxious.
>
> **Your task:** Is to inform his sister (Miss Ayesha) about the death of her brother (Mr Yasir)
> and address any concerns she may have.

Approach

Always read the scenario carefully and make sure you understand the instructions before
you start. All information provided is important. Make notes and a framework for your
discussion. Sometimes, a hidden agenda is incorporated; pay attention to that.

Introduction and identification

- **Prepare the environment**
  Sit at the same level as the relative with comfort and avoid barriers like tables.

- **Introduce yourself to the relative**
  Shake hands.
  Hello Miss Ayesha, I am Dr X, working in the oncology ward.

- **Enquire from the relative if they would like someone else to be present during
  discussion**
  Can I confirm that I am talking to Miss Ayesha?
  Would you like to invite anybody else to this discussion?

- **Confirm the objective of the interview**
  We are here today to discuss Mr Yasir's condition. Is that alright?

Check relative's understanding and expectation

Tell me Miss Ayesha, how much do you know about Mr Yasir's illness?

Discussion with the relative (information giving)

- **Give the relative the information (avoid medical jargon)**
  As you know Miss Ayesha, Mr Yasir had advanced cancer of the blood. Unfortunately,
  his cancer was very aggressive and despite multiple treatments, it had spread to
  other parts of his body. He also developed complications because of cancer that had
  resulted in multiple admissions to the hospital over the last 6 months. I am sorry to
  inform you that when he was admitted today, he was gravely ill and despite our best
  efforts, his heart stopped and he passed away peacefully, pause...

- **Pause and give her time to express her emotions**
  She will not be able to take more information right now. It will be wise to give her some time to express her emotions and ask questions. At the same time, show empathy to her emotions and offer tissue paper. Wait and let her absorb the grief.
      Doctor, why did you not resuscitate my brother when his heart stopped, he was young?
      Miss Ayesha, we discussed this with your brother, and he had made an advanced directive stating that he did not want to be resuscitated in such a situation. Also given his diagnosis of advanced cancer that was not responding to treatment, I would support his wish for no resuscitation as it would only have prolonged his suffering.

- **Gently explain what steps were taken to alleviate his pain and suffering**
  I am really very sorry to give you such bad news, but I can assure you that we made every effort to minimise his pain and suffering before he passed away.

- **Avoid discussing about what could have been better**
  At this point, it is of no use to discuss that advanced planning such as DNR could have been better.

- **Pause and ask the relative if everything is clear so far**

- **Provide information on the support available to the relatives**
  Miss Ayesha, I understand this must be a huge shock and very painful for you and you may not be aware of burial arrangements. The bereavement office in this hospital and our nursing staff can help you in this regard.
  - This is a map to guide you to where the bereavement office is located
  - The staff there will help you to complete the paper work
  - If you agree, we will invite someone from the spiritual department to talk with you
  - Our nurses and mortuary staff will help you to see your brother
  - I will also leave my contact number if you need any further help.
- **Check her understanding.**
  Is everything clear?

Explore and respond to the relative's concerns

Do you have any further questions or concerns?
- **Why did his cancer not respond to treatment?**
  Although lymphoma is usually a treatable cancer, there are certain types of lymphoma that are very aggressive and do not respond to the treatments that have been developed so far. Unfortunately, Mr Yasir had one of these aggressive lymphomas.

Show empathy

I understand this is a very difficult time for you.

Summarise and confirm understanding

Miss Ayesha, once again I am very sorry to be the one to inform you about the tragic death of your brother.
Do you have any question or concern at this moment?

Offer help and close the discussion

This is my office telephone number in case you have any more questions.
Would you like us to arrange a taxi for you?

Discussion
Ethical principles
- **What are the main ethical principles in this scenario?**
  Autonomy: It is the right of the relatives/next of kin to know the exact circumstances of death and the condition that has led to it.

  Beneficence and non-maleficence: A decision of not to resuscitate is in the best interest of the patient. The patient had a terminal illness. His cancer did not respond to the best available treatment options. Resuscitating him might just prolong his suffering. Every effort should be made to decrease the suffering of the patient.

  Justice: Mr Yasir had received the best available treatments for lymphoma but did not respond. All efforts were made to minimise his pain and suffering.

Hidden agenda (any one possible)
- Breaking bad news (death of family member)
- Explaining circumstances of death
- DNAR decision by the doctor.

DNAR decision by doctor
- **Indications of DNAR**
  - Advance directives (patient will not be resuscitated)
  - Medical futility (such as brain death, advanced cancer, etc.)
  - Patient is likely to be left with a poor quality of life if resuscitated (such as bedridden and demented patients).

- **Important issues regarding DNAR**
  - DNAR does not mean do not care. DNAR order does not affect other treatments received by the patient.
  - DNAR orders should be reviewed regularly particularly if the patient's condition changes or the patient's views change.
  - If the patient has no capacity to make the decision themselves about whether they wish to receive resuscitation, a DNAR decision can be made in the patient's best interests.

- **Which type of deaths should be reported to the coroner in the United Kingdom?**
  The following categories of death should be reported:
  - Death that is sudden
  - Death due to suicide
  - Death due to violence
  - Death from medical interventions or procedures
  - If someone is found dead when they reach hospital
  - Death in prison or after admission from prison
  - Death when the cause cannot be certified by a doctor.

Lymphoma

The WHO 2016 classification of tumours of hematopoietic and lymphoid tissue:
- **Myeloid neoplasms:**
  Tumours from bone marrow progenitor cells:
  - Erythrocyte
  - Granulocyte
  - Monocyte
  - Megakaryocyte.

- **Lymphoid neoplasms:**
  - B cell tumours
  - T cells tumours.

- **Histiocytic/dendritic neoplasms:**
  Tumour from macrophage (histiocytes) and antigen-presenting cells (dendritic cells).

WHO 2016 classification of mature lymphoid, histiocytic, and dendritic neoplasms:

- Mature B cell neoplasms
- Mature T cell and NK neoplasms
- Hodgkin lymphoma:
  - Nodular lymphocyte predominant Hodgkin lymphoma
  - Classical Hodgkin lymphoma:
    - Nodular sclerosis classical Hodgkin lymphoma
    - Lymphocyte-rich classical Hodgkin lymphoma
    - Mixed cellularity classical Hodgkin lymphoma
    - Lymphocyte-depleted classical Hodgkin lymphoma.

- Post-transplant lymphoproliferative disorders (PTLD)

- Histiocytic and dendritic cell neoplasms

- *Non-Hodgkin lymphoma:* Mature B and mature T cell neoplasm come under non-Hodgkin lymphoma. Subtypes of non-Hodgkin lymphoma have different characteristics and treatment:
  - Follicular lymphoma
  - Mantle cell lymphoma
  - Diffuse large B cell lymphoma
  - Primary cutaneous lymphoma
  - Gastric marginal zone lymphoma of the mucosa-associated lymphatic tissue (MALT).

Diagnosis:

- Peripheral smear
- Tissue biopsy is needed for optimal diagnosis (excisional).
- Core needle biopsy is an alternative in certain circumstances.
- Fine needle aspiration (FNA) is not adequate for the initial diagnosis.
- Bone marrow in certain circumstances.

Staging:

A PET-scan is the gold standard for fluorodeoxyglucose (FDG)-avid lymphoma. Cotswold's-modified Ann Arbor classification:

- *Stage I:* One nodal group or lymphoid organ (e.g. spleen).
- *Stage II:* Two or more nodal groups, same side of diaphragm.
- *Stage III:* Nodal groups on both sides of the diaphragm.
- *Stage IV:* Disseminated involvement of one or more extra lymphatic organ (e.g. lung, bone) +/– any nodal involvement.
- *Stage 1 and stage 2 are limited disease.*
- *Stage 3 and stage 4 are advanced disease.*

Additional staging variables:

- **A:** Asymptomatic
- **B:** B symptoms (fever, 10% weight loss, and drenching night sweat)
- **E:** Extra nodal extension or single, isolated site of extra nodal disease
- **X:** Bulky nodal disease; greater than 10 cm in diameter.

Treatment:
There are different treatments for the different stages and types of lymphoma:

- Chemotherapy
- Radiotherapy
- Immunotherapy
- Stem cell transplant
- Surgery in selected cases.

Some of the common chemotherapy regimens are:

- *R-CHOP-21*: Rituximab plus cyclophosphamide, doxorubicin, vincristine, and prednisone with 21 days between cycles *(non-Hodgkin lymphoma)*.
- *CHOP-21*: Cyclophosphamide, doxorubicin, vincristine, and prednisone *(non-Hodgkin lymphoma)*.
- *ABVD*: Doxorubicin plus bleomycin, vinblastine, and dacarbazine *(Hodgkin lymphoma)*.

Further reading

Canellos GP, Anderson JR, Propert KJ, et al. Chemotherapy of advanced Hodgkin's disease with MOPP, ABVD, or MOPP alternating with ABVD. N Engl J Med 1992; 327: 1478–1484.

Coiffier B, Lepage E, Briere J, et al. CHOP chemotherapy plus rituximab compared with CHOP alone in elderly patients with diffuse large-B-cell lymphoma. N Engl J Med 2002; 346:235–242.

General Medical Council (GMC)-UK. Cardiopulmonary resuscitation (CPR). [online] Available from https://www.gmc-uk.org/ethical-guidance/ethical-guidance-for-doctors/treatment-and-care-towards-the-end-of-life/cardiopulmonary-resuscitation-cpr [Last accessed October, 2019].

Gov.UK. When a death is reported to a coroner? [online] Available from https://www.gov.uk/after-a-death/when-a-death-is-reported-to-a-coroner [Last accessed October, 2019].

Swerdlow S, Campo E, Pileri S, et al. The 2016 revision of the World Health Organization classification of lymphoid neoplasms. Blood 2016; 127:2375–2390.

Varney M. A guide for patients and families to Do Not Resuscitate (DNR) decisions. Leigh Day. [online] Available from https://www.leighday.co.uk/LeighDay/media/LeighDay/documents/Guides/DNR-leaflet_final.pdf [Last accessed: October, 2019].

Scenario no. 13

Type of scenario: Discussing unprofessional behaviour with a colleague

Candidate information

Your role: You are the registrar of the medical team.
Problem: Discussing unprofessional attitude with a junior colleague.
Patient: Dr Ahmad, a 30-year-old man.

Please read the scenario printed below. When the bell sounds, enter the room. You have (---) minutes for your consultation with the patient/relative, (---) minutes to collect your thoughts, and (---) minutes for discussion.

Please do not examine the patient
Please do not take a history

You are working as the registrar in the medical ward. Dr Ahmad started his rotation in your team as a senior resident. You have received multiple complaints from nurses and junior colleagues that he has been rude with them. Doctors from the emergency department have also commented that he is not responding to their bleeps, is very rude to them, and does not accept referrals easily. He frequently arrives late to the ward rounds and disappears after the round finishes.

Your task: Is to discuss this issue with Dr Ahmad and answer any question or concern he may have.

Approach

Always read the scenario carefully and make sure you understand the instructions before you start. All information provided is important. Make notes and a framework for your discussion. Sometimes, a hidden agenda is incorporated; pay attention to that.

Introduction and identification

- **Prepare the environment**
  Sit at the same level as the colleague with comfort and avoid barriers like tables.

- **Introduce yourself to the colleague (if no prior relation)**
  Shake hands.
  Hello Dr Ahmad, I am doctor X, the medical registrar on the medical ward.

- **Confirming identification (If no prior relation)**
  Can I confirm that I am talking to Dr Ahmad?

- **Confirm the objective of the interview**
  We are here Dr Ahmad to discuss some work-related issues. Is that alright?
  (Make sure you discuss with Dr Ahmad in a private room and in a non-stress environment).

Check Dr Ahmad's understanding and expectation

Tell me Dr Ahmad how do you feel your work in this hospital is going?
Have you faced any difficulties or problems and want to discuss them?

Discussion with Dr Ahmad (information giving)

- **Emphasise that you are here to help him**
  Dr Ahmad, from time to time, we meet with other colleagues to discuss issues related to work and see if they have encountered any problems.

- **Explain the problems and explore Dr Ahmad's ideas/reasons for his behaviour (be frank and honest)**
  Unfortunately, I have received several complaints from your colleagues that you are coming late to the hospital and going home early as well as leaving many jobs for the on-call team in the evening. Some of the nurses and junior doctors have also complained that you are treating them harshly and recently colleagues from the emergency room have informed me that you do not readily accept referrals and keep arguing with them about straight forward medical cases. I want to hear your views regarding these concerns. Are you facing any problems and need help from our side? *(It would be unfair not to listen to his side of the story. He may have his own reasons for his behaviour. It is important to try to find out what issues may underlie his actions and whether he has considered asking for help from his senior colleagues).*

- **Explain the consequences of his behaviour on patient safety and on the doctor himself**

  Dr Ahmad, patients who come to the hospital are suffering and many of them are in pain and are distressed. Our colleagues from the emergency room are doing their best to help these patients. As physicians, we are obliged to help relieve the patient's suffering without delay. This can only be accomplished through team work. We all need to get along with each other and to help each other. In addition, some of our junior colleagues have less practical knowledge and experience. We have to help and teach them rather than get angry at them. Coming and leaving on time in our profession is very important to prevent any delay in our patient's management and shows respect to other colleagues. Arriving late to the hospital and leaving early with pending issues for the incoming doctor can delay patient care and put their safety at risk and place extra burden on our colleagues. Furthermore, the lack of a prompt response to consultations from other specialties, particularly when we are on call, can adversely affect outcomes for our patients.

  I think you would agree with me, therefore, that such behaviour is unacceptable and continuing this way may affect your career progression and if repeated, may be reported to HR and the GMC (or regulatory body) as unprofessional behaviour.

- **Offer solutions**

  Dr Ahmad, if you feel that you are facing some problems and you need help, we are here to help you.
  - Have you attended any communication skill or professionalism courses? The hospital is very supportive and offers free communication skill and professionalism courses and workshops for junior physicians. If you have not attended any such courses, I strongly recommend that you do.
  - Meanwhile, I will meet you on a daily basis before finishing your duty to discuss the cases that have been referred to you and go over their management.

Explore and respond to the colleague's concerns

Do you have any questions or concerns to discuss?

- **Will this discussion be documented in my file? Is there any disciplinary action to be taken against me?**

  Today, I am only here to make you aware of these concerns so that you can address them. However, if this behaviour continues, then things will be escalated to higher management and potentially the general medical council as this behaviour is outwith the professional values and behaviour expected of a doctor *(as stated in the 2014 good medical practice guidance issued by the GMC-UK).*

Summarise and confirm understanding

Dr Ahmad, I would like to summarise our discussion, as it is important for me to be sure that you understand the information discussed in this meeting. Please make sure that you come and leave the hospital on time, take care of all your patients in a timely manner, and treat your colleagues and other healthcare staff in a respectful manner. I will see you on a daily basis to discuss different cases and work-related issues. I suggest that you attend some communication skill and professionalism courses.

Offer help and follow-up and close the discussion

Dr Ahmad, being your senior colleague, it is always our aim that you progress in your clinical knowledge and career.

You have my telephone number. Please call me any time in case you need help or you have any further questions.

Discussion

Ethical principles

- **What are the main ethical principles in this scenario?**
  Autonomy: It is the right of the junior doctor to express his views regarding the concerns. All the concerns should be raised and explained to the doctor in a frank and honest way.

  Beneficence and non-maleficence: Counselling Dr Ahmad is in the best interest of patient safety and to ensure professional behaviour with colleagues. Continuing such behaviour is harmful to him, patients, and colleagues.

  Justice: It should include justice to colleagues, patients, and other healthcare staff. Dr Ahmad should be counselled to help him identify unacceptable and unprofessional behaviour if he is to continue to practice as a doctor. Correcting his behaviour will be to the benefit of his patients and colleagues.

Hidden agenda (any one possible)

- Identifying hidden reason of non-professional behaviour and correct accordingly.
- Offer solutions such as daily supervision and participation in communication skill and professionalism courses.

- **Which types of problems in doctors need to be reported to the regulatory bodies?**
  Certain regulatory bodies such as the 'General Medical Council (GMC)' in the UK identify certain problems in doctors that need to be reported. These problems include:
  - Poor performance (incompetence)
  - Misconduct
  - Physical or mental health
  - Personality type and behavioural issues.

- **What action should be taken when a doctor with difficulty is identified?**
  - Early remedial action is needed if any behavioural issue is found in a colleague
  - Ensure patient safety
  - Discuss with the doctor in-person
  - Try to find the cause and address it. An investigator is appointed that can:
    - Conclude the case with no action
    - Issue a warning
    - Agree undertaking regular review
    - Refer the case to a fitness to practice panel or committee.

Further reading

General Medical Council (GMC)-UK. Guidance for decision makers on assessing the impact of health in misconduct, conviction, caution and performance cases. [online] Available from https://www.gmc-uk.org/-/media/documents/dc11461-health-and-conduct-guidance_pdf-75637116.pdf [Last accessed October, 2019].

Scenario no. 14

Type of scenario: To discuss live organ donation from an unrelated donor with a patient

Candidate information

Your role: You are the medical registrar in the nephrology unit.
Problem: Mr Mazin has end-stage renal disease (ESRD) requiring a renal transplant from his wife Mrs Ayesha.
Patient: Mr Mazin, a 45-year-old man.

Please read the scenario printed below. When the bell sounds, enter the room. You have (---) minutes for your consultation with the patient/relative, (---) minutes to collect your thoughts, and (---) minutes for discussion.

Please do not examine the patient
Please do not take a history

> Mr Mazin is a 45-year-old man who is suffering ESRD because of long-standing diabetes and hypertension. He is being considered for a renal transplant. His wife who is genetically unrelated wants to discuss with you the possibility of donating her kidney to Mr Mazin. She is 40 years old and has no chronic illnesses.
>
> **Your task:** Is to discuss with Mrs Ayesha about kidney transplantation.

Approach

Always read the scenario carefully and make sure you understand the instructions before you start. All information provided is important. Make notes and a framework for your discussion. Sometimes, a hidden agenda is incorporated; pay attention to that.

Introduction and identification

- **Prepare the environment**
  Sit at the same level as the relative with comfort and avoid barriers like tables.

- **Introduce yourself to the patient**
  Shake hands.
  Hello Mrs Ayesha, I am Dr X, working as a medical registrar in the nephrology unit.

- **Confirming identification**
  Can I confirm that I am talking to Mrs Ayesha?

- **Enquire from the patient if she would like anyone else to be present during the discussion**
  Would you like to invite anyone else to this discussion?
  (It would be better to have Mr Mazin present and involved in this discussion as he is central to the management plan).

- **Confirm the objective of the interview**
  Mrs Ayesha, we are here today to discuss about your offer to donate your kidney to your husband, Mr Mazin. Is that alright?

Check Mrs Ayesha's understanding and expectation

Tell me Mrs Ayesha, what do you know about your husband's health status?

Discussion with the relative (information giving)

- **Give the relative the information (avoid medical jargon)**
  As you know Mrs Ayesha, your husband's kidneys are seriously damaged due to long-standing diabetes and hypertension and they are no longer functioning. Kidneys are vital organs as they remove waste products and excess water from the body and retain important salts that help in regulating normal body function. Mr Mazin requires alternative ways to replace the function of his kidneys. The excess waste products and water can be removed by peritoneal or haemodialysis. Both require regular hospital attendance and are not ideal long-term solutions. Transplanting a kidney from another person to his body would be a better solution and Mr Mazin wants to be considered for this.

- **Explore the patient's ideas about kidney transplant**
  Have you ever heard of kidney transplantation before? Pause....

- **Explain to the patient in simple terms about kidney transplantation (avoid medical jargon).**
  I understand that you want to donate one of your kidneys to your husband? Is that correct?
  Are you a blood-relative of your husband?
  Do you suffer any kind of health problem/disease?
  Are you taking any kind of medications?
  Before kidney transplantation: Both of you need to undergo some blood testing to make sure that none of you have serious infections and your kidney matches with your husband's tissues. Matching is important as it predicts how well your kidney will survive in your husband's body after transplantation. For this, you will be referred to a transplant physician who will assess you and have further discussions with you.
  During kidney transplantation: You will also be referred to a transplant surgeon who will discuss possible complications of surgery both for you and your husband (like bleeding, infection, etc.).
  After kidney transplantation: Both of you will have to stay in the hospital after surgery for a short while. After transplantation, your husband will need lifelong medications that reduce his immunity in order to reduce the chance of his body rejecting your kidney. A frequent follow-up with the kidney transplant doctor is also important after kidney transplantation.

- **Pause and ask the relative if everything is clear so far**

- **Outcome of transplantation**
  After you have donated one kidney, you will only have one kidney left. You can live a normal life with only one kidney, but you have to keep this kidney healthy, otherwise you will require dialysis or a transplant. You will have to ensure that you drink enough water and fluids, avoid medications that are toxic to the kidney, avoid contrast material given for medical imaging, and take early antibiotic treatment for urinary tract infections. Of course, there is no guarantee that the kidney transplant will be 100% successful and your husband's body may reject the new kidney, immediately or after several years.

- **Check the relatives understanding.**

Explore and respond to the relative's concerns

Do you have any questions or concerns?
(Do not hesitate to suggest seeking a transplant doctor opinion if you do not have a clear answer to any question).

- **Do I need to take any medication after donating my kidney?**
  No, you do not need to take any medication except those that are needed to heal your wound (which will only be for a few days).

- **Which is better, donating a kidney from a living or dead person?**
  A kidney from a live donor is better and has a better chance of survival without being rejected particularly if the donor is a blood-relative of the recipient.

Show empathy

I understand Mrs Ayesha that it is not an easy situation. It is important that you make sure you understand about kidney donation.

Summarise and confirm understanding

Mrs Ayesha, I would like to briefly summarise our discussion to make sure that you understand important information about kidney donation. We have discussed the treatment options for your husband who has end-stage kidney disease. For kidney transplantation, we have discussed the steps involved in kidney donation. My colleagues from transplant surgery and the transplant physicians will provide further details regarding the tests and procedure as well as the risks that can be associated with kidney donation.

Is everything clear so far?

Please let me know if you want to discuss anything else at this moment.

Offer help and follow-up and close the discussion

This is my telephone number. Please do not hesitate to contact me should you have any further questions.

I will arrange an appointment with our transplant surgeon and transplant physician to further discuss the surgery and post-transplant follow-up.

I will arrange another meeting in 2 weeks in case you have any more questions or concerns.

I will provide you with some website addresses and printed material to read about kidney donation and transplantation.

Discussion

Ethical principles

- **What are the main ethical principles in this scenario?**
  Patient autonomy: It is the right of the donor and recipient to know all the information about organ donation. Organ donation should be done without any pressure from both parties and informed consent obtained can be withdrawn at any time.

  Beneficence and non-maleficence: Kidney transplantation is in the best interest of Mr Mazin, but this should be done only after proper preparation and matching to avoid rejection. Rejection can result in great harm to the patient and his wife.

  Justice: It should include justice to the recipient and donor. Recipient should be treated in a fair manner without discrimination. Kidney transplantation is currently the best option for treating ESRD. The donor should be provided with adequate information on how to keep her other kidney healthy.

Duty of candour (honesty): The doctor should be honest to the patient explaining all possible complications during and after the procedure along with the outcome and survival of a renal transplant.

Hidden agenda

Explaining renal transplant in layman terms.
Explaining possible complications of kidney transplantation.
Live unrelated donor versus live related donor.

- **What do you know about the human tissue act?**
  It is an act that ensures the safe use of human tissue and its use with proper consent. It was implemented in 2004 and is followed in England, Scotland and Northern Ireland.

- **What is elective ventilation and how is it related to organ donation?**
  It means keeping a dying patient alive on ventilation until organ donation can be carried out. Elective ventilation for the sole purpose of organ transplantation allows preservation of the organs till the time of transplant.

- **Is there a role of unrelated relative organ donation?**
  If there is no financial conflict of interest, then organ donation from an unrelated donor may be considered.

- **When to refer for kidney transplantation?**
  Patients with irreversible kidney damage and an estimated glomerular filtration rate (eGFR) less than 15 mL/minute.

- **Live related versus live unrelated versus cadaveric donor for transplant?**
  Live related and living, emotionally attached unrelated donors have almost comparable outcomes and both of them have better outcomes compared to a deceased cadaveric donor.

- **How to evaluate a candidate for transplantation?**
  History and physical examination are the most valuable part of a candidate's evaluation for kidney transplantation. The degree of human leucocyte antigen (HLA) matching correlates with the rapidity and severity of transplant rejection. All the following points should be considered and documented to assess for any contraindication:
  - Cause of renal damage
  - Review renal biopsy
  - Risk of recurrence in transplanted candidate
  - Comorbidities and their control
  - Family history of chronic disease
  - Evidence of CAD, cerebrovascular disease, and peripheral vascular disease
  - Haematological abnormality such as coagulation abnormalities
  - Abnormality in the urinary tract and bladder
  - Financial evaluation to support future lifelong on-going treatment
  - Psychosocial evaluation
  - Assessing the risk of sensitisation from previous blood product transfusion or transplant sensitisation
  - Patient who is for a retransplant needs a more thorough assessment and evaluation.

- **What are the contraindications for renal transplantation?**
  - Severe comorbidities with a decreased life expectancy
  - Untreatable malignancy

- Psychiatric disorder
- Persistent substance abuse
- Non-compliance
- Persistent chronic infection
- Primary oxalosis
- Reversible renal failure
- HIV is not an absolute contraindication for renal transplantation unless the patient has AIDS or CD4 count <200 cells/mL
- No definite cutoff for preferred age for kidney transplantation. General rules are:
  - The preferred age for kidney transplantation is <60 years. Patients >70 years of age are preferred to be kept on other forms of renal replacement therapy.

Organ rejection

- *Hyperacute rejection*: Occurs immediately within minutes and necessitates immediate organ removal.
- *Acute rejection*: Occurs within weeks, is mediated by cellular immunity, and occurs to some extent in all types of transplants, especially highly vascular tissues like the kidney and liver. It is detected by failing organ function and can be confirmed via a renal biopsy of the transplant which will show infiltrating T cells, injury to blood vessels, and histological changes in the transplant organ.
- *Chronic rejection*: May occur after several years and is immune-mediated and due to fibrosis of the transplanted organs blood vessels (chronic allograft vasculopathy).
- *Non-adherence rejection*: Non-adherence to immunosuppressive medication.
- **Disease recurrence in transplant recipient**
  - ANCA-associated vasculitis and anti-GBM
  - Oxalosis
  - Haemolytic uremic syndrome
  - IgA nephropathy
  - Fabry's disease
  - Focal segmental glomerulosclerosis.

Further reading

Bunnapradist S, Danovitch GM. Evaluation of adult kidney transplant candidates. Am J Kidney Dis 2007; 50:890–898.

Legislation.gov.uk. Human Tissue Act 2004. [online] Available from https://www.legislation.gov.uk/ukpga/2004/30/contents [Last accessed October, 2019].

Mathew TH. Recurrence of disease following renal transplantation. Am J Kidney Dis 1988; 12:85–96.

Scenario no. 15

Type of scenario: Information giving/discussing terminal illness/end of life care

Candidate information

Your role: You are the medical registrar on the oncology unit.
Problem: Newly diagnosed terminal illness.
Patient: Mrs Smith, a 76-year-old lady.

Please read the scenario printed below. When the bell sounds, enter the room. You have (---) minutes for your consultation with the patient/relative, (---) minutes to collect your thoughts, and (---) minutes for discussion.

Please do not examine the patient
Please do not take a history

> Mrs Smith is a 76-year-old lady who was admitted to the hospital with cough and fever. She was diagnosed with community-acquired pneumonia and was treated with antibiotics. However, she also complained of recurrent abdominal pain, mild jaundice, and weight loss. An abdominal ultrasound revealed a mass lesion of the head of the pancreas. A staging CT scan confirmed that it was a malignant tumour of the head of the pancreas with metastasis to the liver and lungs. She does not want to have any further tests and does not want any treatment because of side effects.
>
> **Your task:** Is to discuss with the patient about her diagnosis and help her make an informed decision about her management plan.

Approach

Always read the scenario carefully and make sure you understand the instructions before you start. All information provided is important. Make notes and a framework for your discussion. Sometimes, a hidden agenda is incorporated; pay attention to that.

Introduction and identification

- **Prepare the environment**
  Sit at the same level as the patient with comfort and avoid barriers like tables.

- **Introduce yourself to the patient**
  Shake hands.
  Hello Mrs Smith, I am Dr X, working in the oncology unit.

- **Enquire from the patient if she would like someone else to be present during the discussion**
  Can I confirm that I am talking to Mrs Smith?
  Would you like to invite anybody else to this discussion?
- **Confirm the objective of the interview**
  We are here today to discuss the results of your investigations and diagnosis. Is that alright?

Check patient's understanding and expectation

Tell me Mrs Smith, how much do you know about your health status?
Did any of my colleagues discuss with you the results of the ultrasound and CT scan of your tummy?
What do you suspect might be the cause of your tummy pain and weight loss?

Discussion with the patient (information giving)

- **Give the patient the information (avoid medical jargon)**
  As you know Mrs Smith, you came initially with cough and fever and you were diagnosed with pneumonia which was treated successfully. However, because of your recurrent tummy pain, yellow eyes, and weight loss, we requested an ultrasound scan of your tummy which showed that you have a lump in the pancreas. The CT scan of

your tummy confirmed the lump in your pancreas and other shadows in your liver and lungs which suggest that this is likely to be a pancreatic cancer. Pause....

- **Explore the patient ideas about pancreatic cancer**
  Have you heard about cancer of the pancreas before? Pause....

- **Explain to the patient in simple terms about pancreatic cancer (avoid medical jargon).**
  Normally, when we find such a lump in the pancreas, we order further tests to confirm its nature. This can be done by taking a small piece from the lump to examine it under the microscope. Alternatively, some blood tests called tumour markers may help in the diagnosis. Treatment depends on the extent of spread identified in the scan and your body's ability to cope with the treatment which will be assessed by our cancer specialists. Different treatment options are available such as surgery (removal of the lump), chemotherapy (killing the cancer cells with medicine), and radiotherapy (killing cancer cells with radiation). As your CT scan showed abnormalities in your lungs and liver suggesting spread of the cancer to these organs, surgery is not an option and chemotherapy is the only remaining viable option. Unfortunately, Mrs Smith, cancer of the pancreas is a very aggressive cancer and the outcome of treatment, particularly if it has spread to other organs, is not good.

- **Pause and ask the patient if they have understood everything so far**
  I understand Mrs Smith that you do not want to have any treatments for your cancer. Is this decision based on your knowledge of the disease?

- **Provide other support and care (ending cancer treatment does not mean ending patient care)**
  Mrs Smith, your wishes will be respected. However, deciding not to receive chemotherapy or radiotherapy for your cancer does not mean that you will not receive medical care. We have a specialised team of doctors, nurses, psychologists, social workers as well as religious leaders called the 'palliative care team' who can help relieve your suffering and pain and provide the necessary psychological and spiritual support. If you agree, I will invite them to have a discussion with you about the type of help they can provide.

  Discuss DNAR status: Mrs Smith, since you have taken the decision not to start treatment for your pancreatic cancer, I think it is the time to discuss another important issue related to your care.

  As you know, cancer of the pancreas, particularly if it has spread to other parts of the body, is a very aggressive cancer and life expectancy is short. I think it makes sense to discuss how you would like things to go at the time of your death. Do you wish a 'do not resuscitate order' to be documented in your records? A do not attempt resuscitation (DNAR) order means that if your heart stops, we will allow natural death to happen and will not attempt to resuscitate you by applying chest compressions and delivering an electric shock to your heart to try restart it.

- **Check patient understanding and document her reply.**

Explore and respond to patient's concerns

Do you have any questions or concerns at this moment?

- **How long do I have to live?**
  This is a very difficult question to answer, but we know that cancer of the pancreas is very aggressive particularly in the advanced stages. Even with good treatment, the outcomes are not good as most patients survive only for 6–12 months.

Show empathy

I am very sorry to have to talk to you about this, but I hope you understand more about your cancer.

Summarise and confirm understanding

Mrs Smith, I would like to summarise our discussion to be sure that you understand important information about your current illness and plan of care. We have found a lump in your pancreas and the CT scan shows that it has spread to the liver and lungs. This normally needs confirmation by taking a small biopsy from the pancreas, but I understand that you do not wish any further tests or treatment. Our palliative care team will visit you shortly and establish your palliative care plan. You have agreed on a 'do not resuscitate order' and your wish will be respected.

Please let me know if there is anything unclear and you would like to discuss it further.

Offer help and follow-up and close the discussion

This is my telephone number. Please do not hesitate to contact me should you have any further questions or concerns.

I will discuss your case with other colleagues specialised in cancer treatment and pancreatic disease to have their input as well.

Our palliative care team will visit you before you go home and arrange for your home visits or provide their care in the hospice.

I will also provide you with website addresses and printed material to have more information about your diagnosis.

Discussion

Ethical principles

- **What are the main ethical principles in this scenario?**
  Patient autonomy: Patient has the right to refuse treatment and investigations and her decision should be respected. In this case, the most important point is that she understands all the information and makes an informed decision for not having any further treatment.

  Beneficence and non-maleficence: Any decision taken should be in the best interest of the patient and to avoid harm. Pancreatic cancer is an aggressive tumour and life expectancy even with good treatment is limited to 6–12 months. Furthermore, chemotherapy and radiotherapy are not without complications and side effects.

  Justice: Justice to the patient prevails. Despite refusing chemotherapy, other forms of therapy, such as pain relief and palliative care should be offered.

  Duty of candour (honesty): Be honest with the patient as pancreatic cancer is an aggressive tumour and life expectancy even with good treatment is limited to 6–12 months.

Hidden agenda (any one possible)

- Explaining diagnosis and management plan
- Reason why patient does not want any treatment
- Offering palliative care and pain management
- Discussing DNAR and end-of-life issues
- Informed decision-making.

Pancreatic cancer

It is the fourth leading cause of cancer death:
- *75%:* In the head of pancreas
- *15–20%:* In the body of pancreas
- *5–10%:* In the tail of pancreas.

Screening: No screening is recommended.

Clinical features:
- Anorexia
- Fatigue
- Nausea
- Mid epigastric pain radiating to back
- Significant weight loss
- Recent onset of DM
- Painless obstructive jaundice
- Palpable gallbladder (courvoisier's law)
- Migratory thrombophlebitis.

Investigation:
- *CBC:* Anaemia
- *Serum albumin:* Low (malnourished)
- *LFT:* Picture of obstructive jaundice
- *Serum amylase/Lipase:* Raised
- *Tumour marker:* CA 19-9 raised and sometimes CEA raised.

Imaging:
- US abdomen
- CT Scan
- EUS
- MRI
- ERCP
- PET scan.

Further workup

Controversial about doing biopsy before surgery as it will not change further management plan and attempting to take a biopsy or FNA may lead to seeding of malignant cells in the abdomen.
- EUS-guided FNA (preferable)
- CT-guided biopsy.

Pathology

About 80% are pancreatic adenocarcinoma and the rest are from endocrine and exocrine pancreatic cells.

Staging

TNM staging:
T0: No evidence of primary tumour
Tis: Carcinoma *in situ*
T1: Less than or equal to 2 cm limited to pancreas
T2: More than 2 cm limited to pancreas
T3: Tumour spread outside the pancreas (e.g. duodenum, bile duct, portal or superior mesenteric vein) but not involving the celiac axis or superior mesenteric artery
T4: Tumour involves the celiac axis or superior mesenteric arteries.
N0: No lymph node metastasis
N1: Regional lymph node metastasis
M0: No distant metastasis
M1: Distant metastasis.

Treatment

Surgery is the mainstay of treatment with different surgical options like:
- Pancreaticoduodenectomy (whipple procedure)
- Distal pancreatectomy
- Total pancreatectomy

Chemotherapy and radiotherapy are given as adjuvant and neo-adjuvant therapy and for a unresectable tumour. However, survival of patients with pancreatic cancer is very limited even with advanced treatment.

Palliative and end of life care

The World Health Organisation (WHO) defines palliative care as follows: Palliative care is 'an approach that improves the quality of life of patients and their families facing the problem associated with life-threatening illness, through the prevention and relief of suffering by means of early identification and impeccable assessment and treatment of pain and other problems, physical, psychosocial and spiritual'.

Palliative and end of life care will

- Provide relief from pain and other distressing symptoms
- Enhance quality of life
- Provide psychological and spiritual care
- Provide continuous support to patients and their families
- Incorporate a team approach to address the needs of patients and their families, including bereavement counselling, if indicated
- Should be provided by a team of skilled healthcare providers
- Should be applied early in the course of illness in conjunction with other therapies.

Which patients fulfil the criteria of 'end of life'?

The following definition of 'end of life' has been accepted in a number of countries: 'People are approaching the 'end of life' when they are likely to die within the next 12 months. This includes patients with one or more of the following:

- Death is imminent (expected within a few hours or days).
- Advanced, progressive and incurable conditions.
- General frailty and co-existing conditions that mean that they are expected to die within 12 months.
- Existing conditions, if they are at risk of dying from a sudden acute crisis in their condition.
- Life-threatening acute conditions caused by sudden catastrophic events.

The Australian Commission on Safety and Quality in Health Care encourages clinicians to use the 'surprise' question as a simple screening mechanism to recognise patients who could benefit from end-of-life care interventions. These surprise questions are:

- Would you be surprised if this patient died in the next 12 months?
- Would you be surprised if this patient died during this admission, or in the next days or weeks?

Important challenges in patients who are for 'end of life' care

- *Deciding to withhold treatment or not to start treatment:* The GMC (UK) states that withdrawing or not starting a treatment when it has the potential to prolong the patient's life as the most challenging decision. Examples are starting antibiotics for life-threatening infection, cardiopulmonary resuscitation (CPR), renal dialysis, 'artificial' nutrition and hydration and mechanical ventilation. The GMC (UK) states that evidence of the benefits, burdens and risks of these treatments is not always clear cut. Clinicians practicing in different countries should seek reassurance from local authorities about what is ethically and legally permissible.
- *Disagreements between the clinician and patient's relatives regarding the overall benefits of certain types of treatments.*
  - Discuss with the relatives the reasons behind your opinion (this is often sufficient to solve the dispute).

- If not, other steps that can be considered are; conducting a case conference, seeking senior colleague opinion or involving an independent advocate.
- If after all this, disagreement is still there, clinicians should consider seeking legal advice.

Further reading

Australian Commission on Safety and Quality in Health Care, National Consensus Statement: Essential Elements for Safe and High-Quality End-of-Life Care, Sydney, ACSQHC, 2015.

DQ Adult Treatment Editorial Board. Pancreatic Cancer Treatment (PDQ®): Health Professional Version. (2019). PDQ Cancer Information Summaries [Internet]. Bethesda (MD): National Cancer Institute (US); 2002. Also available from https://www.ncbi.nlm.nih.gov/books/NBK65957/ [Last accessed October, 2019].

General Medical Council (UK). Treatment and care towards the end of life: good practice in decision making. May, 2010. Available from: https://www.gmc-uk.org/-/media/documents/treatment-and-care-towards-the-end-of-life---english-1015_pdf-48902105.pdf?la=en. [Last accessed: October, 2019].

Kauhanen SP, Komar G, Seppänen MP, et al. A prospective diagnostic accuracy study of 18F-fluorodeoxyglucose positron emission tomography/computed tomography, multidetector row computed tomography, and magnetic resonance imaging in primary diagnosis and staging of pancreatic cancer. Ann Surg 2009; 250:957–963.

Khorana AA, Mangu PB, Berlin J, et al. Potentially curable pancreatic cancer: American Society of Clinical Oncology Clinical Practice Guidelines. J Clin Oncol 2016; 34:2541–2556.

Maisonneuve P, Lowenfels AB. Epidemiology of pancreatic cancer: an update. Dig Dis. 2010;28(4-5):645-56.

National Comprehensive Cancer Network (NCCN). Clinical Practice Guidelines in Oncology. Pancreatic Adenocarcinoma [online] Available from http://www.jnccn.org/content/15/8/1028.full.pdf [Last accessed October, 2019].

Raimondi S, Maisonneuve P, Lowenfels AB. Epidemiology of pancreatic cancer: an overview. Nat Rev Gastroenterol Hepatol 2009; 6:699–708.

World Health Organization. Palliative care. Available from: https://www.who.int/cancer/palliative/definition/en/.[Last accessed October, 2019].

Scenario no. 16

Type of scenario: Breaking bad news (brain death and organ donation)

Candidate information

Your role: You are a medical registrar in critical care.
Problem: Breaking bad news and organ donation.
Patient: Mrs Qazi, a 52-year-old woman.
Relative: Mr Rashid, son of Mrs Qazi.

Please read the scenario printed below. When the bell sounds, enter the room. You have (---) minutes for your consultation with the patient/relative, (---) minutes to collect your thoughts, and (---) minutes for discussion.

Please do not examine the patient
Please do not take a history

> Mrs Qazi is a 52-year-old woman with a past history of hypertension. She was brought to the hospital with a seizure and loss of consciousness. CT brain confirmed a massive ischaemic stroke with haemorrhagic transformation. From the time she was intubated, she has not responded or triggered the ventilator for almost 48 hours, despite sedation being withheld. The apnoea test confirmed brain stem death and was signed by two senior ICU physicians. Her son is aware of his mother's major stroke but does not know about her brainstem death. He is waiting outside.
>
> **Your task:** Is to discuss with the son about his mother's brainstem death and organ donation.

Approach

Always read the scenario carefully and make sure you understand the instructions before you start. All information provided is important. Make notes and a framework for your discussion. Sometimes, a hidden agenda is incorporated; pay attention to that.

Introduction and identification

- **Prepare the environment**
  Sit at the same level as the relative with comfort and avoid barriers like tables.

- **Introduce yourself to the relative**
  Shake hands.
  Hello Mr Rashid, I am Dr X, working in the ICU.

- **Enquire if the relative would like someone else to be present during the discussion**
  Can I confirm that I am talking to Mr Rashid? You are the son of Mrs Qazi. Is that right?
  Would you like to invite anybody else to this discussion?

- **Confirm the objective of the interview**
  We are here today to discuss Mrs Qazi's health status. Is that alright?

Check Mr Rashid's understanding and expectation

Tell me Mr Rashid, how much do you know about Mrs Qazi's health status?
What do you suspect might be wrong with Mrs Qazi?

Discussion with the relative (information giving)

- **Give the relative information (avoid medical jargon)**
  As you know Mr Rashid, Mrs Qazi was brought in an unconscious state to the hospital and she was connected to an artificial breathing machine called a ventilator as she was unable to breathe by herself. The scan of her brain showed a major stroke due to the blood supply to a large part of her brain being cutoff. She also developed bleeding in that area of the brain which made things even worse as we could not give a blood thinner to improve the blocked blood flow.
  Unfortunately, since her admission, Mrs Qazi has been completely unresponsive even to pain and has been unable to breathe by herself. She remains totally dependent on the ventilation machine for breathing which means that if we stop the machine, her breathing will stop. Because of that, two senior colleagues from the ICU have assessed her brain function and I am sorry to inform you she has been confirmed to be brain dead. Pause...

- **Be prepared for reactions such as: anger, tearing and crying**
  (In all cases, stay calm and behave in a professional manner)

- **Let him absorb the grief, show empathy, and provide tissue paper**

- **Explain further to the relative in simple terms the meaning of brain death.**
  Brain death occurs when all brain functions completely stop and this cannot be reversed. This means that the brain has permanently stopped functioning and legally the person is dead. Certain tests were done on your mother that confirmed brain death.

Discussion about organ donation

- Discussing organ donation is a very sensitive issue after breaking bad news of brain death.
- The clinician can often judge if the time is suitable to discuss organ donation or postpone it to another meeting from the relative's reaction.
- If you feel it is an appropriate time to discuss about organ donation, then prepare the ground for the discussion and begin by asking some questions about the patient's life.

Mr Rashid, I would like to ask a few questions about the life of Mrs Qazi. (use the following questions to begin the discussion):

- Has she left any wishes before becoming ill?
- Did she leave any advance directives?
- Did she sign or have a donor card?
- Was she generous to the community?
- Was she involved in any charity?
  If his answer is yes, you may ask if he would like to continue this after her death.

  Continue the discussion : As you may know Mr Rashid, after the death and burial of the body, the organs will decompose and vanish. Every day, many ill patients with organ failure like kidney and liver failure die while waiting for organs that could save their lives. There are hundreds of thousands of people on the transplant waiting lists. A single donor can save as many as 50 lives. As Mrs Qazi used to participate and promote charitable work, do you think she would have wanted to continue this after her death. What do you think?

- **Pause and ask the relative if everything is clear so far**

- **Check the patient understanding.**

Explore and respond to relative's concerns

Do you have any questions or concerns?

- **Doctor, organ donation may be against my religion?**
  Organ donation is encouraged in most major religions. If you are unsure, you may confirm this from your local religious leaders. Certainly, from an Islamic perspective organ donation is encouraged.

- **Doctor, I am concerned that her body will be disfigured if her organs are removed.**
  Any incisions made during the removal of organs and tissues are always closed after the procedure, so the body is not disfigured and is ready for burial. Organ removal will be done by expert surgeons.

Show empathy

I understand Mr Rashid it must be very difficult to hear about all this.

Summarise and confirm understanding

Mr Rashid, I would like to briefly summarise our discussion, as it is important for me to be sure that you understand important information about your mother's condition. Your mother was brought to the hospital because of sudden collapse at home. Her brain scan confirmed that she had a major stroke. Since her admission she had not responded and further tests showed that she is brain-dead. The brain death was confirmed by two senior consultants. We have discussed about organ donation. If you agree on organ donation, then the ventilator machine will be kept on until her organs have been removed by the transplant team.

Would you like to discuss anything else at this moment?

Offer help and follow-up and close the discussion

This is my office number, please do not hesitate to contact me should you have any further questions or concerns.

I will also provide you with some website addresses and printed material on organ donation.

Discussion

Ethical principles

- **What are the main ethical principles in this scenario?**

    Patient autonomy: Patient has the right to make a decision about his treatment. As the patient in this situation is unable to make a decision, the decision will be taken in the best interest of the patient by the treating medical team after discussing with the relative.

    Beneficence and non-maleficence: A decision will be taken in the best interest of the patient, as a part of providing optimal care and to avoid harm. In this scenario, the patient is brainstem dead and keeping her on a ventilator is not in the best interest of the patient. Every effort should be made to decrease the suffering of the patient.

    Justice: It should include justice to the patient and community. The patient should be treated in a fair manner without discrimination. In this scenario, justice to the patient was done as she was provided with all the necessary treatment without discrimination. Justice to the community is an important issue in this scenario as keeping her on a ventilator imposes unnecessary cost and may prevent another patient from receiving ventilator support. Furthermore, discussing organ donation is considered just to the community.

Hidden agenda

- Explaining brainstem death
- Consent for organ donation
- Decision to stop the ventilator.

Brainstem death

Death diagnosed after irreversible cessation of brainstem function and confirmed using neurological criteria. The diagnosis of brain death is made while the body of the person is attached to an artificial ventilator and the heart is still beating.

Cardiac death

Death diagnosed and confirmed by a doctor after cardiorespiratory arrest.

Brainstem death criteria

Coma

Patient should lack all evidence of responsiveness with absent eye opening or movement to noxious stimuli and absent motor responses (other than spinally mediated reflexes).

Absence of brainstem reflexes

- Absence of pupillary response to light.
- Absence of ocular movements using oculocephalic testing and oculovestibular reflex testing.

- Absence of corneal reflex.
- Absence of facial muscle movement to noxious stimulus.
- Absence of the pharyngeal and tracheal reflexes.

Apnoea test
- Absence of a respiratory drive
- Absence of a breathing drive is tested with a CO_2 challenge.

Ancillary tests
In clinical practice, EEG, cerebral angiography, nuclear scan, transcranial Doppler ultrasonography, CTA, and MRI/MRA are currently used as ancillary tests in adults.

Prerequisites before applying the criteria
- Exclude the presence of a CNS-depressant drug effect.
- No recent administration or continued presence of neuromuscular blocking agents.
- No severe electrolyte, acid–base, or endocrine disturbance.
- Achieve normal core temperature.
- Achieve normal systolic blood pressure.
- Perform two neurologic examinations (by expert clinicians).

Further reading

Mayo Clinic. Organ donation: Don't let these myths confuse you. [online] Available from https://www. mayoclinic.org/healthy-lifestyle/consumer-health/in-depth/organ-donation/art-20047529 [Last accessed October, 2019].

National Institute for Health and Clinical Excellence (NICE)-UK. Organ donation for transplantation: improving donor identification and consent rates for deceased organ donation. [online] Available from https://www. nice.org.uk/guidance/cg135/documents/organ-donation-final-scope3 [Last accessed October, 2019].

Wijdicks EF, Varelas PN, Gronseth GS, et al; American Academy of Neurology. Evidence-based guideline update: determining brain death in adults: report of the Quality Standards Subcommittee of the American Academy of Neurology. Neurology 2010; 74:1911–1918.

Scenario no. 17

Type of scenario: Obtaining informed consent from patient's son for insertion of feeding gastric tube

Candidate information

Your role:	You are the registrar on the medical ward.
Problem:	To take consent from patient's son.
Relative:	Mr Salem, son of Mrs Noof.

Please read the scenario printed below. When the bell sounds, enter the room. You have (---) minutes for your consultation with the patient/relative, (---) minutes to collect your thoughts, and (---) minutes for discussion.

Please do not examine the patient
Please do not take a history

Mrs Noof is a 75-year-old woman. She was admitted to the hospital with fever and cough and was diagnosed with severe aspiration pneumonia that was treated with antibiotics. Last year, she suffered a major ischaemic stroke that rendered her hemiplegic and aphasic, with impaired cognition and she became fully dependent on her family. She has long-standing type 2 diabetes mllitus (T2DM) and hypertension. She has good family support. She has suffered from significant muscle wasting since her last stroke because of poor oral intake and was assessed during this admission by speech and swallowing specialists and declared unfit for oral feeding due to poor swallowing and risk of aspiration. Her son says that she repeatedly coughs and chokes after feeding her. Nasogastric tube insertion has been attempted, but the patient pulled it out on two occasions.

Your task: Your task is to explain to Mr Salem, the need for gastric tube feeding and obtain informed consent from him.

Approach

Always read the scenario carefully and make sure you understand the instructions before you start. All information provided is important. Make notes and a framework for your discussion. Sometimes, a hidden agenda is incorporated; pay attention to that.

Introduction and identification

- **Prepare the environment**
  Sit at the same level as the relative with comfort and avoid barriers like tables.

- **Introduce yourself to the patient's relative**
  Shake hands.
  Hello Mr Salem, I am Dr X, working in the medicine department.

- **Enquire from the relative if he would like someone else to be present during the discussion**
  Can I confirm that I am talking to Mr Salem, the son of Mrs Noof?
  Would you like to invite anybody else to this discussion?

- **Confirm the objective of the interview**
  We are here to discuss ways of safely feeding your mother, Mrs Noof. Is that alright?

Check patient's son understanding and expectation

  Tell me Mr Salem how much do you know about the current health status of Mrs Noof?
  Do you know about the results of her swallowing assessment?
  Do you know why she developed pneumonia?

Discussion with the patient's son (information giving)

- **Explain the current situation and problem in her care (avoid medical jargon)**
  As you know Mr Salem, Mrs Noof had a stroke 2 years ago that limited her movement and ability to communicate. The stroke has affected her ability to swallow due to weakness of the swallowing muscles. Some of the food she swallows may pass into her lungs rather than the stomach and this explains why Mrs Noof gets cough and choking when she eats. This is called 'food aspiration' and is very serious because it can result in chest infection and 'aspiration pneumonia'. Furthermore, Mrs Noof has lost significant weight and muscle because of her poor food intake. This can further weaken her immunity to fight infections and worsen

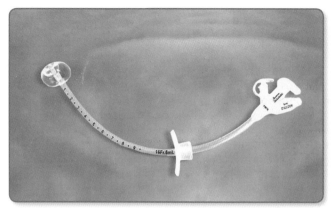

Figure 1 PEG tube. (*See colour plate 2*)

her nutritional status. Because of this, we are here today to discuss the best way to feed her to try improving her nutritional status as well as reduce the risk of developing aspiration pneumonia.

- **Explain about the various methods of tube feeding (Figure 1)**
  There are three main ways of providing tube feeding for patients like Mrs Noof. The first one is to pass a tube through her nose to the stomach. Although this method is easy as it can be done without the need to cut the skin and takes the shortest time, it is a temporary solution. Many patients cannot tolerate the tube in their nose, and it can cause ulceration in the nose and colonisation of bacteria around the tube with recurrent sinus infection. It also does not reduce the risk of aspiration. I understand that this tube was tried previously for Mrs Noof but she could not tolerate it and pulled the tube out. The other method is called 'Percutaneous Endoscopic Gastrostomy' or PEG. In this procedure, a flexible feeding tube is placed through the tummy wall into the stomach. PEG allows nutrition, fluids, and/or medications to be put directly into the stomach. We use a flexible tube with a camera called an endoscope to guide the creation of a small opening through the skin of the tummy. If the tube is placed into the stomach, we call this a gastrostomy tube and if it is placed in the small intestine, we call it a jejunostomy tube. A jejunostomy tube is preferred in patients who are at risk of recurrent aspiration.

- **Explain how the PEG/PEJ tube is inserted**
  Before the procedure: We need to temporarily stop blood thinning medications such as aspirin and optimise diabetes control as this will help minimise the risk of infection. The patient should abstain from taking food by mouth for about 8 hours before the procedure.

  During the procedure: Local anaesthesia, medication to make the patient relax, and sedation will be given to Mrs Noof to make her more comfortable for the procedure. While your mother is lying on her back, a specialist doctor will place the endoscope in her mouth and down her food pipe. After visualising the stomach from inside with the help of a camera, a small cut is made in her tummy wall and the feeding tube is inserted through that cut into the stomach. The tube will be fixed in place and a sterile dressing will be placed around the site. The whole procedure usually takes about an hour.

  After the procedure: After the procedure, feeding initiation through the PEG tube will be delayed for 12–24 hours to allow for healing. The tube area should be kept dry and clean to avoid skin irritation or infection. A dietician will see your mother to prescribe a special feeding formula and also educate you on how to care for the tube. Most patients can return home the same day as the procedure.

Explore and respond to Mr Salem's concerns

Do you have any questions or concerns at this moment?

- **Doctor, what are the complications of PEG/PEJ?**
  This is a good question. A few patients with PEG placement experience minor complications such as inflammation and pain around the tube due to leakage of stomach contents. Less than 5% of patients may develop serious complications such as continuous leakage of stomach content, infection of the inner lining of the abdomen (peritonitis), infection of the anterior abdominal wall, bleeding, or extremely rarely, injury to internal organs.

- **Doctor, how long is the tube kept in her stomach?**
  PEG tubes can last for months or years. However, because they can break down or become clogged over extended periods of time, they might need to be replaced. Your doctor can easily remove or replace a tube without sedatives or anaesthesia.

- **Doctor, what should I do if the tube comes out of its place?**
  This is again a very important question. PEG sites close quickly (within hours) once the tube is removed or dislodged. Therefore, accidental dislodgment requires immediate attention. You must immediately call your doctor or bring your mother to the hospital to reinsert it before the opening closes.

Show empathy

I understand how difficult it is for you to hear about all this. We are here to help you.

Summarise, confirm understanding and obtain consent

Mr Salem, I would like to summarise our discussion as it is important for me to be sure that you understand important information about tube feeding. Because of her stroke, your mother, Mrs Noof, has poor swallowing, which has led to recurrent aspiration pneumonia. She is also malnourished because of poor oral intake. Therefore, we need to place a tube called a PEG tube to feed her. I have explained to you how the procedure is done, and the advantages and possible complications of tube feeding.

If you agree on the PEG, could you kindly sign the consent form?

Offer help and follow-up plan and close the discussion

This is my contact number. Please do not hesitate to contact me if you have any further questions. I will also provide you with some printed material to read about PEG tube feeding.

Discussion

Ethical principles

- **What are the main ethical principles in this scenario?**
  Patient autonomy: The patient in this scenario does not have the capacity to decide. The next of kin is her son who should know about the condition and the procedure to be performed for his mother. The doctor should be honest and truthful in discussing the risks and complications.
  Beneficence and non-maleficence: PEG tube insertion will be in the best interest of the patient. It will improve her nutritional status. PEJ tube feeding may help reduce the risk of recurrent aspiration. The patient should be prepared for the procedure and all

anticipated risks for complications should be addressed before the procedure such as withholding antiplatelet medication.

Justice: Patient should be treated in a fair manner without discrimination.

Hidden agenda

- Steps of discussing a procedure (pre-during-post)
- Understanding the indications and care for tube feeding
- Advantage and disadvantages of different types of tube feeding.

What are the types of enteral tube feeding?

- Nasoenteric tube feeding
- Gastrostomy tube feeding
- Jejunostomy tube feeding.

  Gastrostomy and jejunostomy tubes can be placed under endoscopic guidance, radiologic guidance or surgically. They are commonly performed under endoscopic guidance and hence called 'PEG' or 'PEJ'.

Advantages and disadvantages of nasoenteric tube feeding

- *Advantages*: Nasal tubes are mainly used for short-term enteral feeding (4-6 weeks) and in situations where other methods of enteral feeding are contraindicated. They are easy to insert and do not require a surgical endoscopic procedure.
- *Disadvantages*:
  - Poorly tolerated by the conscious patient, as they elicit a foreign body sensation in the pharynx.
  - May cause reflux esophagitis and pressure ulcers in the nose.
  - May lead to sinusitis and colonisation of bacteria around the tube.
  - Have a tendency to dislocate.
  - Can be a source of psychological stress to the patient, the presence of the tube being a visible sign of his/her illness.
  - Aspiration is reported in up to 89% of patients, with no clear advantage of nasoenteric over gastroenteric feeding.

Indications for enteral tube feeding

- Unconscious patient (e.g. head injury, stroke)
- Neuromuscular swallowing disorder (e.g. post-CVA, multiple sclerosis, motor neurone disease, Parkinson's disease)
- Physiological anorexia (e.g. cancer, sepsis, liver disease)
- Upper GI obstruction (e.g. oropharyngeal or oesophageal stricture or tumour)
- Severe mental health (e.g. dementia, severe depression).

Advantages of jejunostomy tube feeding

- Appropriate for patients at risk of recurrent aspiration (lower risk for aspiration compared to PEG).
- Appropriate in patients with recurrent vomiting and severe gastroesophageal reflux, gastroparesis, gastric outlet obstruction, or total or partial gastrectomy.

Complications of PEG/PEJ

About 13-40% of patients with PEG placement experience minor complications such as maceration due to leakage of gastric contents around the tube, and peristomal pain. Serious complications requiring further intervention have been reported in 0.4-4.4% of procedures and include peristomal leakage with peritonitis, necrotizing fasciitis of the anterior abdominal wall, gastric bleeding, injury to internal organs, tumour seeding at the PEG site, and death. The incidence of clogged feeding tubes in PEG is reported to be as high as 23–35%. Clogging is especially common when thick enteral feeds, bulking agents, and medications are delivered through relatively small PEG tubes.

Further reading

American Society for Gastrointestinal Endoscopy (ASGE). Understanding Percutaneous Endoscopic Gastrostomy (PEG). Information for patients. [online] Available from https://www.asge.org/home/for-patients/patient-information/understanding-peg. [Last accessed October, 2019].

Blumenstein I, Shastri YM, Stein J. Gastroenteric tube feeding: techniques, problems and solutions. World J Gastroenterol 2014; 20:8505–8524.

Healthline. Feeding tube insertion (Gastrostomy). [online] Available from https://www.healthline.com/health/feeding-tube-insertion-gastrostomy. [Last accessed October, 2019].

National Collaborating Centre for Acute Care (UK). Nutrition Support for Adults: Oral Nutrition Support, Enteral Tube Feeding and Parenteral Nutrition. London: National Collaborating Centre for Acute Care (UK); 2006 Feb. (NICE Clinical Guidelines, No. 32.) 9. Enteral tube feeding in hospital and the community. Also Available from https://www.ncbi.nlm.nih.gov/books/NBK49253/ [Last accessed October, 2019].

Scenario no. 18

Type of scenario: Discussing fitness to drive

Candidate information

Your role: You are the medical registrar in the medical outpatient clinic.
Problem: To counsel Mr Aziz about his fitness to drive.
Patient: Mr Aziz.
Please read the scenario printed below. When the bell sounds, enter the room. You have (---) minutes for your consultation with the patient/relative, (---) minutes to collect your thoughts, and (---) minutes for discussion.

Please do not examine the patient
Please do not take a history

You were requested by a junior colleague to help in the case of Mr Aziz who is a 50-year-old gentleman with type 2 diabetes mellitus (T2DM). He was initially treated with oral drugs for 4 years and was recently started on insulin therapy because of poor glycaemic control. He has experienced 6 hypoglycaemic episodes during the last 3 months and 2 of them required medical assistance. Your junior colleague is finding it difficult to convince Mr Aziz to inform the 'Driver and Vehicle Licensing Agency (DVLA)'.

Your task: Is to discuss with Mr Aziz the issue of driving in view of his recurrent hypoglycaemic episodes and respond to his concerns.

Approach

Always read the scenario carefully and make sure you understand the instructions before you start. All information provided is important. Make notes and a framework for your discussion. Sometimes, a hidden agenda is incorporated; pay attention to that.

Introduction and identification

- **Prepare the environment**
  Sit at the same level as the patient with comfort and avoid barriers like tables.

- **Introduce yourself to the patient's relative**
  Shake hands.
  Hello Mr Aziz, I am Dr X working in the medical outpatient clinic.

- **Enquire if the patient would like someone else to be present during the discussion**
  Can I confirm that I am talking to Mr Aziz?
  Would you like to invite anyone else to this discussion?

- **Confirm the objective of the interview**
  We are here to discuss regarding your driving and diabetes. Is that alright?

Check patient's understanding and expectation

Tell me Mr Aziz, how much do you know about diabetes and your ability to drive?
Which type of vehicle are you driving?
Do you have any warning symptoms or signs when your blood sugar levels go low (hypoglycaemia)?

Discussion with the patient (information giving)

- **Explain the current situation (avoid medical jargon)**
  Mr Aziz, it appears that your diabetes control is not optimal. Since starting insulin therapy 3 months ago, you have had several readings of low blood sugar and on two occasions, you required medical assistance for that. Low blood sugar or hypoglycaemia may lead to loss of consciousness and this is particularly dangerous when you are driving. It may lead to a serious accident that may harm yourself or other people on the road. This is more serious as you lack awareness of hypoglycaemia and your body does not show warning symptoms or signs when your sugar goes low. All these are important reasons for you to stop driving until your sugar is well controlled without having low sugar episodes. As you know Mr Aziz, you are legally required to inform the DVLA about any change in your illness that might affect your ability to drive. Recurrent episodes of low sugar readings are one of the conditions that necessitate informing the DVLA. Failure to inform the DVLA may pose a legal risk to you and is also important for your car and health insurance in case any road traffic accident happens while driving.

Explore and respond to the patient's concerns

Does that make sense to you?
Do you have any questions or concerns at this moment?
- Doctor, it is very difficult for me to stop driving. I am the only one in my family who has a driving licence. I need to drive to my work that is far from home.
- I am sorry about that Mr Aziz. I understand it must be a difficult situation for you. Have you thought of other ways to reach work such as public transport using a bus or train? What about discussing the issue with your employer to make reasonable adjustments such as flexible working hours or moving you to a near workplace until you can go back to driving? In addition, the DVLA will re-evaluate your ability to drive once your sugar levels are controlled and you do not have any more low sugar episodes.

Show empathy

Mr Aziz, I understand how difficult the current situation is for you. We are here to help.

Summarise and confirm understanding

Mr Aziz, I would like to summarise our discussion as it is important for me to be sure that you understand important information about your current condition. Your current blood sugar control is not optimal as you suffer frequent episodes of low sugar readings and you lack warning symptoms and signs for these low sugar readings. Therefore, you are required to inform the DVLA and have a regular follow-up with your doctor to improve your blood sugar control. I would like to inform you also that as doctors, we are required to document this discussion in your records.

Offer help and follow-up plan and close the discussion

This is my contact number. Please do not hesitate to contact me should you have any further questions or concerns. I will also provide you with the website address of the DVLA.

Discussion

Ethical Principles

- **What are the ethical principles involved in this case?**
  Autonomy: The patient should know about the risks of continuing to drive. The doctor should be honest and truthful in discussing the risks and complications.

  Beneficence and non-maleficence: It is in the best interest of the patient to quit driving given his recurrent hypoglycaemic attacks. It is also in the best interest of the patient to know how to prevent recurrent hypoglycaemia, whilst improving his glycaemic control. The patient's confidentiality should be maintained, unless the risks to the community outweigh the benefits of divulging confidentiality.

  Justice: Justice in this scenario is applicable to the patient as well as the community. For the patient, all possible treatments to better monitor (continuous glucose monitoring) control of his blood sugar should be offered without discrimination. For the community, all possible interventions to avoid harm and risks to other people from continuing to drive should be made.

Hidden agenda

- Diabetes and driving.
- Duties of health care professionals in cases of fitness to drive.
- Explaining to the patient the consequences of continuing to drive.

In some countries, the responsibility of the medical practitioner with regard to assessing and discussing fitness to drive is not well established.

In the UK, two groups of licence holders are identified:

- Group 1 includes cars and motorcycles.
- Group 2 includes large lorries (category C) and buses (category D).

In most cases, the medical standards for Group 2 drivers are substantially higher than for Group 1 drivers.

The following criteria must be met for the DVLA to license the person with insulin-treated diabetes for 1, 2, or 3 years (Group 1):

- Adequate awareness of hypoglycaemia
- No more than 1 episode of severe hypoglycaemia while awake in the preceding 12 months and the most recent episode occurred more than 3 months ago.

Lack of awareness of hypoglycaemia is defined as 'inability to detect the onset of hypoglycaemia because of total absence of warning symptoms'.

- **Who should notify the DVLA about change in health status?**
  Licence holders (patients) have a legal duty to notify the DVLA of any injury or illness that would have a likely impact on safe driving.

- **Who should decide about fitness to drive?**
  The DVLA is the one to decide, but they base it on a report from the consultant looking after the patient.

- **What are the duties of the doctors or healthcare professionals in cases of fitness to drive? [GMC (UK)/DVLA (UK)]**
  - Advise the individual of the impact of their medical condition for safe driving.
  - Advise the individual of their legal requirement to notify the DVLA of any relevant condition.
  - Treat, manage, and monitor the individual's condition with on-going consideration of their fitness to drive.
  - Notify the DVLA when fitness to drive requires notification but an individual cannot or will not notify the DVLA themselves.
- **What if the patient cannot or will not notify the DVLA?**
  - Ask for a patient's consent to disclose information for the protection of others.
  - If it is not practicable to seek consent or the patient has refused consent, disclosing personal information may be justified in the public interest.
  - If you consider that failure to disclose the information would leave individuals or society exposed to a risk so serious that it outweighs patients' and the public interest in maintaining confidentiality, you should disclose relevant information promptly to an appropriate person or authority. You should inform the patient before disclosing the information, if it is practicable and safe to do so, even if you intend to disclose without their consent.

Further reading

Driving and Vehicle Licensing Agency (UK). (2016). Assessing fitness to drive–a guide for medical professional. [online] Available from https://www.gov.uk/government/publications/assessing-fitness-to-drive-a-guide-for-medical-professionals [Last accessed October, 2019].

General Medical Council (UK). Confidentiality: good practice in handling patient information 2017. [online] Available from https://www.gmc-uk.org/ethical-guidance/ethical-guidance-for-doctors/confidentiality [Last accessed October, 2019].

Scenario no. 19

Type of scenario: Ethical considerations/refusal to disclose HIV status to sexual partner

Candidate information

Your role: You are the doctor on the medical ward.
Problem: Encouraging a patient to disclose his HIV status to his sexual partner.
Patient: Mr Eddie, a 26-year-old man.

Please read the scenario printed below. When the bell sounds, enter the room. You have (---) minutes for your consultation with the patient/relative, (---) minutes to collect your thoughts and (---) minutes for discussion.

Please do not examine the patient
Please do not take a history

Mr Eddie is a 26-year-old man who was admitted to the hospital 2 weeks ago with acute hypoxemic respiratory failure and found to have *Pneumocystis jirovecii* pneumonia. His blood tests confirmed HIV infection. He was treated with Trimethoprim-Sulfamethoxazole and steroids. His condition improved and he is now fit for discharge. Mr Eddie admitted that he had shared heroin needles and had multiple sexual partners in the past. For the last 3 months, he has had only one female sexual partner. Your junior colleague found difficulty in persuading Mr Eddie to disclose his HIV status to his sexual partner.

Your task: Is to encourage Mr Eddie to disclose his HIV status to his sexual partner.

Approach

Always read the scenario carefully and make sure you understand the instructions before you start. All information provided is important. Make notes and a framework for your discussion. Sometimes, a hidden agenda is incorporated; pay attention to that.

Introduction and identification

- **Prepare the environment**
  Sit at the same level as the patient with comfort and avoid barriers like tables.

- **Introduce yourself to the patient**
  Shake hands
  Hello Mr Eddie, I am Dr X, the medical registrar on the team looking after you.

- **Enquire if the patient would like someone else to be present during the discussion**
  Can I confirm that I am talking to Mr Eddie?
  Would you like to invite anybody else to this discussion?

- **Confirm the objective of the interview**
  We are here to discuss some issues regarding your HIV status. Is that alright?

Check patient's understanding and expectation

Mr Eddie, I have been informed that you do not want your current sexual partner to know about your HIV status, is that correct?

Discussion with the patient (information giving)

- **Enquire about the reasons behind his decision (avoid medical jargon)**
  Could you tell me the reasons behind this decision?

- **Patient's concerns**
  Doctor, I am concerned that my partner will leave me if she knows that I have HIV. In addition, as you know, having HIV is a social stigma in this community.

  Reply: I understand Mr Eddie and these are very important concerns to anyone who is newly diagnosed with HIV. As you know, HIV can be transmitted to others via the blood and semen. Your sexual partner will be at risk of acquiring the infection from you if she has not already acquired it and therefore, informing her about your current HIV status may help protect her from acquiring the infection. In addition, if we find that she has already acquired the infection, starting her on HIV treatment will help her avoid serious infections like the one that resulted in your hospital admission.

- **Reassure the patient that effective treatment for HIV is now available**
  Mr Eddie, the treatment of HIV has now advanced significantly. Nowadays, we have very effective drugs that can maximally suppress the HIV virus and stop the

progression of HIV disease. These drugs can also prevent transmission of HIV. Huge reductions have been seen in the rates of death and infections when HIV medications are given particularly in the early stages of the disease.

- **If the patient is still not willing to inform his sexual partner**
  I am sorry to say that continuing to have sexual relations with your partner and not informing her while knowing that you have HIV makes you legally liable.

- **Encourage the use of protective measures**
  Mr Eddie, are you using protective measures, such as condoms, during sexual activity with her?
  Patient's answer: No

  Doctor's reply: Well Mr Eddie, it is very important to use condoms and other protective measures to minimise the chances of giving your partner HIV until we can test her and determine her HIV status.

- **Ask if the sexual partner is or may be pregnant**
  Is there a possibility that your partner may be pregnant?
  If this is a possibility then there is a risk that she may transmit the infection to her baby if she is HIV positive. Treatment for her becomes more urgent to stop transmission of the infection to the baby.

- **Emphasise the importance of informing his sexual partner**
  For these reasons, I would strongly advise you to inform your partner about your HIV status.

Explore and respond to patient's concerns
Already discussed

Show empathy
I understand this is a very difficult situation for you. We are here to help.

Summarise and confirm understanding
Mr Eddie, I would like to summarise our discussion as it is important for me to be sure that you understand important information discussed in this meeting. The tests show that you have HIV infection and therefore your sexual partner will be at risk of acquiring the infection from you if she has not already acquired it. Informing her about your current HIV status may help protect her from acquiring the infection. In addition, if we find that she has already acquired the infection, starting her on HIV treatment will help her avoid serious infections like the one that led to your hospital admission. Continuing to have sexual relations with your partner while knowing that you are infected with HIV and not informing her may make you legally liable. Using protective measures such as condoms during sexual intercourse may help reduce the risk of infection to your partner.

- **Inform the patient that you will document this discussion**
  Mr Eddie, as doctors, we are required to document this discussion in your medical records.

- **Suggest inviting both the patient and his sexual partner to a meeting**
  Mr Eddie, if you agree, we can invite your partner to a meeting and discuss the situation with both of you.

- **If the patient is still insisting on not informing his sexual partner**
  Inform him that as a doctor you are obliged to protect other people in the community, and you are going to discuss this issue with your seniors and his sexual partner will be informed.

Offer help and follow-up plan and close the discussion

This is my contact number. Please do not hesitate to contact me should you have any further questions or concerns. I will also provide you with some useful website addresses related to HIV.

Discussion

Ethical principles

- **What are the ethical principles involved in this case?**

  Patient's autonomy: The patient has the right to know about his HIV status. The doctor should be honest and truthful in discussing the risks and complications.

  Beneficence and non-maleficence: Patient should be offered treatment of HIV without discrimination. Early disclosure and screening as well as early diagnosis of HIV carry a better prognosis for his sexual partner. Patient's confidentiality should be maintained unless risks to the community outweigh the benefit of maintaining confidentiality.

  Justice: Justice in this scenario is applicable to the patient as well as community. For the patient, all possible treatments to better control his HIV should be offered without discrimination. For the community (his partner), all possible interventions should be made to avoid risks of transmitting HIV to her. Also using protective measures such as condoms may help reduce this risk.

Hidden agenda

- Use of barrier methods such as condoms.
- Steps to encourage patient with communicable disease to disclose information to people at risk.
- Discuss increased risk to the baby during pregnancy.

Important points related to confidentiality

- Confidentiality is a crucial aspect to maintain trust between doctors and their patients.
- Patient confidentiality is not absolute.
- Legitimate conditions to disclose patient's information are:
  - Disclosures with patient consent
  - When required by law
  - When maintaining confidentiality carries a serious risk to the public or other party.
- When deciding to breach patient confidentiality based on the above, use the minimum necessary patient identifiable information.
- Access to personal information should be on a strict need-to-know basis.
- If patient consent cannot be obtained, you may seek advice from senior colleagues or a medical defence union.
- Always document your reasons clearly.

Patients with serious communicable diseases should be informed about the possible risk to other people in the community. You should explain to patients with serious communicable diseases how they can protect others from infection, including from sexually transmitted diseases. This includes practical measures to avoid transmission, and the importance of informing people with whom they have sexual contact. Disclosing information to a person who has close contact with a patient who has a serious communicable disease may be considered if the person is at risk of infection that is likely to result in serious consequences and the patient has not informed them and cannot be persuaded to do so. You should tell the patient before you disclose the information if it is practicable and safe to do so.

Further reading

Blightman K, Griffiths SE, Danbury C. Patient confidentiality: when can a breach be justified? Continuing Education in Anaesthesia Critical Care & Pain 2014; 14:52–56.

Epstein R, Thomas JC, Rotek GW. Please don't say anything: partner notification and the patient-physician relationship. Virtual Mentor 2003:5.

General Medical Council (UK). Confidentiality: disclosing information about serious communicable diseases. [online] Available from https://www.gmc-uk.org/-/media/documents/confidentiality---disclosing-information-about-serious-communicable-diseases_pdf-70061396.pdf. [Last accessed October 2019].

World Health Organization. (2018). Viral suppression for HIV treatment success and prevention of sexual transmission of HIV. [online] Available from http://www.who.int/hiv/mediacentre/news/viral-supression-hiv-transmission/en/ [Last accessed October 2019].

Scenario no. 20

Type of scenario: Information giving/consent for haemodialysis procedure

Candidate information

Your role: You are the nephrology registrar in the outpatient clinic.
Problem: Informing patient about haemodialysis.
Patient: Mr Bahadur, a 50-year-old man.

Please read the scenario printed below. When the bell sounds, enter the room. You have (---) minutes for your consultation with the patient/relative, (---) minutes to collect your thoughts, and (---) minutes for discussion.

Please do not examine the patient
Please do not take a history

Mr Bahadur is a 50-year-old man with chronic kidney disease (CKD) secondary to polycystic kidney disease. His CKD has progressed significantly over the past 3 years. His latest serum creatinine level is 1,400 µmol/L, HCO_3—13 mmol/L, Na—132 mmol/L, K—5.0 mmol/L, and Hb—7 g/dL. His GFR is 10 mL/min. He is complaining from easy fatigue and lethargy for the past 1 month. A diagnosis of end-stage renal disease was made and the plan is to start haemodialysis until he is prepared for kidney transplantation. He wants to know more about haemodialysis.

Your task: Is to explain to the patient about haemodialysis and answer his questions.

Approach

Always read the scenario carefully and make sure you understand the instructions before you start. All information provided is important. Make notes and a framework for your discussion. Sometimes, a hidden agenda is incorporated; pay attention to that.

Introduction and identification

- **Prepare the environment**
  Sit at the same level as the patient with comfort and avoid barriers like tables.

- **Introduce yourself to the patient**
  Shake hands
  Hello Mr Bahadur, I am Dr X, the nephrology registrar.

- **Enquire if the patient would like someone else to be present during the discussion**
  Can I confirm that I am talking to Mr Bahadur?
  Would you like to invite anybody else to this discussion?

- **Confirm the objective of the interview**
  I understand Mr Bahadur that you want to know more about haemodialysis. I am here to discuss this issue with you. Is that alright?

Check patient's understanding and expectation

Mr Bahadur how much do you know about your kidney status and haemodialysis?

Discussion with the patient/information giving (avoid medical jargon)

- **Explain what end-stage kidney disease is.**
  As you know Mr Bahadur, your kidney function has been deteriorating over the past few years and now you have reached an advanced stage such that your kidneys are no longer able to work to meet your body needs. This condition is called 'end-stage kidney disease'. Pause...

  Your kidneys filter wastes and excess fluids from your blood, which are then excreted in your urine. When your kidneys lose their function, dangerous levels of fluid, electrolytes, and wastes can accumulate in your body. Accumulation of fluids in your body can cause difficulty in breathing and accumulation of wastes in your body can cause tiredness, nausea, and vomiting. The accumulation of electrolytes can cause serious heart and brain abnormalities and can also lead to death if not corrected.
  Does that make sense to you?

- **Explain the procedure of haemodialysis (Figure 2)**
  There are different ways to remove the waste products and excess electrolytes from your blood when the kidneys are no longer functioning. One way is called haemodialysis in which your blood will be diverted to an external dialysis machine which will purify and filter your blood, remove the waste substances, and return the purified blood back to your body.

  Before the haemodialysis: The haemodialysis machine has to be connected to one of your blood vessels each time you undergo dialysis. This is to allow blood flow to and from the machine. Therefore, before starting haemodialysis, suitable access to your blood vessels has to be created in your body. There are three ways to create this access. A surgeon specialised in blood vessels may create a special blood vessel in your arm by connecting an artery to a vein called an AV fistula. An AV fistula is considered to be the best permanent access but it requires at least 4–8 weeks for the fistula to get strong enough before we can initiate haemodialysis. Some patients may have narrow blood vessels and, in that case, an AV graft may be established by connecting the artery and vein via synthetic tubing. A third but usually short-term measure is by inserting a central line in one of your neck veins.

  Haemodialysis procedure: During haemodialysis, the dialysis machine is connected to the AV fistula via two needles. The blood will be withdrawn from one of the vessels,

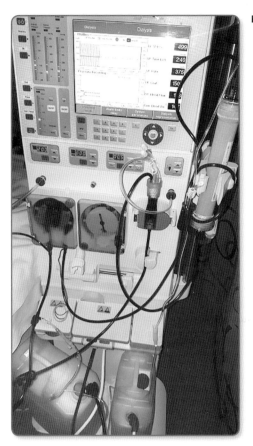

Figure 2 Haemodialysis machine. (*See colour plate 2*)

passes through the dialysis machine and gets filtered there and then returns back to your body through the other vessel. There are multiple filtering membranes that filter the blood and remove its toxins and waste substances in the dialysis machine. You will need about three sessions of haemodialysis a week, with each session lasting around 4 hours. This can be done in the hospital or at home if you are trained to do it and have your own machine.

After haemodialysis: After the dialysis session, the needles are removed, and a plaster is applied to prevent bleeding.

If haemodialysis is done in hospital, you can usually go home shortly afterward.

- **Care of your access**

Every now and then, you should feel your access after washing your hands. You should be able to feel vibration over your access. If you do not feel such vibration you must inform your doctor.

Your access should be kept clean at all times. Please wash the area with soap and water every day and before each haemodialysis session.

Avoid scratching your access as this may cause bleeding.

Please do not allow hospital staff to extract blood or measure blood pressure from the arm that contains the access.

Do not carry anything heavy or do anything that would put pressure on the access.

- **Fluid restriction**
  If you are having haemodialysis, the amount of fluid you can drink will be restricted.
       This is because the dialysis machine will not be able to remove all the fluid accumulated in your body over 2–3 days in 4 hours if you drink too much.
       This can lead to serious problems where excess fluid builds up in your blood, tissues, and lungs.
       The amount of fluid you will be allowed to drink will depend on your size and weight. Most people are only allowed to drink 1,000–1,500 mL of fluid a day.

- **Diet**
  You will also need to be careful about what you eat while having haemodialysis.
       This is because minerals such as sodium (salt), potassium, and phosphorus, which would normally be filtered out by your kidneys, can build up to dangerous levels quickly between treatment sessions.
       You will be referred to a dietician for a suitable diet plan to be drawn up for you.
       Diet plans differ from person to person, but it is likely you will be asked to avoid eating foods high in potassium and phosphorus and cut down the amount of salt you eat.

Explore and respond to patient's concerns

Do you have any questions or concerns?
- **Is haemodialysis painful? What are the complications of haemodialysis?**
  Haemodialysis is usually not painful, but some people feel a bit sick and dizzy, and may have muscle cramps during the procedure. This is caused by the rapid changes in blood fluid levels that occur during the treatment. Because blood pressure and heart rate can fluctuate as excess fluid is drawn from your body, your blood pressure and heart rate will be checked several times during each treatment.

Show empathy

I can understand it must be difficult to hear about all this. We are here to help.

Summarise and confirm understanding and obtain consent

Mr Bahadur, I would like to summarise our discussion as it is important for me to be sure that you understand important information about haemodialysis. Your kidneys are no longer able to work as they should to meet your body's needs. This condition is called 'end-stage kidney disease' and can lead to serious consequences if not appropriately treated. Haemodialysis is a procedure to purify and filter your blood and remove the waste substances and excess salt and water. Before haemodialysis can start, you will need to have a special blood vessel called an arteriovenous fistula (AV fistula) created in your arm. You will have a haemodialysis session 3 days per week with each session lasting 3–4 hours. If you agree to start haemodialysis, could you kindly read and sign this consent form?

Offer help and follow-up plan and close the discussion

This is my contact number with you in case you have any further question. You will also be seen by our dialysis team and nurse to further discuss haemodialysis. I will also provide you with some useful website addresses related to dialysis.

Discussion

Ethical principles

- **What are the ethical principles involved in this case?**
  Autonomy: The patient has the right to know about his end-stage kidney disease and haemodialysis. The doctor should be honest and truthful in discussing the risks and complications.

Beneficence and non-maleficence: Haemodialysis is an important treatment for end-stage kidney disease. Leaving a patient with end-stage kidney disease without renal replacement therapy is dangerous. The risks of not having renal replacement therapy should be explained to the patient.

Justice: Justice in this scenario is applicable. The best treatment for end-stage kidney disease should be offered without discrimination.

Hidden agenda

- Steps of discussing a procedure (pre, during and post).
- Discussing post-haemodialysis care.

Definition of chronic kidney disease (CKD)

Chronic kidney disease is defined by the presence of kidney damage or decreased kidney function for 3 or more months, irrespective of the cause.

Classification of CKD stages

The new classification of CKD depends on glomerular filtration rate (GFR) and presence of albuminuria. The recent incorporation of albuminuria in the staging of CKD is because of the graded increase in risk for mortality, progression of CKD, and ESRD at higher levels of albuminuria, independent of GFR.

GFR stages of CKD [according to GFR (mL/min/1.73 m^2)]:

- G1: GFR >90
- G2: GFR 60–89
- G3a: GFR 45–59
- G3b: GFR 30–44
- G4: GFR 15–29
- G5: GFR <15.

Albuminuria stages (albumin/creatinine ratio in mg/g)

- A1: ACR <30 mg/g (<3.4 mg/mmol)
- A2: ACR 30–299 mg/g (3.4–34.0 mg/mmol)
- A3: ACR ≥300 mg/g (>34.0 mg/mmol).

Management of CKD

- Control blood pressure:
    - <140/90 mmHg in nondiabetic and <130/80 mmHg in diabetic persons.
    - Use ACE inhibitor if there is albuminuria.
- Control blood sugar.
- Antiplatelet drugs for the secondary prevention of cardiovascular disease (Caution regarding the increased risk of bleeding).
- If vitamin D deficiency has been corrected and symptoms of CKD—mineral and bone disorders persist, offer alfacalcidol (1-alpha-hydroxycholecalciferol) or calcitriol (1,25-dihydroxycholecalciferol) to people with a GFR of less than 30.
- Oral sodium bicarbonate supplementation for people with both: A GFR less than 30 (GFR category G4 or G5) and a serum bicarbonate concentration of less than 20 mmol/L.
- Manage anaemia with erythropoietin treatment after correction of iron (goal is a haemoglobin level of 10–12 g/dL); avoid raising haemoglobin >12 g/dL in patients with CKD stages 4 and 5.
- Correct hypophosphatemia with dietary phosphate restriction and the use of phosphate binders (calcium acetate or sevelamer carbonate).
- Encourage people with CKD to take exercise, achieve a healthy weight, and stop smoking.
- Offer dietary advice about potassium, phosphate, calorie, and salt intake appropriate to the severity of CKD.
- Do not offer low-protein diets (dietary protein intake less than 0.6–0.8 g/kg/day) to people with CKD.

When to refer to a specialist?

People with CKD in the following groups should normally be referred for specialist assessment:

- GFR less than 30 mL/min/1.73 m^2 (GFR category G4 or G5), with or without diabetes
- ACR 70 mg/mmol or more, unless known to be caused by diabetes and already appropriately treated.
- ACR 30 mg/mmol or more (ACR category A3), together with haematuria.
- Sustained decrease in GFR of 25% or more, and a change in GFR category or sustained decrease in GFR of 15 mL/min/1.73 m^2 or more within 12 months.
- Hypertension that remains poorly controlled despite the use of at least four antihypertensive drugs at therapeutic doses.
- Known or suspected rare or genetic causes of CKD.
- Suspected renal artery stenosis.

When to refer for haemodialysis?

The clinical guidelines differ with regard to consideration for dialysis based on the GFR. With a GFR <15, nephrologists should evaluate the benefits, risks, and disadvantages of beginning kidney replacement therapy.

Further reading

Andrassy KM. Comments on 'KDIGO 2012 Clinical Practice Guideline for the Evaluation and Management of Chronic Kidney Disease'. Kidney Int 2013; 84:622–623.

Improving Global Outcomes (KDIGO) CKD Work Group. KDIGO 2012 clinical practice guideline for the evaluation and management of chronic kidney disease. Kidney Int Suppl 2013; 3:1–150.

Nasrallah GE, Mustafa RA, Clark WF, et al. Canadian Society of Nephrology 2014 clinical practice guideline for timing the initiation of chronic dialysis. CMAJ 2014; 186:112–117.

National Institute for Health and Care Excellence (NICE). Clinical guideline [CG182]. Chronic kidney disease in adults: assessment and management. [online] Available from https://www.nice.org.uk/guidance/cg182 [Last accessed October, 2019].

National Kidney Foundation. Haemodialysis Access. [online] Available from https://www.kidney.org/atoz/content/hemoaccess [Last accessed October, 2019].

NHS (UK). How it's performed? Dialysis. [online] Available from https://www.nhs.uk/conditions/dialysis/what-happens/ [Last accessed October, 2019].

Scenario no. 21

Type of scenario: Dealing with angry patient/relative

Candidate information

Your role: You are the on-call doctor on the medical floor.
Problem: To discuss with an angry relative.
Relative: Mr Nasser, son of Mr Khalifa.

Please read the scenario printed below. When the bell sounds, enter the room. You have (---) minutes for your consultation with the patient/relative, (---) minutes to collect your thoughts, and (---) minutes for discussion.

Please do not examine the patient
Please do not take a history

You are requested by the nurse on the medical floor to speak to Mr Nasser (son of Mr Khalifa) as he is very angry and requesting to speak to a doctor immediately. Mr Khalifa was admitted to the medical floor 5 days ago for cough and haemoptysis. A CT scan of the chest revealed a right upper lobe peripheral lung mass with multiple osteolytic lesions in the spine. A report of the CT-guided biopsy result released today confirmed the diagnosis of adenocarcinoma of the lung. Three months ago, Mr Khalifa was admitted to the medical floor for acute kidney injury due to the use of NSAID for new onset back pain. A routine chest radiograph done at that time revealed a small right pulmonary nodule. An appointment was arranged in the chest clinic but he did not attend as he went on holiday. Mr Nasser is now very angry and he thinks there was a delay in the diagnosis of his father's lung cancer during the previous admission. He feels doing a CT scan of the lungs at that time could have diagnosed the cancer at an earlier stage.

Your task: Is to discuss with Mr Nasser and answer his questions and concerns.

Approach

Always read the scenario carefully and make sure you understand the instructions before you start. All information provided is important. Make notes and a framework for your discussion. Sometimes, a hidden agenda is incorporated; pay attention to that.

Introduction and identification

- **Prepare the environment**
  Sit at the same level as the patient's son with comfort and avoid barriers like tables.

- **Introduce yourself to the patient's relative**
  Shake hands.
  Hello Mr Nasser, I am Dr X, working in the medical department.

- **Enquire from the relative if he would like someone else to be present during the discussion**
  Can I confirm that I am talking to Mr Nasser, the son of Mr Khalifa?
  I understand that Mr Khalifa is aware of this discussion. Would you like to invite anybody else to this discussion?

- **Confirm the objective of the interview**
  I understand Mr Nasser that you have concerns about the management of you father's illness. I am here to help.

Check patient's son concerns and expectation

Could you kindly tell me about your concerns/questions?

Discussion with the patient's son

Listen carefully to the concerns of the patient's son.
  Stay calm and professional when encountering difficult patients/relatives.
  Never confront patients or their relatives or blame them; arguing, blaming or confronting patients is unprofessional behaviour and may worsen a difficult situation.
  Never talk badly about your colleagues or criticise them or give your judgement.
  If there is a misunderstanding from the patient or his/her relative, politely correct the misunderstanding.

Son's concerns: Today, I came to know that my father has lung cancer which has already spread to his bones. It means that it is at an advanced stage. Three months ago, the doctors found a small shadow in his lung, but it seems to me that they did not pay much attention to that shadow otherwise; they should have ordered a CT scan of his lungs. They just sent him home after his kidney function got better. I am sure if they had requested a CT scan at that time, his lung cancer could have been discovered at an earlier stage and he could have been treated.

Doctor's reply: I am sorry to hear that Mr Nasser and I understand your frustrations. We are here to help you. Could you tell me more about the previous admission of Mr Khalifa? What was the reason for admission? Was he suffering from any illness before that? Was he a smoker?

Son's reply: My father was admitted because of poor kidney function which improved with fluids and stopping his ibuprofen, which he had been taking for back pain. The doctors informed him that the cause of poor kidney function was ibuprofen. They saw the abnormal chest X-ray but did not request a CT scan and they sent him home. My father never smoked.

Doctor's reply: Mr Nasser, I agree with you that the early diagnosis of lung cancer or any type of cancer can make the treatment easier and the outcome better. I am sorry; I do not know why the doctors did not order a lung CT scan during his first admission. Your concerns can be directed to the hospital committee concerned with patient's complaints. However, I understand that your father had poor kidney function at that time. As you may know, in order for a CT scan to better show a lung shadow, a contrast material has to be injected in the veins of the patient. This contrast material can be very harmful to the kidneys particularly if the kidney function is already poor. I assume that this was one of the reasons the doctors postponed the CT scan. Of course, there are many causes of lung shadows on chest radiograph and being a non-smoker; a doctor may assume the shadow is a benign lesion.

I understand that your father was also suffering back pain during the previous admission for kidney failure and he used ibuprofen for that pain. Do you know what the cause of his back pain was at that time? Has it been investigated before? Was it a long-standing pain or new one?

Son's reply: No, it was not investigated and it was a new pain.

Doctor's reply: As the current CT scan showed that the cancer has spread to the bones, one of the possibilities is that the cancer had already spread to the bones at that time and was the cause of his back pain.

Was your father given any follow-up appointment with a chest doctor?

Son's reply: Yes doctor, however, he could not make it as he was on holiday outside the country.

Explore and respond to patient's concerns

Done.

Show empathy

I understand Mr Nasser it must be very difficult to hear that your father has advanced cancer. We are here to help you.

Summarise, confirm understanding, and obtain consent

Mr Nasser, I would like to summarise our discussion as it is important for me to be sure that you have understand important information about your father's illness. The diagnosis of lung cancer that has spread to other parts of his body has been confirmed during this admission. I do not know the exact reason that made the doctors not to request a lung CT during his previous admission for kidney failure. I assume that the fear of contrast toxicity on the kidneys was one of the reasons. There is also a possibility that the cancer had already spread to the bones in his previous admission as your father had back pain at that time.

Does that make sense to you?

Offer help and follow-up plan and close the discussion

Mr Nasser, we have a committee that is assigned to investigate the complaints of patients and their families. If you want to make a formal complaint, I can guide you through the procedure to do that. Meanwhile, I will provide you with my contact number in case you have any further questions or concerns.

Discussion

Ethical principles

- **What are the main ethical principles in this scenario?**
  Patient autonomy: The patient has provided consent to his son to discuss his health status. The doctor should be honest and truthful in discussing the patient's management.

  Beneficence and non-maleficence: Giving IV contrast to a patient with kidney failure could further worsen his kidney function.

  Justice: The patient should be treated in a fair manner without discrimination.

Hidden agenda

- Presence of misunderstanding
- Referral to complaint committee
- Avoid criticising or judging colleagues or the system.

About 15% of patient encounters are experienced as difficult. Factors contributing to difficult clinical encounters may be related to the physician, patient, situation, or a combination. Physician's background, skill level, and personality are important and may contribute to the frequency of difficult patient encounters. Patient's and environmental factors may include excessive anxiety about their current illness, extended waiting time, underlying mood disorders, alcohol abuse, lack of health facilities, poor healthcare system, low literacy etc. Difficult patient encounters include dealing with an angry patient, dealing with an anxious patient, dealing with an overconfident patient, dealing with a calm patient, and dealing with a violent patient. The doctors have a moral and ethical obligation to help patients and answer their questions and concerns in a professional manner. The majority of patients who may seem initially to be difficult will calm down with simple statements such as 'I am sorry to hear that this is happening to you', 'I understand your frustration; we are here to help you'. Always remain calm and maintain a professional demeanour. Show empathy and an understanding of the patient's emotional responses to the condition. Never confront patients, argue with or blam patients. Such behaviour is unprofessional and could worsen the situation. Do not react defensively when the patient expresses concerns. Never criticise your colleague or the health system or try to judge their actions.

Further reading

Cannarella Lorenzetti R, Jacques CH, Donovan C, et al. Managing difficult encounters: understanding physician, patient, and situational factors. Am Fam Physician 2013; 87:419–425.

Hinchey SA, Jackson JL. A cohort study assessing difficult patient encounters in a walk-in primary care clinic, predictors and outcomes. J Gen Intern Med 2011; 26:588–594.

Scenario no. 22

Type of scenario: Information giving/discharge management plan

Candidate information

Your role: You are a doctor on the medical floor.
Problem: Explanation of new diagnosis/discharge plan.
Patient: Mr Naif, a 62-year-old.

Please read the scenario printed below. When the bell sounds, enter the room. You have (---) minutes for your consultation with the patient/relative, (---) minutes to collect your thoughts, and (---) minutes for discussion.

Please do not examine the patient
Please do not take a history

> Mr Naif is a 60-year-old accountant. He was admitted 1 week ago to the hospital with left-sided body weakness and found to have right middle cerebral artery ischaemic stroke. He received thrombolytic therapy and his weakness improved. Now, he is able to walk with minimal support using a walker. He has had type 2 diabetes mellitus (T2DM) for 20 years and hypertension for 10 years and has smoked 15 cigarettes per day for the last 20 years. His HbA1$_c$ on admission was 10%. He is living with his family and wants to be discharged home. He was assessed by the stroke team today who decided to discharge him home.
>
> **Your task:** Is to help him understand his further plan of management and answer his questions and concerns.

Approach

Always read the scenario carefully and make sure you understand the instructions before you start. All information provided is important. Make notes and a framework for your discussion. Sometimes, a hidden agenda is incorporated; pay attention to that.

Introduction and identification

- **Prepare the environment**
  Sit at the same level of the patient with comfort and avoid barriers like tables.

- **Introduce yourself to the patient**
  Shake hands
  Hello Mr Naif, I am Dr X, working in the medical unit.
  Can I confirm that I am talking to Mr Naif?

- **Enquire if the patient would like someone else to be present during the discussion**
  Would you like to invite anybody else to this discussion?

- **Confirm the objective of the interview**
  We are here to discuss about your stroke and further discharge plan. Is that alright?

Check patient's understanding and expectation

Tell me Mr Naif, how much do you know about your health status?

Has any of my colleagues discussed with you about stroke?

Discussion with the patient

- **Give the patient the information (avoid medical jargon and explain what they mean)**

  As you know Mr Naif, you came initially with weakness of the left side of your body. A CT scan of your brain confirmed that the blood supply to the right side of your brain was reduced due to a blockage in your main carotid artery and you had a stroke. I assume one of my colleagues from the stroke team has already explained to you what a stroke is. If you like, I can explain it further. Is that alright?

  Stroke results from a blockage of one of the blood vessels to the brain due to a narrowing or clot in that vessel. Because of this blockage, blood flow to the part of the brain supplied by that vessel will stop or diminish resulting in death of that part of the brain. This may result in weakness or numbness of the parts of the body controlled by that part of the brain.

- **Giving information about what happened in the hospital**

  As you know Mr Naif, when you were admitted to the hospital, doctors treated your stroke with medication to open the blocked vessel called 'thrombolytic therapy' and now you are on other medications to prevent further clots and narrowing in your vessels. These medications are the aspirin and cholesterol lowering tablet called a statin. In addition, you have had extensive physiotherapy and occupational therapy and your weakness has improved significantly.

- **Discussion about further management plan/discharge planning**

  Mr Naif, as you will go home today, it is very important that we discuss your further treatment plan. Is that alright?

- **Medications**

  There are important medications that you need to take after discharge to keep your blood vessels open and avoid the formation of new clots inside the vessels. It is very important that these medications are used as directed and not to skip any dose. Medications that need to be taken lifelong post ischaemic stroke:

  – Aspirin

  – High-intensity statin.

- **Explain the importance of controlling risk factors**

  Mr Naif, it is very important that the risk factors that caused your stroke are controlled in order to prevent another stroke. These risk factors are diabetes, hypertension, smoking, and a high cholesterol level. Smoking plays a major role in causing a stroke; therefore, quitting smoking is a crucial step in managing your illness and to reduce the chances of a second stroke or heart attack. Are you willing to discuss smoking cessation now and the kind of help we can offer to help you quit smoking? (If he agrees, discuss with him the benefits of smoking cessation and the type of help which can be offered such as referring to the smoking cessation clinic. If he is not willing to discuss this issue now, consider discussing it in a separate meeting and provide some information regarding the importance of smoking cessation). Diabetes and hypertension are major risk factors for stroke, and you should make sure that your sugar and blood pressure readings are optimal. I am going to update your GP about your stroke and emphasise the need for optimal control of diabetes and blood pressure.

- **Lifestyle modification**
    - *Fall precautions:* You need to take care while moving or standing to avoid falls. Our physiotherapy and occupational therapy teams will inform you about how to avoid falls.
    - *Diet:* You need a proper diet and I will refer you to a dietician to explain to you about what food to eat and what to avoid. Generally speaking, you need to reduce sugary and high fat food and to avoid greasy, fried and fatty foods. Eat more vegetables and fruits.
    - *Alcohol:* You need to limit your alcohol intake [maximum of 2 glasses (20 g of alcohol) daily for men and one for women].
    - *Stroke rehabilitation program and exercise:* The stroke rehabilitation program is a special program for patients with stroke. It helps you to perform the exercise and physical activity that suits you, avoid the risk factors that caused the stroke and manage your stress. It also helps you to cope with psychological stress.
    - *Blood pressure control:* Your blood pressure should be well-controlled. Your systolic blood pressure (SBP) target should be < 140 mmHg.
    - *Lipid control:* Your LDL cholesterol should be < 1.8 mmol/L (70 mg/dL).
    - *Air travel:* Patients who have recovered from a stroke and are able to move independently can usually travel safely as long as necessary precautions are taken. However, we generally advise that you avoid travel for the first 2 weeks until your condition stabilises. During the flight, please ensure that you move and walk every now and then to avoid a DVT in your legs.
    - *Driving:* I am sorry Mr Naif, it will not be possible for you to drive for at least one month after your stroke and you need to inform the DVLA and insurance company.
- **Check patient understanding.**

Explore and respond to patient's concerns

Do you have any questions or concerns?

- **When can I resume sexual activity?**
  Sexual activity can be resumed once you feel you are *okay* to perform it.

- **When can I return to work?**
  Our stroke rehabilitation team will assess your improvement and will be able to advise you on the appropriate time you can return to work.

- **When can I travel by air after stroke?**
  Already discussed

Show empathy

I understand Mr Naif how difficult it must be to hear about all this. We are here to help you.

Summarise and confirm understanding

Mr Naif, I would like to briefly summarise our discussion as it is important for me to be sure that you understand important information about your stroke. You were admitted to the hospital with weakness of the left side of your body due to a stroke. You received thrombolytic therapy and underwent extensive physiotherapy and occupational therapy during your stay in the hospital and your muscle strength is now better. I have explained to you regarding regular medication use and lifestyle changes to stay healthy and prevent another stroke. We have also discussed the importance of controlling the risk factors for stroke and the need for a proper diet, attending the stroke rehabilitation program, smoking cessation, air travel, and driving.

Please let me know if you want to discuss anything more at this moment.

Offer help and follow-up

This is my telephone number. Please do not hesitate to contact me if you have any questions or concerns.

You will be contacted shortly to start your stroke rehabilitation program.

You will also have an appointment in our stroke clinic in 1 week.

I will arrange another meeting with you in 2 weeks.

If at any time if you feel the weakness comes back, please call our emergency telephone number.

I will also provide you with some website addresses and printed material to read about stroke.

Discussion

Ethical principles

* **What are the main ethical principles in this scenario?**
  Patient's autonomy: The patient has the right to know about the diagnosis and prognosis of his disease. The doctor should provide the patient with the necessary information to help him make his decisions. The doctor should be honest and truthful in discussing the risks and advice regarding the diagnosis and treatment. The patient has the right to refuse or accept the advice or other forms of therapy.

  Beneficence and non-maleficence: In this scenario, controlling risk factors and taking the recommended medications are in the best interest of the patient and should be encouraged. The patient should also be informed about the possible side effects of medications. Advice regarding driving is also in the best interest of the patient.

  Justice: The patient has the right to receive medication and treatment that are important to him without any discrimination. The stroke rehabilitation program is expensive but is important to him.

Hidden agenda

* Explaining the management plan.
* Stroke and air travel.
* Stroke and driving.

Secondary prevention, medications, and lifestyle interventions for patients after stroke should always be monitored and emphasised.

Falls are common after stroke. As some falls can lead to fracture, measures should be taken to minimise the risk of falling.

Patients with stroke should be advised not to drive for at least 1 month after their stroke. Patients with residual limitations in activity at 1 month must inform the DVLA (particularly if there are visual problems, motor weakness or cognitive deficits) and can only resume driving if their physician/GP agrees, or after formal assessment.

Persons who have had a recent stroke or near stroke should avoid air travel until the acute phase has passed and the condition is stable as determined by the managing physician. However, once stable, travel can be considered. Travelling with a companion is advisable for some. Most airlines will provide assistance for disabled passengers with a stroke.

Further reading

Bagshaw M, DeVoll J, Jennings R, et al. Medical Guidelines for Airline Passengers. Aerospace Medical Association Alexandria, VA (2002). Available from https://www.asma.org/asma/media/asma/Travel-Publications/paxguidelines.pdf/ [Last accessed October, 2019].

Scottish Intercollegiate Guidelines Network (SIGN). (2010). Management of patients with stroke: Rehabilitation, prevention and management of complications, and discharge planning. A national clinical guideline. [online] Available from https://www.sign.ac.uk/assets/sign118.pdf [Last accessed October, 2019].